VENOUS
THROMBOEMBOLISM

LUNG BIOLOGY IN HEALTH AND DISEASE

Executive Editor

Claude Lenfant
Director, National Heart, Lung, and Blood Institute
National Institutes of Health
Bethesda, Maryland

ADDITIONAL VOLUMES IN PREPARATION

The opinions expressed in these volumes do not necessarily represent the views of the National Institutes of Health.

VENOUS THROMBOEMBOLISM

Edited by

James E. Dalen
University of Arizona
Tucson, Arizona, U.S.A.

MARCEL DEKKER, INC.

NEW YORK · BASEL

Cover: Rudolph Virchow (1821-1902), the great German pathologist of the 19th century, was called the "father of modern pathology" by William Osler. Virchow described the factors that cause blood to coagulate: stasis, trauma, and hypercoagulability ("Virchow's triad"). He was the first to recognize that venous thrombi in peripheral veins could migrate into the circulation, through the heart and into the lungs, where they would become emboli (a term he invented).

Library of Congress Cataloging-in-Publication Data
A catalog record for this book is available from the Library of Congress.

ISBN: 0-8247-4287-7

This book is printed on acid-free paper.

Headquarters
Marcel Dekker, Inc., 270 Madison Avenue, New York, NY 10016, U.S.A.
tel: 212-696-9000; fax: 212-685-4540

Distribution and Customer Service
Marcel Dekker, Inc., Cimarron Road, Monticello, New York 12701, U.S.A.
tel: 800-228-1160; fax: 845-796-1772

Eastern Hemisphere Distribution
Marcel Dekker AG, Hutgasse 4, Postfach 812, CH-4001 Basel, Switzerland
tel: 41-61-260-6300; fax: 41-61-260-6333

World Wide Web
http://www.dekker.com

The publisher offers discounts on this book when ordered in bulk quantities. For more information, write to Special Sales/Professional Marketing at the headquarters address above.

Current printing (last digit):

10 9 8 7 6 5 4 3 2 1

PRINTED IN THE UNITED STATES OF AMERICA

INTRODUCTION

Venous thromboembolic disease is a very frequent condition with major short- and long-term consequences. For example, annual cases of pulmonary embolism have been reported to exceed 600,000, and, among them, 50,000 to 200,000 are said to be fatal. Furthermore, pulmonary embolism is only one of the consequences of venous thromboembolism, albeit the most frequent and the most serious.

Economists and cost-effectiveness experts have studied the impact of this disease, and their conclusions are alarming, to say the least.

Ever since the importance of the venous system was recognized in the 1600s, anatomists, clinicians, and investigators have studied this system and the diseases that are related to it. One would expect to find even more activity today, since vascular biology is an area of considerable interest. However, it seems that vascular biologists are focusing most of their attention on the arterial side of the vascular bed, particularly on atherosclerosis and its consequences. In no way should this interest diminish, but the venous side should receive equal attention. Vascular biology is, after all, an all-encompassing study that includes the blood and the vessel wall, their interplay, and the consequences of alterations in one or both of them. Venous thromboembolism is really a prototype for such study, as it results from both venous damage and hypercoagulability.

In his preface, the editor, Dr. James E. Dalen, makes the aforementioned very clear. He also delivers an important and essential message: "Therapy for venous embolism is effective, but [it is] of no value unless the diagnosis is suspected and confirmed." Of course, this is easier said than done because tests to detect venous thromboembolism lack sensitivity. Nevertheless, it is within our power to enhance diagnostic alertness, as we know quite well what conditions may lead to venous thromboembolism. In addition, blood coagulability can be monitored very easily.

Pulmonary embolism has been presented and discussed in several of the monographs in the Lung Biology in Health and Disease series, but never before have the condition and its cause, venous thromboembolism, been a primary focus. Dr. Dalen's acceptance of my invitation to undertake the editing of a volume entirely devoted to this condition and its consequences was indeed a marvelous happening. He himself has been a career-long pioneer in studies of venous thromboembolism. Furthermore, the roster of contributors is a true asset to this volume and to the entire series; the authors, who hail from the United States and other countries, bring years of experience and work in venous thrombosis.

I cannot emphasize enough how pleased I am to introduce this volume to the readership of the series. Investigators and clinicians alike will find its contents fascinating and challenging. Should the medical community take advantage of what we know about venous thromboembolism and apply what is reported in this volume, the patients will greatly benefit and the reported staggering statistics about this disease and its consequence will diminish.

Claude Lenfant, M.D.
Bethesda, Maryland

PREFACE

The purpose of this volume is to present our current understanding of venous thromboembolism (VTE). We will review the evolution of our understanding of this disease since it was first described by Virchow nearly a century and a half ago.

Therapy for venous thromboembolism is effective, but it is of no value unless the diagnosis is suspected and confirmed. Unfortunately, the clinical diagnosis of VTE continues to lack sensitivity and specificity. Pulmonary embolism is confirmed in only one-third of the patients in whom it is clinically suspected. Clinical prediction models have been developed that increase the specificity of the clinical diagnosis of VTE, thereby avoiding unnecessary diagnostic testing. However, these clinical prediction models can be used only if the diagnosis of VTE is suspected. Unfortunately, the sensitivity of the clinical diagnosis of VTE continues to be very low. In patients who die of pulmonary embolism, the diagnosis was suspected and treatment was initiated in only one-third of the patients.

Until the accuracy of the clinical recognition of VTE is greatly improved, improved therapy will not have a major impact on the number of patients dying of pulmonary embolism.

Our ability to identify patients at risk of VTE because of recently recognized hypercoagulable conditions and/or acquired risk factors continues to improve. This, along with the availability of new and more effective anticoagulants will have a major impact on preventing VTE and its fatal complication of pulmonary embolism.

It is the hope of the authors that this volume will increase the understanding of VTE, and thereby help to improve its prevention, diagnosis, and treatment.

James E. Dalen

CONTRIBUTORS

Joseph S. Alpert, M.D. Robert S. and Irene P. Flinn Professor and Head, Department of Medicine, University of Arizona College of Medicine, Tucson, Arizona, U.S.A.

John Bonnar, M.D., F.R.C.P.I., F.R.C.O.G. Emeritus Professor, Department of Obstetrics and Gynecology, Trinity College, and St. James's Hospital, Dublin, Ireland

Henri Bounameaux, M.D. Professor and Chairman, Division of Angiology and Hemostasis, Department of Internal Medicine, University of Geneva, and University Hospitals of Geneva, Geneva, Switzerland

J. Jaime Caro, M.D.C.M., F.R.C.P.C., F.A.C.P. Scientific Director, Caro Research Institute, Concord, Massachusetts, U.S.A., and Adjunct Professor, Department of Medicine, McGill University, Montreal, Quebec, Canada

Richard N. Channick, M.D. Associate Professor, Division of Pulmonary and Critical Care Medicine, Department of Medicine, University of California San Diego Medical Center, La Jolla, California, U.S.A.

James E. Dalen, M.D., M.P.H. Professor Emeritus, University of Arizona College of Medicine, Tucson, Arizona, U.S.A.

Peter F. Fedullo, M.D. Professor, Division of Pulmonary and Critical Care Medicine, Department of Medicine, University of California San Diego Medical Center, La Jolla, California, U.S.A.

William R. Flinn, M.D. Professor and Chief, Department of Surgery, University of Maryland, Baltimore, Maryland, U.S.A.

William H. Geerts, M.D., F.R.C.P.C. Consultant, Clinical Thromboembolism and Respirology, Department of Medicine, University of Toronto, and Sunnybrook & Women's College Health Sciences Centre, Toronto, Ontario, Canada

Samuel Z. Goldhaber, M.D. Staff Cardiologist, and Director, Venous Thromboembolism Research Group and Anticoagulation Service, Cardiovascular Division, Department of Medicine, Brigham & Women's Hospital, and Harvard Medical School, Boston, Massachusetts, U.S.A.

Robin L. Gross, M.D. Assistant Professor, Department of Medicine, University Medical Center, University of Medicine and Dentistry of New Jersey–Robert Wood Johnson Medical School, and Cooper Hospital, Camden, New Jersey, U.S.A.

Jack Hirsh, C.M., M.D., F.R.C.P.(C), F.R.A.C.P., F.R.S.C., D.Sc. Professor Emeritus, Department of Medicine, McMaster University, Hamilton, Ontario, Canada

Russell D. Hull, M.B.B.S., M.Sc., F.R.C.P.C., F.A.C.P. Professor, Department of Medicine, and Director, Thrombosis Research Unit, University of Calgary, Calgary, Alberta, Canada

Thomas M. Hyers, M.D. Clinical Professor, Department of Internal Medicine, St. Louis University School of Medicine, St. Louis, Missouri, U.S.A.

Richard S. Irwin, M.D. Professor and Chief, Division of Pulmonary, Allergy, and Critical Care Medicine, Department of Medicine, University of Massachusetts Medical School, Worcester, Massachusetts, U.S.A.

Bruce E. Jarrell, M.D., F.A.C.S. Professor and Chairman, Department of Surgery, University of Maryland, Baltimore, Maryland, U.S.A.

Hylton V. Joffe, M.D. Department of Medicine, Brigham & Women's Hospital, and Harvard Medical School, Boston, Massachusetts, U.S.A.

Judith A. O'Brien, R.N., B.S.P.A. Director of Cost Development, Caro Research Institute, Concord, Massachusetts, U.S.A.

John A. Paraskos, M.D. Professor, Department of Medicine, University of Massachusetts Medical School, Worcester, Massachusetts, U.S.A.

Arnaud Perrier, M.D., F.C.C.P. Assistant Professor, Department of Internal Medicine, University of Geneva, and University Hospitals of Geneva, Geneva, Switzerland

Graham F. Pineo, M.D., F.R.C.P.C. Professor, Departments of Medicine and Oncology, University of Calgary, Calgary, Alberta, Canada

Melvin R. Pratter, M.D., F.C.C.P. Head, Division of Pulmonary and Critical Care Medicine, and Professor and Associate Chief, Department of Medicine, Robert Wood Johnson School of Medicine, and Cooper Hospital, Camden, New Jersey, U.S.A.

Rita Selby, M.B.B.S., F.R.C.P.C. Assistant Professor, Departments of Medicine and Clinical Pathology, University of Toronto, and Sunnybrook & Women's College Health Sciences Centre, Toronto, Ontario, Canada

Paul D. Stein, M.D. Director of Research, St. Joseph Mercy Oakland Hospital, Pontiac, Michigan, U.S.A.

Dennis A. Tighe, M.D. Associate Professor, Department of Medicine, University of Massachusetts Medical School, Worcester, Massachusetts, U.S.A.

Jeffrey I. Weitz, M.D., F.R.C.P.(C), F.A.C.P. Professor, Department of Medicine, McMaster University, Hamilton, Ontario, Canada

CONTENTS

1

Venous Thromboembolism
Past, Present, and Future

JAMES E. DALEN

University of Arizona College of Medicine
Tucson, Arizona, U.S.A.

The purpose of this volume is to present our current understanding of venous thromboembolism (VTE). We will review the evolution of our understanding of this disease, and we will speculate about future developments in the prevention, diagnosis, and treatment of VTE.

Rudolph Virchow, in 1859 (1), was the first to recognize that blood clots found in the pulmonary artery at post mortem examination originated as venous thrombi. He reported that, "the detachment of larger or smaller fragments from the end of the softening thrombus are carried along by the current of blood and driven into remote vessels. This gives rise to the very frequent process upon which I have bestowed the name of Embolia" (1). Virchow was also the first to describe the pathogenesis of venous thrombosis. He described a triad of factors that lead to venous thrombosis: hypercoagulability, stasis, and injury to the vessel wall (2). In Chapter 2, Joffe and Goldhaber discuss the risk factors for venous thrombosis that we now recognize; nearly all fall into one of the three factors that comprise Virchow's triad.

Hypercoagulability has emerged as the most critical risk factor. A hypercoagulable state may be acquired, as in pregnancy, with cancer, or with the use of oral contraceptive agents, or it may be inherited. The first inherited hypercoagulopathies to be described, antithrombin III deficiency, protein C deficiency, and protein S deficiency, are uncommon in the general population, and are present in less than 5% of patients with VTE (3). The most recently described inherited hypercoagulable states are far more frequent, and are present in more than 25% of patients with VTE (3). The prevalence of inherited hypercoagulable states is even higher in patients with idiopathic VTE and in patients with recurrent VTE.

Acquired risk factors such as immobility and trauma precipitate venous thrombosis in patients with inherited thrombophilia. Identification of patients with inherited thrombophilia will permit targeted prophylactic therapy when additional risk factors such as surgery, cancer, or immobility occur in these patients.

The pathogenesis of venous thrombosis is outlined by Weitz and Hirsh in Chapter 3. They explain how fibrin plays a dominant role in venous thrombosis, whereas platelets are critical to the formation of arterial thrombi. Venous thrombosis occurs when inherited and/or acquired factors activate the coagulation system and overwhelm the natural anticoagulant mechanisms. Our understanding of these factors and their interactions has led to the development of effective new anticoagulants that are described in Chapters 4 and 11.

Owing to the difficulty in recognizing pulmonary embolism, most patients who die of pulmonary embolism die because the diagnosis was not suspected and, as a result, they did not receive therapy (4). The most effective way to prevent fatal pulmonary embolism is to recognize patients at risk of VTE and then treat them with prophylactic therapy. The first prophylactic therapy to be reported in the 1930s was intravenous unfractionated heparin in postoperative surgical patients (5,6). Oral anticoagulants were introduced in the 1940s (7), and in 1959, they were shown to be effective in preventing VTE by a randomized, controlled clinical trial (8). Subcutaneous low-dose unfractionated heparin was introduced in 1962 (9), and was shown to be effective by a randomized clinical trial in 1972 (10).

As discussed by Hull and Pineo in Chapter 4, subcutaneous low molecular weight heparin, first introduced in 1982 (11), has been shown to be remarkably effective in patients at high risk of VTE. As they discuss, there are a number of new antithrombotic agents, including a pentasaccharide, fondaparinax, that are very promising. Specific direct thrombin inhibitors such as melagatran and ximelagatran are also being evaluated in clinical trials.

If patients with risk factors for venous thrombosis are not treated with prophylactic therapy when they undergo surgery or are immobilized by other illness, thrombosis in the deep veins (DVT) of the lower extremities may occur. DVT may cause unilateral leg swelling, but in the majority of cases it is asymptomatic. The occurrence of signs or symptoms suggestive of pulmonary embolism may be the first evidence that DVT is present. The most definitive diagnostic test for DVT, ascending contrast venography, is the "gold standard" as discussed by Geerts and Selby in Chapter 5.

Venography, an invasive procedure that is not available in all hospitals, has been used to validate noninvasive tests for DVT. Impedance plethysmography was widely used in the 1970s and 1980s, but it has been largely replaced by Doppler ultrasound imaging, which has been shown to be more accurate. Other noninvasive tests for DVT that are being evaluated are computed tomographic venography and magnetic resonance venography.

Geerts and Selby show how the use of a clinical probability model can be used to assess the probability of DVT. The model includes risk factors for thrombosis, physical signs, and the presence of a possible alternate diagnosis. Although the clinical model itself can not be used to exclude the diagnosis of DVT, if the clinical probability is shown to be low, and the results of a d-dimer assay (discussed in Chap. 7) are negative, further testing for DVT may not be necessary.

The clinical recognition of pulmonary embolism is discussed in Chapter 6. Although Virchow noted that PE might or may not cause pulmonary infarction, as evidenced by necrosis of alveolar walls at post mortem, he did not discuss the clinical presentation of PE. Osler, in 1899 (12), reported that the "symptoms of pulmonary infarction are by no means definite, but it may be suspected when hemoptysis occurs, particularly in mitral stenosis." The clinical findings in patients with pulmonary infarction—hemoptysis, pleuritic chest pain, pleural friction rub, and signs of consolidation—were well described by Graham Steell in 1906 (13). PE without pulmonary infarction was poorly understood until the classic study of McGinn and White in 1935 (14) demonstrated that massive PE may cause acute cor pulmonale with specific electrocardiographic findings and signs and symptoms of acute right ventricular failure.

The two most frequent findings in acute PE are dyspnea and chest pain. When either of these symptoms occurs in a patient with risk factors for VTE, PE should be suspected. Several clinical prediction models are available to assess the probability of PE (15,16). As with clinical prediction models for DVT, the PE prediction model can not be used to exclude PE. However, in patients with a predicted low probability of PE, further testing for PE may be avoided if the d-dimer assay is negative (15).

Clinical findings lead to the suspicion of PE, but they are not diagnostic of PE. The diagnosis of PE must be confirmed. The tests that are available to confirm the diagnosis of PE once it has been suspected are presented in Chapter 8 by Gross et al.

The chest radiograph was the first imaging test for PE. In 1924, Kohlman reported that pulmonary infarction may cause a "triangular or rounded massive shadow" by chest radiography (17). The pioneering postmortem studies of Hampton and Castleman (18) confirmed the correlation of chest radiographic findings and the presence of pulmonary infarcts at post mortem. Unfortunately, the radiographic findings in pulmonary infarction are not diagnostic, and in patients without infarction, the radiographic findings are even less specific or normal.

The development of selective pulmonary angiography in the 1960s had a major impact on our understanding of PE. Prior to pulmonary angiography, the definitive diagnosis of PE could only be made at post mortem or at the time of pulmonary embolectomy. The availability of pulmonary angiography to confirm the diagnosis of PE allowed the development and validation of noninvasive tests for the diagnosis of PE. Perfusion lung scanning and subsequently the addition of ventilation scans rapidly became the diagnostic test of choice in patients suspected of having PE (19). Correlation with pulmonary angiograms demonstrated that lung scans are very sensitive but not specific (20). A normal perfusion scan can be used to exclude PE, and high probability scans have approximately 90% accuracy for the diagnosis of PE. Unfortunately, in the majority of patients with suspected PE, the findings are nondiagnostic. When the results of lung scanning are nondiagnostic, the clinician has several options. If the d-dimer assay is negative and/ or the probability of PE by a clinical prediction model is low, therapy may be withheld (15,21). An alternative in the presence of nondiagnostic lung scan results is to perform Doppler ultrasound of the lower extremities. If the Doppler ultrasound is negative, therapy for PE may be withheld (3).

The diagnosis of PE by chest computed tomography (CT) was reported in 1978 (22), and chest CT findings were correlated with pulmonary angiography in 42 patients in 1992 (23). Chest CT has been shown to detect PE accurately in the central pulmonary arteries, but it is less accurate in the detection of PE in smaller, subsegmental arteries. The sensitivity and specificity of chest CT in the diagnosis of PE is currently being assessed in a cooperative clinical trial comparing chest CT, pulmonary angiography, and lung scans in patients suspected of PE. The results of this trial will determine if chest CT will replace lung scans as the noninvasive test of choice in patients suspected of PE.

The role of echocardiography in the diagnosis of PE is presented in Chapter 9 by Paraskos and Tighe. The first report of the diagnosis of PE by echocardiography appeared in 1978 (24). In 1980, Kasper et al. (25) reported the findings by M mode echo in 18 patients with angiographically documented PE. The most common finding was right ventricular dilatation. Subsequent reports of two-dimensional (2D) echo have confirmed that dilatation of the right ventricle and the right pulmonary artery are the most common findings in acute PE.

The echocardiogram is normal in 20% of cases (26). Echocardiography may visualize a clot in the right atrium or right ventricle. Echocardiographic evidence of right ventricular dysfunction secondary to major pulmonary vascular obstruction is present in approximately half of patients with acute PE (27). Transesophageal echocardiography may visualize emboli in the main or in the proximal right or left pulmonary arteries in patients with massive PE. Doppler echocardiography can estimate pulmonary artery and right heart pressures and detect tricuspid insufficiency in patients with major PE.

Echocardiography, which can be performed at the bedside, may provide important information in patients with major PE.

The special problems associated with venous thromboembolism occurring during pregnancy are presented by Bonnar in Chapter 10. PE is the leading cause of maternal death. The incidence of PE is increased in patients undergoing cesarean section and in patients with a past history of VTE. Patients with inherited hypercoagulable states (see Chap. 2) are at particular risk of VTE during pregnancy. Duplex ultrasound of the legs and V/Q lung scans can be used to document VTE during pregnancy. d-Dimer assay is not useful, because it is usually raised in normal pregnancy and the puerperium. Warfarin, which crosses the placenta and can cause warfarin embryopathy, should be avoided in pregnancy. Heparin, unfractionated or low molecular weight heparin, is the treatment of choice for VTE occurring during pregnancy. Bonnar presents guidelines for thrombophylaxis in patients at increased risk of VTE during pregnancy and the puerperium.

Anticoagulation, the cornerstone of therapy for VTE, is discussed by Hyers in Chapter 11. The first reports of the treatment of pulmonary embolism with heparin was by Murray and Best in 1938 (5) and by Craaford in 1939 (28). The first use of an oral anticoagulant (dicumarol) was reported by Allen et al. in 1947 (7). The first (and only) randomized clinical trial demonstrating the efficacy of heparin followed by oral anticoagulation was reported by Barritt and Jordan in 1960 (29). This was a very small trial by current standard; only 35 patients were randomized, but the results were striking. Recent reviews indicate that the mortality of PE treated with unfractionated heparin followed by oral anticoagulation is less than 5% (30). Earlier studies, before the advent of heparin, reported a mortality of 20–30% in patients with a clinical diagnosis of PE who were not treated (30).

Unfractionated heparin (UF) is rapidly being replaced by low molecular weight heparin (LMWH) for the treatment of VTE. LMWH has a predictable dose response, which permits a fixed dose that does not require laboratory monitoring. It can be given subcutaneously once daily, making it possible to treat VTE out of hospital. Fondaparinux, an indirect factor Xa inhibitor, which has been approved for VTE prevention, is currently being tested for the treatment of PE. Several direct thrombin inhibitors are available for the treatment of the heparin-induced thrombocytopenia thrombosis syndrome.

Thrombolytic therapy of PE with streptokinase or urokinase has been available for more than 25 years, and rt-PA was approved for the treatment of acute PE in 1990. Despite more than 25 years of experience with thrombolytic therapy, its role in the treatment of PE remains uncertain (31). As Stein and Dalen point out in Chapter 12, there is clear evidence by angiography, lung scans, and hemodynamic findings that thrombolytic therapy causes more rapid early resolution of pulmonary embolic resolution than heparin. However, the resolution is incomplete, and within 1–2 weeks of therapy, the degree of resolution in patients treated with heparin is the same as those treated with thrombolytics. In the majority of studies, the confirmed rate of recurrent PE is the same in those treated with heparin or thrombolytics. There is no evidence that thrombolytic agents decrease the mortality of PE. The risk of major bleeding in patients treated with thrombolytics is formidable. The risk of intracranial bleeding is 2–3%; much higher than in patients with acute myocardial infarction who are treated with rt-PA (31). Stein and Dalen conclude that thrombolytic therapy should be considered in patients with massive PE who are hemodynamically unstable even though its efficacy has not been documented.

The role of vena cava interruption is discussed by Jarrell and Flinn in Chapter 13. Homans, in 1934, was the first to recommend and perform "venous ligation above the thrombus" in patients with deep vein thrombosis (32). Since heparin and oral anticoagulants were not available, this became the first treatment to prevent pulmonary embolism. In the 1940s and 1950s, bilateral femoral vein ligation became the treatment of choice. There was a substantial incidence of PE after bilateral femoral vein ligation. Homans, in 1944, had suggested ligation of the inferior vena cava (IVC) if there was reason to suspect the source of emboli was above the inguinal ligament (33). IVC ligation, which replaced bilateral femoral vein ligation, had significant morbidity and some mortality, especially in patients with congestive heart failure.

In the 1960s, a variety of surgical procedures were used to plicate rather than ligate the IVC. All of these procedures required a direct approach to the IVC under general anesthesia. A report in 1969 by Mobin-Uddin et al. (34) described an IVC umbrella filter which could be placed transvenously. Since then a variety of IVC filters have been introduced. The most widely utilized filter is the Greenfield filter (35).

In Chapter 13, Jarrell and Flinn describe new temporary filters that are retrievable. These filters may be useful in patients with a short-term risk of

PE, avoiding the risk of late DVT that is associated with permanent IVC filters (36).

Pulmonary embolectomy, the first definitive therapy for PE, and the only available therapy until the introduction of heparin in 1938 (5), is discussed in Chapter 14. Pulmonary embolectomy, as first described and first performed (unsuccessfully) by Trendelenburg in 1908 (37), was a heroic and dramatic procedure that was rarely successful until it was performed in patients on cardiopulmonary bypass in whom the diagnosis of PE was confirmed by pulmonary angiography. In the largest series reported from one hospital, embolectomy was performed in 96 patients with documented PE with an overall mortality of 38% (38).

As an alternative to embolectomy by means of thoracotomy, embolectomy can be performed with a specially designed catheter introduced by Greenfield et al. (39). Recent reports have demonstrated that modified angiographic catheters can fragment emboli in patients with massive PE complicated by shock. The outcomes in these, as yet, small series seem to be comparable to the reports of surgical embolectomy (40,41).

The most accepted indication for pulmonary embolectomy is documented massive PE complicated by shock. The mortality in these patients, who make up approximately 10% of all patients with documented PE, is approximately 30% (30). A randomized clinical trial will be required to determine if heparin, thrombolytic therapy, or pulmonary embolectomy is the most effective therapy in this subset of patients with PE.

In the majority of patients treated for acute pulmonary embolism, clot lysis leads to near complete or partial resolution of embolic obstruction and pulmonary artery pressure returns to normal (3). In less than 1% of patients, the embolic obstruction fails to resolve, with resultant chronic pulmonary hypertension. In Chapter 15 Channick and Fedullo discuss how to recognize this entity, which in many cases can be corrected with surgical thromboendarterectomy. More than 1100 patients with chronic thromboembolic pulmonary hypertension have undergone thromboendarterectomy at the University of California at San Diego with an operative mortality of less than 10%; the majority of patients have a favorable hemodynamic and symptomatic outcome.

The costs of venous thromboembolism in the United States are discussed by Caro and O'Brien in Chapter 16. They estimate that more than 210,000 cases of DVT and more than 220,000 cases of PE are diagnosed each year in the United States. The total incidence of DVT and PE is much higher, since most cases are not recognized (4). They estimate that the cost of treating DVT as an outpatient ranges from $2400 to $3370 per case. The cost of in-hospital treatment of DVT is much higher: ranging from $3486 in the absence of complications to $11,189 in patients who have a major bleed. The average cost for all patients treated for DVT in hospital is $5779. The total cost of treating DVT per year ranges from a half a billion if all patients were treated as outpatients to $2.1 billion if all were treated in hospital. The mean cost for the treatment of an episode of PE is estimated to be $15,137. Their estimate of the total cost of treating PE per year is $3.4 billion. These costs are only the direct costs; they do not include lost wages and patients' out-of-pocket expenses. When the costs of "ruling out" PE and DVT are added to the direct costs of treating VTE, the total costs of VTE are even more formidable, and highlight the importance of recognizing patients who are at risk of VTE and implementing prophylactic therapy.

References

1. Virchow RLK. Cellular Pathology. 1859 Special edition. London: John Churchill, 1978, pp 204–207.
2. Virchow RLK. Cellular pathology as based upon Physiological and Pathohistology. 7th American edition. Chance F, DeWitt RM (trans.) New York 1860, p 236.
3. Dalen JE. Pulmonary embolism: what have we learned since Virchow? 1. Natural history, pathophysiology, and diagnosis. Chest 2002; 122:1440–1456.
4. Dalen JE, Alpert JS. Natural history of pulmonary embolism. Prog Cardiovasc Dis 1975; 17:259–270.
5. Murray GDW, Best CH. Heparin and thrombosis: the present situation. JAMA 1938; 110:118–122.
6. Crafoord C. Preliminary report on post-operative treatment with heparin as a preventive of thrombosis. Acta Chir Scand 1937; 79:407–426.
7. Allen EV, Hines EA, Kvale WF, et al. The use of dicumarol as an anticoagulant: experience in 2,307 cases. Ann Intern Med 1947; 27:371–381.
8. Sevitt S, Gallagher NG. Prevention of venous thrombosis and pulmonary embolism in injured patients. Lancet 1959; 2:981–989.
9. Sharnoff JG, Kass HH, Mistica BA. A plan of heparinization of the surgical patient to prevent postoperative thromboembolism. Surg Gynecol Obstet 1962; 115:75–79.
10. Kakkar VV, Corrigan T, Spindler J, et al. Efficacy of low doses of heparin in prevention of deep-vein thrombosis after major surgery: a double blind, randomized trial. Lancet 1972; 101–106.
11. Kakkar VV, Djazaeri B, Fok J, et al. Low-molecular-weight heparin and prevention of postoperative deep vein thrombosis. BMJ 1982; 284:375–379.
12. Osler W. The Principles and Practice of Medicine. 1 ed. New York: Appleton, 1899, pp 638–639.
13. Steell G. Textbook on Diseases of the Heart. Special edition. Manchester, UK: University Press, 1906, pp 36–37.

14. McGinn S, White PD. Acute cor pulmonale resulting from pulmonary embolism. JAMA 1935; 104:1473–1480.
15. Wells PS, Ginsberg JS, Anderson DR, et al. Use of a clinical model for safe management of patients with suspected pulmonary embolism. Ann Intern Med 1998; 129:997–1005.
16. Wicki J, Perneger TV, Junod AF, et al. Assessing clinical probability of pulmonary embolism in the emergency ward. Arch Intern Med 2001; 161:92–97.
17. Kohlman G. Dic klinik and rontgendiagnose des lungeninfarkfes. Fortschr. A.D. Geb. D. Rontgenstrahlen 1924; 32:1–12.
18. Hampton AO, Castleman B. Correlation of postmortem chest teleroentgenograms with autopsy findings. Am J Roentgenol Radium Ther 1940; 43:305–326.
19. Wagner HN, Sabiston DC, McAfee JG, et al. Diagnosis of massive pulmonary embolism in man by radioisotope scanning. N Engl J Med 1964; 271:377–384.
20. PIOPED Investigators. Value of the ventilation/perfusion scan in acute pulmonary embolism. JAMA 1990; 263:2753–2759.
21. Wells PS, Anderson DR, Rodger M, et al. Excluding pulmonary embolism at the bedside without diagnostic imaging: management of patients with suspected pulmonary embolism presenting to the emergency department by using a simple clinical model and d-dimer. Ann Intern Med 2001; 135:98–107.
22. Sinner WN. Computer tomographic patterns of pulmonary thromboembolism and infraction. J Comput Assist Tomogr 1978; 2:395–399.
23. Remy-Jardin M, Remy J, Wattine L, et al. Central pulmonary thromboembolism: diagnosis with spiral volumetric CT with the single-breath-hold technique—comparison with pulmonary angiography. Radiology 1992; 185:381–387.
24. Steckley R, Smith CW, Robertson RM. Acute right ventricular overload: an echocardiographic clue to pulmonary thromboembolism. Johns Hopkins Med J 1978; 143:122–125.
25. Kasper W, Meinertz T, Kersting F, et al. Echocardiology in assessing acute pulmonary hypertension due to pulmonary embolism. Am J Cardiol 1980; 45:567–572.
26. Kasper W, Meinertz T, Henkel B, et al. Echocardiographic findings in patients with proved pulmonary embolism. Am Heart J 1986; 112:1284–1290.
27. Ribeiro A, Lindmarker P, Juhlin-Dannfelt A, et al. Echocardiography doppler in pulmonary embolism: right ventricular dysfunction as a predictor of morality rate. Am Heart J 1997; 134:479–487.
28. Crafoord C. Heparin and post-operative thrombosis. Acta Chir Scand 1939; 82:319–335.
29. Barritt DW, Jordan SC. Anticoagulant drugs in treatment of pulmonary embolism: controlled trial. Lancet 1960; 1:1309–1312.
30. Dalen JE. Pulmonary embolism: what have we learned since Virchow? 2. Treatment and prevention. Chest 2002; 122:1801–1817.
31. Dalen. J.E. The uncertain role of thrombolytic therapy in the treatment of PE. Arch Intern Med 2002; 162:2521–2523.

32. Homans J. Thrombosis of the deep veins of the lower leg, causing pulmonary embolism. N Engl J Med 1934; 211:993–997.
33. Homans J. Deep quiet venous thrombosis in the lower limb. Surg Gynecol Obstet 1944; 79:70–82.
34. Mobin-Uddin K, McLean R, Bolooki H, et al. Caval interruption for prevention of pulmonary embolism. Arch Surg 1969; 99:711–715.
35. Greenfield LJ, McCurdy JR, Brown PP. A new intracaval filter permitting continued flow and resolution of emboli. Surgery 1973; 73:599–606.
36. Decousus H, Leizorovicz A, Parent F, et al. A clinical trial of vena caval filters in the prevention of pulmonary embolism in patients with proximal deep-vein thrombosis. N Engl J Med 1998; 338:409–415.
37. Trendelenburg F. Ueber die operative behandlung der embolie der lungenarterie. Arch Klin Chir 1908; 86:686–700.
38. Meyer G, Tamisier D, Sors H, et al. Pulmonary embolectomy: a 20-year experience at one center. Ann Thorac Surg 1991; 51:232–236.
39. Greenfield LJ, Kimmell GO, McCurdy WC. Transvenous removal of pulmonary emboli by vacuum-cup catheter technique. J Surg Res 1969; 9:347–352.
40. Schmitz-Rode T, Janssens U, Duda S, Erley CM, Gunther RW. Massive pulmonary embolism: percutaneous emergency treatment by pigtail rotation catheter. J Am Coll Cardiol 2000; 36:375–379.
41. Fava M, Soledad L, Flores P, Huete I. Mechanical fragmentation and pharmacologic thrombolysis in massive pulmonary embolism. J Vasc Inter Radiol 1997; 8:261–266.

2

Hypercoagulable States and Other Risk Factors for Venous Thromboembolism

HYLTON V. JOFFE and SAMUEL Z. GOLDHABER

Brigham & Women's Hospital
and Harvard Medical School
Boston, Massachusetts, U.S.A.

I. Introduction

In the 19th century, Virchow defined three mechanisms of thrombosis that hold true today: venous stasis, vessel wall injury, and hypercoagulability (or thrombophilia). Acquired and inherited conditions (Table 1) predispose to these processes and disrupt the delicate balance between pro-thrombotic and antithrombotic mechanisms. Venous stasis occurs during long-haul flights, surgery, pregnancy, and immobilization. Tobacco, chemotherapy, and indwelling central venous catheters cause endothelial injury. Inherited thrombophilias, especially factor V Leiden and the pro-thrombin gene mutation have been increasingly recognized in patients with venous thromboembolism (VTE). Acquired causes of thrombophilia, such as hyperhomocysteinemia, hypertension, exogenous estrogen use, cigarette smoking, and advancing age, frequently coexist with other risk factors for VTE.

Table 1 Acquired and Inherited Causes of Hypercoagulability

Acquired thrombophilias	Inherited thrombophilias
Long-haul flights	Factor V Leiden
Age	Prothrombin gene mutation
Obesity	Antithrombin III deficiency
Hypertension	Protein C deficiency
Tobacco use	Protein S deficiency
Immobilization	Plasminogen deficiency
Surgery	Dysfibrinogenemia
Cancer	Elevated factor VIII levels
Medical illness	Elevated factor IX levels
Critical illness	Elevated factor XI levels
Oral contraceptives	Elevated lipoprotein (a) levels
Pregnancy	
Hormone replacement therapy	
Antiphospholipid antibodies	
Hyperhomocysteinemia	

II. Acquired Risk Factors for Venous Thromboembolism

A. Long-Haul Flights

Air travel is a remarkable advance of the modern world that allows travelers to journey great distances within hours. However, long-haul flights are an emerging risk factor for VTE, especially when travel time exceeds 6 hr or distance exceeds 5000 km (3125 miles) (1). Restricted space in economy class limits mobility ("economy class syndrome") and predisposes to venous stasis. Other factors, such as water loss in the dry cabin, changes in cabin pressure, and hemoconcentration from alcohol consumption or reduced fluid intake probably also increase VTE risk. Therefore, we recommend avoidance of alcohol and adequate fluid intake, and we encourage minor physical activity, such as occasionally walking around the cabin. Below-knee stockings have also been shown to reduce the risk of deep vein thrombosis (DVT) in this setting (2,3). Prophylaxis with low molecular weight heparin should be considered for travelers at high risk for VTE (4).

B. Age, Obesity, Hypertension, and Cigarette Smoking

Data from the Nurses' Health Study, a large prospective cohort of women, have shown that the acquired factors of obesity, cigarette smoking, and hypertension increase the risk for VTE. Hypertensive patients have a 50% higher risk of pulmonary embolism (PE) compared to normotensive controls. Patients with a body mass index (BMI, a standard measure of obesity calculated as weight in kilograms divided by the square of height in meters) of 29 or greater have a threefold higher risk of PE compared to those with a BMI of less than 21 (Fig. 1). Obesity probably causes venous stasis and increases levels of several procoagulants, such as factor VII and fibrinogen (5).

Although prior tobacco use is not a risk factor for VTE, patients who currently smoke are at increased risk for PE, probably as a result of increased fibrinogen levels and direct toxic effects of tobacco on the vascular endothelium (Fig. 2) (5).

The Physicians' Health Study has demonstrated that advancing age also increases the risk for VTE, especially when patients are more than 70 years old and a coexisting thrombophilia, such as factor V Leiden, is present (Fig. 3) (6,7).

C. Surgery

As many as one-third of patients who undergo general surgery develop DVT, although most do not have apparent symptoms (8). Postoperative

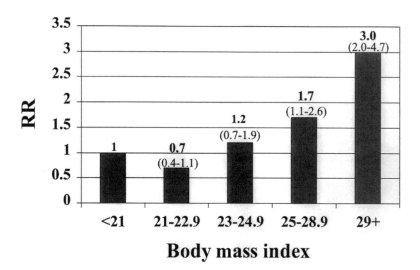

Figure 1 Relative risk (RR) for pulmonary embolism according to body mass index (BMI). Values in parentheses are 95% confidence intervals. Subjects with a BMI < 21 were used for the reference category. Patients with a BMI ≥25 have a significantly higher risk of pulmonary embolism compared to those with a BMI < 21. (From Ref. 5.)

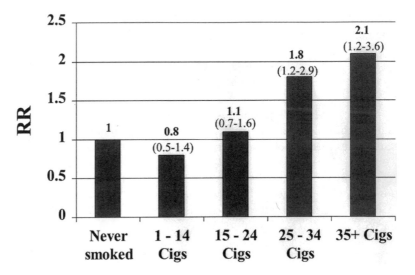

Figure 2   Relative risk (RR) for pulmonary embolism according to number of cigarettes (Cigs) currently smoked per day. Values in parentheses are 95% confidence intervals. Subjects who never smoked were used for the reference category. Patients who smoke at least 25 cigarettes per day have a significantly higher risk of pulmonary embolism compared to nonsmokers. (From Ref. 5.)

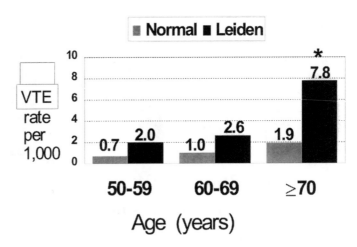

Figure 3   Incidence of venous thromboembolism (VTE) according to age and the presence of factor V Leiden (FVL). The incidence rate among men with FVL ≥70 years of age was significantly greater than that among men in the same age group without this mutation. (From Ref. 6.)

venous thrombosis occurs more frequently in cancer patients compared to those without malignancy (9). The supine position on the operating table and vasodilatory effects of anesthesia reduce venous return and predispose to stasis (10). Patient age and the type and duration of surgery strongly influence the mortality rate from PE in the first few weeks following surgery. Patients at low risk for postoperative VTE are under 40 years of age, require general anesthesia for less than 30 min, and are undergoing minor elective surgery. Moderate-risk patients are over 40 years of age, require general anesthesia for more than 30 min, and have other risk factors for VTE, including obesity, malignancy, estrogen use, or paralysis. High-risk patients are over 40 years of age, are undergoing surgery for cancer or an orthopedic procedure of the legs lasting more than 30 min, have a personal history of VTE, or have risk factors for VTE, including thrombophilias (Table 2) (11). Although one-third of DVTs are diagnosed within the first 2 postoperative days, most DVTs are diagnosed during the third to sixth postoperative days. The mean time between surgery and clinically detected PE was 14 days in patients not receiving prophylaxis in the landmark International Multicenter Trial (12). Furthermore, approximately one-fourth of postoperative PE occurs after hospital discharge. Presumably, risk factors for VTE persist or increase after discharge when patients who are stimulated to walk during the hospital stay become less mobile upon returning home (13).

Asymptomatic DVT following total knee replacement, especially isolated calf DVT, has been reported in at least half of the patients not receiving prophylaxis and occurs more often than after primary total hip arthroplasty (14). Venous stasis and direct endothelial injury are important factors that contribute to this high incidence of DVT during total hip and knee arthroplasty (15). In addition to the thrombogenic effects of the supine position and anesthesia, the use of a thigh tourniquet to create a bloodless field and flexion of the limb further promote venous stasis (10).

During orthopedic procedures, transesophageal echocardiography commonly detects echogenic masses in the right heart chambers within 1 min of tourniquet release and knee manipulation (16,17). Usually this embolic material, which may represent thrombus, air, fat, marrow content, or cement, causes no readily apparent adverse clinical sequelae. Longer tourniquet times are associated with larger number of emboli (17).

D. Cancer

Cancer has long been recognized as a risk factor for VTE. Thrombosis is especially frequent in patients with mucin-secreting adenocarcinomas, brain tumors, myeloproliferative disorders, and some leukemias (18). Prothrom-

Table 2 Levels of Venous Thromboembolism Risk in Surgical Patients Without
Prophylaxis

Levels of risk with examples	Calf DVT (%)	Proximal DVT (%)	Clinical PE (%)	Fatal PE (%)
Low	2	0.4	0.2	0.002
Minor surgery in patients less than 40 years old without risk factors				
Moderate	10–20	2–4	1–2	0.1–0.4
Minor surgery in patients with risk factors				
Major surgery in patients less than 40 years old without risk factors				
High	20–40	4–8	2–4	0.4–1.0
Major surgery in patients over 40 years old or anyone with risk factors				
Highest	40–80	10–20	4–10	0.2–5
Major surgery in patients over 40 years old with prior VTE, cancer, or thrombophilia				
Hip/knee arthroplasty or hip fracture surgery				
Major trauma				
Spinal cord injury				

DVT, deep vein thrombosis; PE, pulmonary embolism; VTE, venous thromboembolism.
Source: Ref. 11.

botic mechanisms in cancer patients include tumor cell activation of clotting,
vessel wall injury by chemotherapy or direct invasion of tumor cells, and
stasis. Chemotherapy also causes cytokine and procoagulant release from
damaged tumor cells and reduces levels of protein C and S, and antithrombin
III partially as a result of hepatotoxicity (9). Some breast, colon, prostatic,
and lung cancers can directly activate coagulation factors, such as factor X,
and cause thrombin generation. Alternatively, cancers may stimulate monocytes and macrophages to synthesize procoagulants, such as tissue factor.
Immobility in debilitated cancer patients or venous compression by extrinsic
masses promotes venous stasis and may also predispose to VTE (19).

Most studies have shown that idiopathic VTE increases the risk of a subsequent diagnosis of cancer, especially within the first year following the thrombotic event (Fig. 4) (18–21). The risk of cancer is highest for patients with recurrent, idiopathic DVT compared to those with an identified triggering factor (Fig. 5) (19). Virtually any cancer can present with DVT, but typical sites of malignancy include the pancreas, ovary, liver, and brain (21,22). The benefit of searching for cancer in patients with primary VTE is unclear and has not been shown to be cost effective. It is uncertain whether early diagnosis would change outcome (especially in patients with lung, brain, prostatic, or pancreatic cancer), because these tumors are often of advanced stage and carry a poor prognosis (22,23).

Less is known about the association between upper extremity DVT (UEDVT) and cancer. One study reported a subsequent diagnosis of mostly lung cancer or lymphomas in approximately one-fourth of patients presenting with idiopathic UEDVT (24).

Trousseau's syndrome, a recurrent, migratory thrombophlebitis of the deep and superficial veins, typically involves unusual sites, such as the upper extremity vasculature. Many patients have an underlying adenocarcinoma of the pancreas, gastrointestinal tract, lung, or prostate (25). Improvement may occur with treatment of the underlying cancer, although most patients

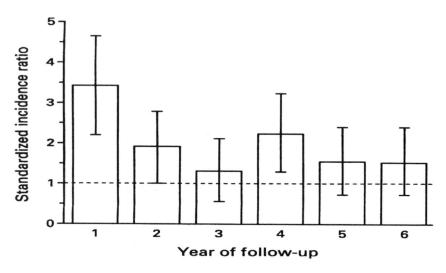

Figure 4 Standardized incidence ratios (with 95% confidence intervals) for newly diagnosed cancers after a first episode of venous thromboembolism. (From Ref. 21.)

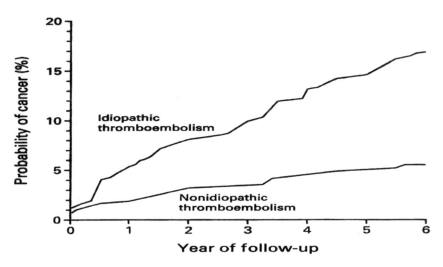

Figure 5 Cumulative probability of newly diagnosed cancer after a first episode of venous thromboembolism according to whether the thromboembolism was idiopathic or nonidiopathic. (From Ref. 21.)

require long-term anticoagulation with heparin. For unknown reasons, warfarin is usually ineffective for this disorder (26).

E. Medical Illness

A variety of medical illnesses increase the risk for VTE, including stroke with extremity paresis, the nephrotic syndrome, chronic obstructive pulmonary disease, and congestive heart failure (Table 3) (27,28). Heart failure is associated with impaired release of endothelium-derived nitric oxide, which may contribute to peripheral vasoconstriction and promote platelet adhesion to the endothelium. Also, low cardiac output and poor forward flow predispose to venous stasis, especially in the setting of right heart failure (29).

Hospitalization increases the risk for VTE, probably because of relative immobilization and the acuity and severity of illness. Nursing home and chronic care facility confinement also increase the risk for VTE. Significant liver disease decreases the risk for VTE, probably because these patients have underlying coagulopathy, thrombocytopenia, and reduced clearance of fibrin degradation products (28).

Critically ill patients are at high risk for VTE. At least one-third of medical and surgical intensive care unit patients without prophylaxis will

Table 3 Medical Illnesses Associated
with Venous Thromboembolism

Cancer
Chronic obstructive pulmonary disease
Congestive heart failure
Hypertension
Nephrotic syndrome
Polycythemia vera
Stroke with extremity paresis
Thoracic outlet syndrome

develop VTE. Approximately two-thirds of patients with multisystem trauma, especially orthopedic trauma (lower extremity fractures), major head injury, or spinal trauma who do not receive prophylaxis develop VTE. The highest incidence of VTE in critically ill patients not receiving prophylaxis occurs in acute spinal cord patients (30).

Most DVTs originate in the lower extremities. However, more frequent use of central venous catheters for dialysis, parenteral nutrition, and chemotherapy has increased the incidence of UEDVT over the past several decades. UEDVT has been reported in up to one-fourth of patients with these catheters (31). The catheter predisposes to thrombosis by impeding blood flow through the vein or causing injury to the vessel wall during catheter insertion or infusion of medication. Catheter tips should be positioned in the lower superior vena cava, because the rapid blood flow may sufficiently dilute the infusate and reduce the risk of thrombophlebitis (32).

A more rare but important cause of UEDVT is the Paget-Schroetter syndrome (also known as "effort thrombosis"), which is characterized by spontaneous UEDVT after strenuous activity such as baseball pitching, rowing, wrestling, or weight lifting in young and otherwise healthy individuals (33). Some of these patients have thoracic outlet syndrome, which refers to compression of the neurovascular bundle (brachial plexus, subclavian artery, and subclavian vein) by hypertrophied muscles, cervical ribs, or other skeletal abnormalities, causing intermittent, positional vessel compression further predisposing to UEDVT (34).

F. Oral Contraceptives

Oral contraceptives predispose to thrombosis by inducing acquired resistance to activated protein C and increasing levels of some procoagulants, such as fibrinogen and factors VII, VIII, and X (35,36). The first-generation oral contraceptives contained at least 50 μg of ethinylestradiol and substantially increased the risk for VTE (37). They have been withdrawn from the market because of their high VTE risk. The newer second-generation oral contraceptives contain lower doses of estrogen with consequent lower risk of VTE, approximately 3 per 10,000 person-years (35). Past use of oral contraceptives is not associated with PE (38). The risk of VTE largely disappears by about 6 weeks after oral contraceptives are discontinued.

Women suffering with acne or hirsuitism are often prescribed third-generation oral contraceptives, which contain a new, less androgenic progestin such as desogestrel, gestodene, or cyproterone. However, these oral contraceptives have a higher risk of VTE compared with the second-generation formulations, indicating that some progestins contribute to thrombosis risk (39–41).

Oral contraceptives increase the risk for VTE most profoundly during the first year and especially within the initial 6 months when used by patients with inherited thrombophilias (42). Oral contraceptives increase the risk for VTE more than 30-fold in patients with coexisting factor V Leiden, but even these patients have a low absolute risk for VTE (Fig. 6) (43).

G. Pregnancy

Pregnant women have a higher risk of VTE than age-matched controls. Prothrombotic mechanisms include venous stasis secondary to prolonged

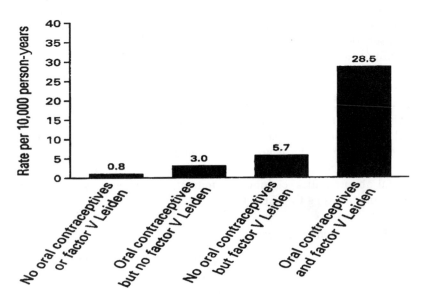

Figure 6 Cases of deep vein thrombosis per 10,000 person-years according to the use of oral contraceptives and the presence of factor V Leiden. (From Ref. 43.)

bed rest and compression of the inferior vena cava by the gravid uterus. Furthermore, there are changes in plasma concentrations of several coagulation factors that predispose to VTE, including a decrease in protein S levels and increased levels of factors II, VII, and X (44). The risk of VTE is higher for cesarean sections than vaginal deliveries, especially when emergency surgery is performed. Advancing maternal age is also associated with a higher risk of VTE (Fig. 7) (45). Although factor V Leiden and/or the prothrombin gene mutation predispose to a high relative risk of VTE, there is a low absolute risk of VTE with these thrombophilias (46).

H. Hormone Replacement Therapy

Approximately one-third of postmenopausal American women use hormone replacement therapy (HRT). HRT increases bone mineral density and decreases the risk of fracture in patients with osteoporosis. HRT is also highly effective for reducing symptoms of menopause such as hot flashes, night sweats, vaginal dryness, and mood changes. There are insufficient data to conclude whether HRT reduces the risk of colorectal cancer and Alzheimer's disease. However, several emerging risks of HRT have reduced enthusiasm for using HRT (47).

Although more than 40 observational studies have suggested reductions in cardiac risk, possibly related in part to decreasing low-density lipoprotein and increasing high-density lipoprotein levels, randomized trials among

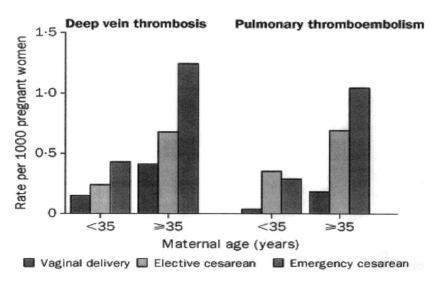

Figure 7 Incidence of postpartum deep vein thrombosis and pulmonary thromboembolism by maternal age and method of delivery. (From Ref. 45.)

women with preexisting heart disease have not confirmed this benefit. Furthermore, the estrogen plus progestin arm of the Women's Health Initiative was recently stopped prematurely. This randomized, placebo-controlled trial of hormone replacement therapy in healthy postmenopausal women found an increased risk of invasive breast cancer, coronary artery disease, stroke, and pulmonary embolism in the group receiving estrogen with progestin. Therefore, HRT should not be prescribed for the purpose of preventing heart disease (47).

The estrogen content of HRT preparations is much lower than that of the oral contraceptive formulations, but the risk of VTE is similar (approximately threefold) (48,49). The risk of VTE is highest near the start of therapy. This is an important consideration when recommending a short course of HRT for relief of menopausal symptoms. The mechanism by which HRT increases VTE risk is uncertain, but like oral contraceptives, HRT may change clotting factor concentrations and cause acquired resistance to activated protein C (50). There is a trend toward higher VTE risk in patients using higher estrogen dose preparations (51). HRT is contraindicated in patients with a personal history of VTE, because HRT confers a higher risk of VTE in these patients (52). Other risk factors for VTE, such as a family history of VTE, morbid obesity, or prolonged immobilization, should be considered when weighing the risks and benefits of HRT in the individual patient. Past HRT use does not increase the risk for VTE (51). HRT substantially increases the risk of VTE in women with coexisting thrombophilias, such as factor V Leiden, antithrombin III deficiency, or protein C deficiency (49).

Raloxifene, a selective estrogen receptor modulator (SERM), competitively inhibits estrogen-induced DNA transcription in the breast and endometrium. Therefore, raloxifene has a lower risk of breast and uterine cancer than estrogen and is sometimes substituted for estrogen for the treatment of osteoporosis. Like estrogen, raloxifene reduces low-density lipoprotein levels, but its effect on cardiovascular risk is uncertain. The risk of VTE is similar for HRT and raloxifene. Therefore, raloxifene is also contraindicated in women with a personal history of VTE (53).

I. Antiphospholipid Antibodies

Antiphospholipid antibodies comprise a family of autoantibodies, including lupus anticoagulant and anticardiolipin antibodies, that bind phospholipids or phospholipid-binding proteins. Antiphospholipid antibodies may occur as a primary thrombotic or obstetrical disorder known as the antiphospholipid antibody syndrome or can be seen in association with other medical disorders, such as systemic lupus erythematosus (54).

Antiphospholipid antibodies predispose to arterial and venous thrombosis and recurrent pregnancy loss. The risk of recurrent thrombosis appears to be higher in patients with antibodies to beta-2-glycoprotein I or those with high IgG anticardiolipin titers (Fig. 8) (54–56). Several hypotheses have been proposed to explain the mechanism by which antiphospholipid antibodies mediate thrombosis. These antibodies may cause oxidant injury to the vascular endothelium or interfere with the regulation of coagulation by altering the function of phospholipid-binding proteins (57). Arnout has postulated that the mechanism of the antiphospholipid antibody syndrome may parallel that of heparin-induced thrombocytopenia (58). In this model, binding proteins, such as beta-2-glycoprotein I or prothrombin, cover damaged phospholipids on blood or endothelial cells. If antiphospholipid antibodies are present, they will concentrate on these cell surfaces, bind to cellular receptors, and induce strong thrombosis-promoting modifications, such as the release of serotonin, thromboxane A_2, and tissue factor.

Clinical Features

Antiphospholipid antibodies are acquired in a small percentage of young and otherwise healthy patients. Therefore, a definitive diagnosis of the antiphospholipid antibody syndrome requires the presence of clinical criteria in addition to laboratory findings (Table 4). Pregnancy complications include spontaneous abortions before the tenth week of gestation (often attributed to placental vein thrombosis), premature births of normal infants

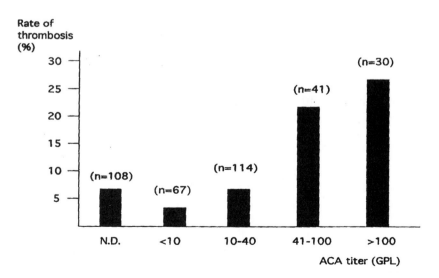

Figure 8 Rate of thrombosis in patients with antiphospholipid antibodies according to the titer of anticardiolipin (ACA) IgG, expressed as GPL units. GPL = IgG phospholipid units; N.D. = not determined. (From Ref. 56.)

Table 4 Criteria for the Antiphospholipid Antibody Syndrome[a]

Clinical criteria
Arterial, venous, or small vessel thrombosis
Pregnancy complications
≥1 unexplained deaths of morphologically normal fetuses ≥10th week of gestation
or
≥1 premature births of morphologically normal fetuses ≤34th week of gestation
or
≥3 unexplained consecutive spontaneous abortions ≤10th week of gestation
Laboratory criteria[b]
Anticardiolipin IgM or IgG antibodies[c]
≥15–20 international "phospholipid" units
or
≥2.0–2.5 times the median level
or
≥99th percentile
Lupus anticoagulant antibodies

[a] Diagnosis requires the presence of at least one of the clinical and one of the laboratory criteria.
[b] Antibodies must be present on two or more occasions at least 6 weeks apart.
[c] The threshold for significant anticardiolipin antibodies has not been standardized so any of the three definitions can be used.
Source: Ref. 57.

at or before the thirty-fourth week of gestation, and unexplained deaths of morphologically normal fetuses at or after the tenth week of gestation (57). Antiphospholipid antibodies increase mortality by causing fatal episodes of myocardial infarction and pulmonary embolism (Fig. 9) (55).

Diagnostic Testing

Testing for antiphospholipid antibodies should be performed on two or more occasions at least 6 weeks apart to exclude the presence of transient, nonconsequential antiphospholipid antibodies (57).

Lupus anticoagulant is detected when an inhibitor is present that increases clotting time in at least two phospholipid-dependent coagulation tests, such as the activated partial thromboplastin time, dilute Russell's viper venom time, or kaolin clotting time (59). Anticardiolipin antibodies are most commonly detected using an enzyme-linked immunosorbent assay (ELISA) (57).

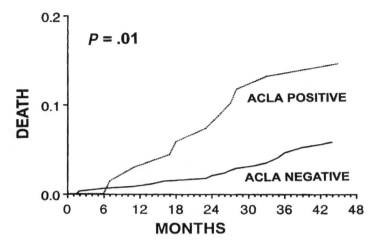

Figure 9 Mortality in patients with a first episode of venous thromboembolism, anticoagulated for 6 months by anticardiolipin antibody (ACLA) status. (From Ref. 55.)

J. Hyperhomocysteinemia

Hyperhomocysteinemia is typically defined as fasting homocysteine levels greater than 15 μmol/L (greater than the 95th percentile of the general population). The true prevalence of this condition is unknown, because there are many methods for measuring levels but no standardization between techniques or laboratories (60). Hyperhomocysteinemia is a well-known risk factor for arterial thrombosis, but has only recently been recognized as a predisposing factor for initial and recurrent VTE (Fig. 10) (61–63). The mechanism of thrombosis is unknown.

Hyperhomocysteinemia occurs when acquired or genetic abnormalities of the homocysteine metabolism pathway are present. Methionine, an essential amino acid occurring abundantly in animal protein, is a precursor for homocysteine. Reconversion of homocysteine to methionine occurs when protein intake is low. However, this pathway requires a sufficient supply of cobalamin (vitamin B_{12}) and dietary folate, as well as properly functioning N^5,N^{10}-methylenetetrahydrofolate reductase (MTHFR) and methionine synthase enzymes. Therefore, cobalamin or folate deficiency or abnormalities of the MTHFR or methionine synthase enzymes will cause hyperhomocysteinemia. In a distinct pathway, homocysteine is also metabolized to cysteine, but this requires pyridoxine (vitamin B_6) and a properly functioning cystathionine beta-synthase enzyme. Therefore, deficiencies of

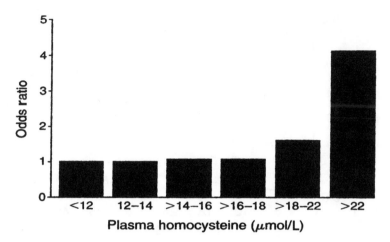

Figure 10 Odds ratio for thrombosis according to plasma homocysteine level. Subjects with plasma homocysteine values <12 μmol/L were used for the reference category. (From Ref. 63.)

pyridoxine will also cause hyperhomocysteinemia. Homozygous deficiency of cystathionine beta-synthase, a rare autosomal recessive trait, causes congenital severe hyperhomocysteinemia that is characterized by premature atherosclerosis. Half of these untreated patients suffer an atherothrombotic event before the age of 30 years (60,64).

Most commonly, an acquired nutritional deficiency of folate causes hyperhomocysteinemia; inadequate intake of vitamin B_{12} and/or vitamin B_6 may exacerbate this condition. Folate antagonists, such as methotrexate and phenytoin or vitamin B_6 antagonists, such as estrogens, tobacco, and theophylline, will also raise homocysteine levels. Reduced renal function may cause hyperhomocysteinemia, because the kidneys predominantly metabolize homocysteine (60).

Diagnosis

High-performance liquid chromatography is usually used to measure plasma homocysteine levels. A methionine load slightly improves sensitivity by stressing the homocysteine pathway but is not routinely used in clinical practice because of inconvenience and expense (65).

Treatment

Regardless of etiology, most patients with hyperhomocysteinemia respond to multivitamin treatment. Folic acid is the most effective therapy and will reduce homocysteine levels even when patients are not obviously folate deficient (60). Clinical trials are currently underway to determine whether these therapies ultimately reduce the frequency of thrombosis.

III. Inherited Risk Factors for Venous Thromboembolism

A. Factor V Leiden

Protein C is a powerful, endogenous anticoagulant that limits thrombosis by cleaving and inactivating the procoagulant factors Va and VIIIa. Less than one decade ago, an adenine for guanine substitution at position 1,691 in the factor V gene was discovered in some patients susceptible to venous thrombosis (66). Autosomal dominant transmission of this single point mutation causes a glutamine for arginine substitution at the initial cleavage site for protein C, rendering factor Va relatively resistant to degradation by protein C (67). Therefore, factor V persists in the activated form, increases thrombin generation, and predisposes to thrombus formation. This abnormal factor V protein, also known as factor V Leiden (FVL) or FV Q506, is the most common cause of activated protein C resistance and the most common genetic mutation predisposing to VTE (67,68). FVL predominantly affects whites of northern European descent and rarely occurs in Africans and Asians (69,70).

Clinical Features

FVL increases the risk for a first episode of VTE and probably contributes to recurrent pregnancy loss by causing placental thrombosis (71,72). The risk of recurrent VTE in patients with FVL is unknown, because studies report varying results (73–75). FVL is not a risk factor for arterial thrombosis, such as stroke or acute myocardial infarction (72).

Some studies suggest that the prevalence of FVL is lower in patients presenting with PE than in those presenting with DVT (76–78). This discrepancy is biologically plausible, because FVL promotes thrombin formation, which may improve thrombus adherence to the vein wall and reduce embolism.

Diagnostic Testing

Functional, plasma-based testing uses a dilution technique or modified activated partial thromboplastin time assay as the initial diagnostic test for resistance to activated protein C. Both tests are relatively easy to perform and have acceptable sensitivity and specificity. The dilution technique is not affected by the presence of exogenous anticoagulants, which may alter the activated partial thromboplastin time. The dilution test measures clotting times after the patient's plasma has been diluted with factor V–deficient plasma. FVL patients have persistently activated factor V, which stimulates thrombin formation and reduces clotting times compared to controls (79). The diagnosis should be confirmed with genetic testing. Screening for FVL is not routinely performed (80).

B. Prothrombin Gene Mutation

After FVL, the prothrombin gene mutation is the second most common genetic abnormality predisposing to VTE (68). Prothrombin (factor II) is a precursor of thrombin. Autosomal dominant transmission of an adenine for guanine substitution at position 20,210 in an untranslated region of the prothrombin gene results in higher plasma prothrombin levels and increases the risk for VTE about threefold, probably by increasing thrombin levels (81). The prothrombin gene mutation is diagnosed with genetic testing. Like FVL, the prothrombin gene mutation is most prevalent in whites and rare among Africans and Asians. Whereas FVL is more prevalent in northern Europeans, the prothrombin gene mutation is more common in southern Europeans (82).

Like FVL, the prothrombin gene mutation increases the risk for a first episode of VTE and does not predispose to arterial thrombosis (83). The risk of recurrent VTE in patients with the prothrombin gene mutation is unknown, because varying results have been reported (68,82,84). The prothrombin gene mutation appears to increase the risk for cerebral vein thrombosis, which presents with a wide range of symptoms ranging from headache to impaired consciousness and has a high mortality rate (85).

C. Antithrombin III Deficiency

Antithrombin III (ATIII), a naturally occurring anticoagulant, limits thrombosis by inactivating procoagulant factors, including thrombin and factors Xa and IXa. ATIII deficiency may be acquired in patients with certain medical conditions, such as cirrhosis, or can be inherited as an autosomal dominant trait (86). Heterozygous ATIII deficiency is classified as type I or II based on the nature of the mutation and the results of three different functional assays that assess the level of ATIII antigen and the ability of ATIII to inhibit coagulation factors in the presence and absence of heparin. Type I deficiency is characterized by reduced levels of ATIII antigen and activity. Type II deficiency, characterized by the presence of a poorly functioning ATIII variant, is further classified as RS (effect on reactive site), HBS (effect on heparin-binding site), or PE (pleiotropic effect). Type II RS defects reduce the ability of ATIII to inhibit the coagulation factors in the absence of heparin. Type II HBS mutations alter ATIII-heparin binding and limit the ability of heparin to catalyze ATIII inhibition of the coagulation factors. Type II PE mutations produce variant ATIII antigen with multiple functional defects. Heterozygotes with type II HBS appear to be at lower risk for VTE than those with type I or type II RS, but their risk for VTE may still be somewhat greater than that of the normal population (87).

Inherited ATIII deficiency increases the risk for initial and recurrent VTE, but the clinical significance of acquired ATIII deficiency is less well defined (86). The risk of VTE in surgical patients with ATIII deficiency is extremely high; in part because surgery further reduces ATIII levels (88). Failure to prolong the activated partial thromboplastin time may occur when heparin is administered to patients with ATIII deficiency. The extent of this resistance to heparin depends on the severity of the deficiency (87). Both concurrent heparin administration and acute VTE reduce ATIII levels even in patients without ATIII deficiency. Therefore, ATIII deficiency cannot be reliably diagnosed in these settings.

D. Protein C and Protein S Deficiencies

Protein C, a naturally occurring anticoagulant, limits thrombosis by inactivating the procoagulant factors Va and VIIIa. Protein S is a cofactor for these reactions (89). More than 100 autosomal dominant mutations in the protein C or protein S genes have been detected that reduce protein level or function and predispose to VTE (68,90).

Protein C and S deficiencies, diagnosed with functional and immunological assays, are rare causes of VTE (89,91). Warfarin inhibits the synthesis of all vitamin K–dependent proteins, including factors II, VII, IX, and X and proteins C and S. Therefore, protein C or S deficiency cannot be reliably diagnosed during concurrent warfarin use. Pregnancy and oral contraceptives also reduce protein S levels.

The half-life of protein C is very short compared to that of the procoagulants. Therefore, protein C levels plummet when warfarin is initiated in patients with protein C deficiency. In the absence of concurrent heparin administration, these patients develop a transient hypercoagulable state, which may progress within days to warfarin-induced skin necrosis (92). This rare condition is characterized by painful necrotic lesions in fatty tissue areas, such as the breast or buttocks, and also may involve the penis, nipples, fingers, or toes. Treatment includes immediate discontinuation of warfarin followed by administration of heparin and vitamin K. Case reports of warfarin-induced skin necrosis have also been described with protein S deficiency and FVL (93).

E. Other Hypercoagulable Disorders

Rare causes of VTE include plasminogen deficiency, dysfibrinogenemia, and elevated levels of some procoagulants, which are not routinely measured in clinical practice. For example, factor XI levels above the 90th percentile increase the risk for VTE about twofold (94). Factor VIII levels increase in patients with inflammatory conditions, cancer, or pregnancy. When these conditions are excluded, factor VIII levels above the 90th percentile increase the risk for VTE approximately sevenfold (95). Increased lipoprotein (a), a known risk factor for arterial thrombosis, has recently been identified as a risk factor for VTE, especially when levels exceed 30 mg/dL. Lipoprotein (a), which is structurally similar to fibrinogen, competes for fibrin binding, causing impaired fibrinolysis and predisposing to VTE (96).

IV. Coexisting Thrombophilias

The risk of VTE is synergistically increased in patients with FVL who also have hyperhomocysteinemia or the prothrombin gene mutation (97–99). Therefore, patients diagnosed with one type of thrombophilia should be screened for coexisting coagulation abnormalities, because long-term anticoagulation may be indicated in these circumstances.

V. Testing for Hypercoagulable States: Recommendations

Screening for thrombophilia is controversial. These tests have the highest yield when patients present with recurrent, idiopathic VTE, a personal or family history of VTE, or a history of recurrent, unexplained pregnancy loss. In our practice, we test for FVL, the prothrombin gene mutation, hyperhomocysteinemia, and antiphospholipid antibodies, because the presence of these conditions may alter medical management. For example, the antiphospholipid antibody syndrome is treated with more intensive, prolonged anticoagulation than are other causes of VTE (100). Hyperhomocysteinemia is easily corrected with folate administration (60). FVL is the most prevalent inherited thrombophilia and synergistically increases the risk of VTE in patients with the prothrombin gene mutation, hyperhomocysteinemia, or concurrent oral contraceptive use. We do not routinely test for protein C or S deficiency or antithrombin III deficiency, because these abnormalities are rare.

VI. Conclusions

Many acquired and inherited risk factors predispose to VTE. Acquired conditions may be transient (such as trauma or pregnancy) or lifelong (such as antiphospholipid antibodies or incurable cancer). Some acquired factors, such as obesity, smoking, hypertension, and hyperhomocysteinemia, can be modified with lifestyle changes or aggressive medical management. The constant lifelong increase in VTE risk due to an inherited defect must be combined with the dynamic risks of advancing age and other acquired conditions. These factors, when taken together, may sufficiently disrupt the net balance between prothrombotic and antithrombotic mechanisms and precipitate an acute thrombotic event. Identifying these factors is an important first step toward prevention.

References

1. Lapostolle F, Surget V, Borron SW, Desmaizieres M, Sordelet D, Lapandry C, Cupa M, Adnet F. Severe pulmonary embolism associated with air travel. N Engl J Med 2001; 345:779–783.
2. Belcaro G, Geroulakos G, Nicolaides AN, Myers KA, Winford M. Venous thromboembolism from air travel: the LONFLIT study. Angiology 2001; 52:369–374.
3. Scurr JH, Machin SJ, Bailey-King S, Mackie IJ, McDonald S, Smith PD. Frequency and prevention of symptomless deep-vein thrombosis in long-haul flights: a randomised trial. Lancet 2001; 357:1485–1489.
4. Belcaro G, Geroulakos G, De Sanctis M, Nicolaides AN, Incandela L, Cesarone MR, Bucci M, Lennox A. Prevention of deep venous thrombosis on long-haul flights. J Am Coll Cardiol 2002; 39: 212A.
5. Goldhaber SZ, Grodstein F, Stampfer MJ, Manson JE, Colditz GA, Speizer FE, Willett WC, Hennekens CH. A prospective study of risk factors for pulmonary embolism in women. JAMA 1997; 277:642–645.
6. Ridker PM, Glynn RJ, Miletich JP, Goldhaber SZ, Stampfer MJ, Hennekens CH. Age-specific incidence rates of venous thromboembolism among heterozygous carriers of factor V Leiden mutation. Ann Intern Med 1997; 126:528–531.
7. Silverstein MD, Heit JA, Mohr DN, Petterson TM, O'Fallon WM, Melton LJ III. Trends in the incidence of deep vein thrombosis and pulmonary embolism: a 25-year population-based study. Arch Intern Med 1998; 158:585–593.
8. Collins R, Scrimgeour A, Yusuf S, Peto R. Reduction in fatal pulmonary embolism and venous thrombosis by perioperative administration of subcutaneous heparin. Overview of results of randomized trials in general, orthopedic, and urologic surgery. N Engl J Med 1988; 318:1162–1173.
9. Donati MB. Cancer and thrombosis. Haemostasis 1994; 24:128–131.

10. Merli GJ. Update. Deep vein thrombosis and pulmonary embolism prophylaxis in orthopedic surgery. Med Clin North Am 1993; 77:397–411.

11. Geerts WH, Heit JA, Clagett GP, Pineo GF, Colwell CW, Anderson FA Jr, Wheeler HB. Prevention of venous thromboembolism. Chest 2001; 119:132S–175S.

12. Prevention of fatal postoperative pulmonary embolism by low doses of heparin. An international multicentre trial. Lancet 1975; 2:45–51.

13. Huber O, Bounameaux H, Borst F, Rohner A. Postoperative pulmonary embolism after hospital discharge. An underestimated risk. Arch Surg 1992; 127:310–313.

14. Fitzgerald RH Jr, Spiro TE, Trowbridge AA, Gardiner GA Jr, Whitsett TL, O'Connell MB, Ohar JA, Young TR. Prevention of venous thromboembolic disease following primary total knee arthroplasty. A randomized, multicenter, open-label, parallel-group comparison of enoxaparin and warfarin. J Bone Joint Surg Am 2001; 83–A:900–906.

15. Stamatakis JD, Kakkar VV, Sagar S, Lawrence D, Naim D, Bentley PG. Femoral vein thrombosis and total hip replacement. BMJ 1977; 2:223–225.

16. Parmet JL, Berman AT, Horrow JC, Harding S, Rosenberg H. Thromboembolism coincident with tourniquet deflation during total knee arthroplasty. Lancet 1993; 341:1057–1058.

17. Hirota K, Hashimoto H, Kabara S, Tsubo T, Sato Y, Ishihara H, Matsuki A. The relationship between pneumatic tourniquet time and the amount of pulmonary emboli in patients undergoing knee arthroscopic surgeries. Anesth Analg 2001; 93:776–780.

18. Piccioli A, Prandoni P, Ewenstein BM, Goldhaber SZ. Cancer and venous thromboembolism. Am Heart J 1996; 132:850–855.

19. Prandoni P, Piccioli A, Girolami A. Cancer and venous thromboembolism: an overview. Haematologica 1999; 84:437–445.

20. Baron JA, Gridley G, Weiderpass E, Nyren O, Linet M. Venous thromboembolism and cancer. Lancet 1998; 351:1077–1080.

21. Schulman S, Lindmarker P. Incidence of cancer after prophylaxis with warfarin against recurrent venous thromboembolism. Duration of Anticoagulation Trial. N Engl J Med 2000; 342:1953–1958.

22. Sorensen HT, Mellemkjaer L, Steffensen FH, Olsen JH, Nielsen GL. The risk of a diagnosis of cancer after primary deep venous thrombosis or pulmonary embolism. N Engl J Med 1998; 338:1169–1173.

23. Fennerty T. Screening for cancer in venous thromboembolic disease: The incidence is higher but intensive screening isn't warranted. BMJ 2001; 323: 704–705.

24. Girolami A, Prandoni P, Zanon E, Bagatella P, Girolami B. Venous thromboses of upper limbs are more frequently associated with occult cancer as compared with those of lower limbs. Blood Coagul Fibrinolysis 1999; 10: 455–457.

25. Goad KE, Gralnick HR. Coagulation disorders in cancer. Hematol Oncol Clin North Am 1996; 10:457–484.

26. Moody J, Scott B. Trousseau's syndrome. Iowa Med 1991; 81:303–304.
27. Cogo A, Bernardi E, Prandoni P, Girolami B, Noventa F, Simioni P, Girolami A. Acquired risk factors for deep-vein thrombosis in symptomatic outpatients. Arch Intern Med 1994; 154:164–168.
28. Heit JA, Silverstein MD, Mohr DN, Petterson TM, O'Fallon WM, Melton LJ III. Risk factors for deep vein thrombosis and pulmonary embolism: a population-based case-control study. Arch Intern Med 2000; 160: 809–815.
29. Lip GY, Gibbs CR. Does heart failure confer a hypercoagulable state? Virchow's triad revisited. J Am Coll Cardiol 1999; 33:1424–1426.
30. Attia J, Ray JG, Cook DJ, Douketis J, Ginsberg JS, Geerts WH. Deep vein thrombosis and its prevention in critically ill adults. Arch Intern Med 2001; 161:1268–1279.
31. Horattas MC, Wright DJ, Fenton AH, Evans DM, Oddi MA, Kamienski RW, Shields EF. Changing concepts of deep venous thrombosis of the upper extremity—report of a series and review of the literature. Surgery 1988; 104: 561–567.
32. Luciani A, Clement O, Halimi P, Goudot D, Portier F, Bassot V, Luciani J, Avan P, Frija G, Bonfils P. Catheter-related upper extremity deep venous thrombosis in cancer patients: a prospective study based on Doppler US. Radiology 2001; 220: 655–660.
33. Zell L, Kindermann W, Marschall F, Scheffler P, Gross J, Buchter A. Paget-Schroetter syndrome in sports activities: case study and literature review. Angiology 2001; 52:337–342.
34. Parziale J, Akelman E, Weiss AC, Green A. Thoracic outlet syndrome. Am J Orthop 2000; 29:353–360.
35. Vandenbroucke JP, Rosing J, Bloemenkamp KW, Middeldorp S, Helmerhorst FM, Bouma BN, Rosendaal FR. Oral contraceptives and the risk of venous thrombosis. N Engl J Med 2001; 344:1527–1535.
36. Rosing J, Middeldorp S, Curvers J, Christella M, Thomassen LG, Nicolaes GA, Meijers JC, Bouma BN, Buller HR, Prins MH, Tans G. Low-dose oral contraceptives and acquired resistance to activated protein C: a randomised cross-over study. Lancet 1999; 354:2036–2040.
37. Chasan-Taber L, Stampfer MJ. Epidemiology of oral contraceptives and cardiovascular disease. Ann Intern Med 1998; 128:467–477.
38. Grodstein F, Stampfer MJ, Goldhaber SZ, Manson JE, Colditz GA, Speizer FE, Willett WC, Hennekens CH. Prospective study of exogenous hormones and risk of pulmonary embolism in women. Lancet 1996; 348:983–987.
39. Kemmeren JM, Algra A, Grobbee DE. Third generation oral contraceptives and risk of venous thrombosis: meta-analysis. BMJ 2001; 323:1–9.
40. Parkin L, Skegg DC, Wilson M, Herbison GP, Paul C. Oral contraceptives and fatal pulmonary embolism. Lancet 2000; 355:2133–2134.
41. Vasilakis-Scaramozza C, Jick H. Risk of venous thromboembolism with cyproterone or levonorgestrel contraceptives. Lancet 2001; 358:1427–1429.
42. Bloemenkamp KW, Rosendaal FR, Helmerhorst FM, Vandenbroucke JP.

Higher risk of venous thrombosis during early use of oral contraceptives in women with inherited clotting defects. Arch Intern Med 2000; 160:49–52.

43. Vandenbroucke JP, Koster T, Briet E, Reitsma PH, Bertina RM, Rosendaal FR. Increased risk of venous thrombosis in oral-contraceptive users who are carriers of factor V Leiden mutation. Lancet 1994; 344:1453–1457.

44. Toglia MR, Weg JG. Venous thromboembolism during pregnancy. N Engl J Med 1996; 335:108–114.

45. Greer I. Thrombosis in pregnancy: maternal and fetal issues. Lancet 1999; 353:1258–1265.

46. Gerhardt A, Scharf RE, Beckmann MW, Struve S, Bender HG, Pillny M, Sandmann W, Zotz RB. Prothrombin and factor V mutations in women with a history of thrombosis during pregnancy and the puerperium. N Engl J Med 2000; 342:374–380.

47. Manson JE, Martin KA. Clinical practice. Postmenopausal hormone-replacement therapy. N Engl J Med 2001; 345:34–40.

48. Grady D, Wenger NK, Herrington D, Khan S, Furberg C, Hunninghake D, Vittinghoff E, Hulley S. Postmenopausal hormone therapy increases risk for venous thromboembolic disease. The Heart and Estrogen/progestin Replacement Study. Ann Intern Med 2000; 132:689–696.

49. Lowe G, Woodward M, Vessey M, Rumley A, Gough P, Daly E. Thrombotic variables and risk of idiopathic venous thromboembolism in women aged 45–64 years. Relationships to hormone replacement therapy. Thromb Haemost 2000; 83:530–535.

50. Jick H, Derby LE, Myers MW, Vasilakis C, Newton KM. Risk of hospital admission for idiopathic venous thromboembolism among users of post-menopausal oestrogens. Lancet 1996; 348:981–983.

51. Daly E, Vessey MP, Hawkins MM, Carson JL, Gough P, Marsh S. Risk of venous thromboembolism in users of hormone replacement therapy. Lancet 1996; 348:977–980.

52. Hoibraaten E, Qvigstad E, Arnesen H, Larsen S, Wickstrom E, Sandset PM. Increased risk of recurrent venous thromboembolism during hormone replacement therapy—results of the randomized, double-blind, placebo-controlled estrogen in venous thromboembolism trial (EVTET). Thromb Haemost 2000; 84:961–967.

53. Cummings SR, Eckert S, Krueger KA, Grady D, Powles TJ, Cauley JA, Norton L, Nickelsen T, Bjarnason NH, Morrow M, Lippman ME, Black D, Glusman JE, Costa A, Jordan VC. The effect of raloxifene on risk of breast cancer in postmenopausal women: results from the MORE randomized trial. Multiple outcomes of raloxifene evaluation. JAMA 1999; 281: 2189–2197.

54. Greaves M. Antiphospholipid antibodies and thrombosis. Lancet 1999; 353:1348–1353.

55. Schulman S, Svenungsson E, Granqvist S. Anticardiolipin antibodies predict early recurrence of thromboembolism and death among patients with venous

thromboembolism following anticoagulant therapy. Duration of Anticoagulation Study Group. Am J Med 1998; 104:332–338.

56. Finazzi G, Brancaccio V, Moia M, Ciavarella N, Mazzucconi MG, Schinco P, Ruggeri M, Pogliani EM, Gamba G, Rossi E, Baudo F, Manotti C, D'Angelo A, Palareti G, De Stefano V, Berrettini M, Barbui T. Natural history and risk factors for thrombosis in 360 patients with antiphospholipid antibodies: a four-year prospective study from the Italian registry. Am J Med 1996; 100: 530–536.

57. Levine JS, Branch DW, Rauch J. The antiphospholipid syndrome. N Engl J Med 2002; 346:752–763.

58. Arnout J. The pathogenesis of the antiphospholipid syndrome: a hypothesis based on parallelisms with heparin-induced thrombocytopenia. Thromb Haemost 1996; 75:536–541.

59. Brandt JT, Triplett DA, Alving B, Scharrer I. Criteria for the diagnosis of lupus anticoagulants: an update. On behalf of the Subcommittee on Lupus Anticoagulant/Antiphospholipid Antibody of the Scientific and Standardisation Committee of the ISTH. Thromb Haemost 1995; 74:1185–1190.

60. Hankey GJ, Eikelboom JW. Homocysteine and vascular disease. Lancet 1999; 354:407–413.

61. Eichinger S, Stumpflen A, Hirschl M, Bialonczyk C, Herkner K, Stain M, Schneider B, Pabinger I, Lechner K, Kyrle PA. Hyperhomocysteinemia is a risk factor of recurrent venous thromboembolism. Thromb Haemost 1998; 80:566–569.

62. Langman LJ, Ray JG, Evrovski J, Yeo E, Cole DE. Hyperhomocyst(e)inemia and the increased risk of venous thromboembolism: more evidence from a case-control study. Arch Intern Med 2000; 160:961–964.

63. den Heijer M, Koster T, Blom HJ, Bos GM, Briet E, Reitsma PH, Vandenbroucke JP, Rosendaal FR. Hyperhomocysteinemia as a risk factor for deep-vein thrombosis. N Engl J Med 1996; 334:759–762.

64. D'Angelo A, Selhub J. Homocysteine and thrombotic disease. Blood 1997; 90:1–11.

65. Federman DG, Kirsner RS. An update on hypercoagulable disorders. Arch Intern Med 2001; 161:1051–1056.

66. Bertina RM, Koeleman BP, Koster T, Rosendaal FR, Dirven RJ, de Ronde H, van der Velden PA, Reitsma PH. Mutation in blood coagulation factor V associated with resistance to activated protein C. Nature 1994; 369:64–67.

67. Svensson PJ, Dahlback B. Resistance to activated protein C as a basis for venous thrombosis. N Engl J Med 1994; 330:517–522.

68. Franco RF, Reitsma PH. Genetic risk factors of venous thrombosis. Hum Genet 2001; 109:369–384.

69. Ridker PM, Miletich JP, Hennekens CH, Buring JE. Ethnic distribution of factor V Leiden in 4047 men and women. Implications for venous thromboembolism screening. JAMA 1997; 277:1305–1307.

70. Rees DC, Cox M, Clegg JB. World distribution of factor V Leiden. Lancet 1995; 346:1133–1134.

71. Ridker PM, Miletich JP, Buring JE, Ariyo AA, Price DT, Manson JE, Hill JA. Factor V Leiden mutation as a risk factor for recurrent pregnancy loss. Ann Intern Med 1998; 128:1000–1003.
72. Ridker PM, Hennekens CH, Lindpaintner K, Stampfer MJ, Eisenberg PR, Miletich JP. Mutation in the gene coding for coagulation factor V and the risk of myocardial infarction, stroke, and venous thrombosis in apparently healthy men. N Engl J Med 1995; 332:912–917.
73. Ridker PM, Miletich JP, Stampfer MJ, Goldhaber SZ, Lindpaintner K, Hennekens CH. Factor V Leiden and risks of recurrent idiopathic venous thromboembolism. Circulation 1995; 92:2800–2802.
74. Simioni P, Prandoni P, Lensing AW, Scudeller A, Sardella C, Prins MH, Villalta S, Dazzi F, Girolami A. The risk of recurrent venous thromboembolism in patients with an Arg506 Gln mutation in the gene for factor V (factor V Leiden). N Engl J Med 1997; 336:399–403.
75. Eichinger S, Pabinger I, Stumpflen A, Hirschl M, Bialonczyk C, Schneider B, Mannhalter C, Minar E, Lechner K, Kyrle PA. The risk of recurrent venous thromboembolism in patients with and without factor V Leiden. Thromb Haemost 1997; 77:624–628.
76. Turkstra F, Karemaker R, Kuijer PM, Prins MH, Buller HR. Is the prevalence of the factor V Leiden mutation in patients with pulmonary embolism and deep vein thrombosis really different? Thromb Haemost 1999; 81:345–348.
77. Bounameaux H. Factor V Leiden paradox: risk of deep-vein thrombosis but not of pulmonary embolism. Lancet 2000; 356:182–183.
78. Meyer G, Emmerich J, Helley D, Arnaud E, Nicaud V, Alhenc-Gelas M, Aiach M, Fischer A, Sors H, Fiessinger JN. Factors V Leiden and II 20210A in patients with symptomatic pulmonary embolism and deep vein thrombosis. Am J Med 2001; 110:12–15.
79. Le DT, Griffin JH, Greengard JS, Mujumdar V, Rapaport SI. Use of a generally applicable tissue factor–dependent factor V assay to detect activated protein C-resistant factor Va in patients receiving warfarin and in patients with a lupus anticoagulant. Blood 1995; 85:1704–1711.
80. Middeldorp S, Meinardi JR, Koopman MM, van Pampus EC, Hamulyak K, van der Meer J, Prins MH, Buller HR. A prospective study of asymptomatic carriers of the factor V Leiden mutation to determine the incidence of venous thromboembolism. Ann Intern Med 2001; 135:322–327.
81. Poort SR, Rosendaal FR, Reitsma PH, Bertina RM. A common genetic variation in the 3'-untranslated region of the prothrombin gene is associated with elevated plasma prothrombin levels and an increase in venous thrombosis. Blood 1996; 88:3698–3703.
82. Nguyen A. Prothrombin G20210A polymorphism and thrombophilia. Mayo Clin Proc 2000; 75:595–604.
83. Ridker PM, Hennekens CH, Miletich JP. G20210A mutation in prothrombin gene and risk of myocardial infarction, stroke, and venous thrombosis in a large cohort of US men. Circulation 1999; 99:999–1004.
84. Miles JS, Miletich JP, Goldhaber SZ, Hennekens CH, Ridker PM. G20210A

mutation in the prothrombin gene and the risk of recurrent venous thromboembolism. J Am Coll Cardiol 2001; 37:215–218.

85. Martinelli I, Sacchi E, Landi G, Taioli E, Duca F, Mannucci PM. High risk of cerebral-vein thrombosis in carriers of a prothrombin-gene mutation and in users of oral contraceptives. N Engl J Med 1998; 338:1793–1797.

86. Buller HR, ten Cate JW. Acquired antithrombin III deficiency: laboratory diagnosis, incidence, clinical implications, and treatment with antithrombin III concentrate. Am J Med 1989; 87:44S–48S.

87. Lane DA, Bayston T, Olds RJ, Fitches AC, Cooper DN, Millar DS, Jochmans K, Perry DJ, Okajima K, Thein SL, Emmerich J. Antithrombin mutation database: 2nd (1997) update for the plasma coagulation inhibitors subcommittee of the scientific and standardization committee of the international society on thrombosis and haemostasis. Thromb Haemost 1997; 77: 197–211.

88. Lechner K, Kyrle PA. Antithrombin III concentrates—are they clinically useful? Thromb Haemost 1995; 73:340–348.

89. Strickland DK, Kessler CM. Biochemical and functional properties of protein C and protein S. Clin Chim Acta 1987; 170:1–23.

90. Engesser L, Broekmans AW, Briet E, Brommer EJ, Bertina RM. Hereditary protein S deficiency: clinical manifestations. Ann Intern Med 1987; 106:677–682.

91. Bucciarelli P, Rosendaal FR, Tripodi A, Mannucci PM, De Stefano V, Palareti G, Finazzi G, Baudo F, Quintavalla R. Risk of venous thromboembolism and clinical manifestations in carriers of antithrombin, protein C, protein S deficiency, or activated protein C resistance: a multicenter collaborative family study. Arterioscler Thromb Vasc Biol 1999; 19:1026–1033.

92. Harrison L, Johnston M, Massicotte MP, Crowther M, Moffat K, Hirsh J. Comparison of 5-mg and 10-mg loading doses in initiation of warfarin therapy. Ann Intern Med 1997; 126:133–136.

93. Sallah S, Thomas DP, Roberts HR. Warfarin and heparin-induced skin necrosis and the purple toe syndrome: infrequent complications of anticoagulant treatment. Thromb Haemost 1997; 78:785–790.

94. Meijers JC, Tekelenburg WL, Bouma BN, Bertina RM, Rosendaal FR. High levels of coagulation factor XI as a risk factor for venous thrombosis. N Engl J Med 2000; 342:696–701.

95. Kyrle PA, Minar E, Hirschl M, Bialonczyk C, Stain M, Schneider B, Weltermann A, Speiser W, Lechner K, Eichinger S. High plasma levels of factor VIII and the risk of recurrent venous thromboembolism. N Engl J Med 2000; 343:457–462.

96. von Depka M, Nowak-Gottl U, Eisert R, Dieterich C, Barthels M, Scharrer I, Ganser A, Ehrenforth S. Increased lipoprotein (a) levels as an independent risk factor for venous thromboembolism. Blood 2000; 96:3364–3368.

97. Ridker PM, Hennekens CH, Selhub J, Miletich JP, Malinow MR, Stampfer MJ. Interrelation of hyperhomocyst(e)inemia, factor V Leiden, and risk of future venous thromboembolism. Circulation 1997; 95:1777–1782.

98. Margaglione M, D'Andrea G, Colaizzo D, Cappucci G, del Popolo A, Brancaccio V, Ciampa A, Grandone E, Di Minno G. Coexistence of factor V Leiden and Factor II A20210 mutations and recurrent venous thromboembolism. Thromb Haemost 1999; 82:1583–1587.

99. De Stefano V, Martinelli I, Mannucci PM, Paciaroni K, Chiusolo P, Casorelli I, Rossi E, Leone G. The risk of recurrent deep venous thrombosis among heterozygous carriers of both factor V Leiden and the G20210A prothrombin mutation. N Engl J Med 1999; 341:801–806.

100. Khamashta MA, Cuadrado MJ, Mujic F, Taub NA, Hunt BJ, Hughes GR. The management of thrombosis in the antiphospholipid-antibody syndrome. N Engl J Med 1995; 332:993–997.

3

Pathogenesis of Venous Thromboembolism

JEFFREY I. WEITZ and JACK HIRSH

McMaster University
Hamilton, Ontario, Canada

I. Introduction

Although venous thrombosis can develop in any vein, it most commonly occurs in superficial or deep veins of the lower limbs. Thrombosis in superficial veins of the legs often develops in varicosities and usually is a benign, self-limiting disorder. In contrast, thrombosis in the deep leg veins is a more serious condition. Deep vein thrombi usually originate in the calf either in the venous sinuses or in the valve cusp pockets (1,2). Calf vein thrombi are often asymptomatic, but will produce symptoms if they obstruct blood flow or induce inflammation of the vessel wall. Obstruction of venous outflow is more likely to occur when calf vein thrombi extend to involve the popliteal or more proximal veins of the leg. Consequently, proximal deep vein thrombosis is symptomatic more often than calf vein thrombosis (3), and it is the proximal thrombi that are more prone to embolize to the lungs (1,3).

Venous thrombi are composed of fibrin and blood cells (4). Because they form under low shear conditions, venous thrombi consist mainly of red blood cells, large amounts of interspersed fibrin, and relatively few platelets. In contrast, arterial thrombi, which form under high shear conditions, are mainly composed of platelet aggregates held together by small amounts of fibrin (4). Because of the preponderance of fibrin in venous thrombi, anticoagulants represent the cornerstone of their prevention and treatment (5). By contrast, prevention and treatment of platelet-rich arterial thrombi is effected with antiplatelet drugs, which are often used in combination with anticoagulants.

Thrombosis occurs when activation of the coagulation system overwhelms natural anticoagulant pathways and the capacity of the fibrinolytic system to degrade fibrin. In 1860, Virchow proposed a triad of factors involved in the pathogenesis of thrombosis. This triad incorporates the contents of the blood vessel, the vessel wall, and blood flow. Although the principles of the triad remain operative today, our understanding of the molecular mechanisms involved in thrombogenesis has markedly increased (Table 1).

Coagulation is triggered by tissue factor exposed at sites of vascular injury or synthesized by monocytes in response to inflammatory cytokines. This process is modulated by natural anticoagulant pathways and by the fibrinolytic system. Rather than serving as a passive lining of blood vessels, the vessel wall has emerged as a dynamic surface that is thromboresistant under normal conditions but becomes prothrombotic when endothelial cells are activated or damaged. Blood flow is important to prevent accumulation of clotting enzymes at sites of injury and to minimize contact of platelets and leukocytes with the vessel wall.

Because venous thrombosis occurs when thrombogenic stimuli overwhelm natural protective mechanisms, this chapter will (1) describe the pro-

Table 1 Mechanisms by Which Various Stimuli Promote Venous Thrombosis

Stimulus	Mechanism
Vessel wall injury	Exposes tissue factor, which activates coagulation
	Exposes subendothelial matrix proteins to which platelets adhere
	Leukocytes become tethered to activated endothelial cells; activated monocytes express tissue factor, whereas neutrophils promote vascular injury
	Loss of endothelial cell protective mechanisms
Blood components	Elevated levels of clotting factors
	Excessive activation of coagulation
	Impaired regulation of coagulation
	Impaired fibrinolytic mechanisms
Stasis	Promotes accumulation of activated clotting factors
	Hypoxic damage to endothelium

tective mechanisms that prevent thrombosis, (2) review the thrombogenic stimuli that trigger thrombosis, and (3) provide clinical perspective by illustrating how well-recognized risk factors for venous thromboembolism perturb the dynamic balance between procoagulant and protective mechanisms.

II. Protective Mechanisms

Factors that limit thrombosis include the nonthrombogenic properties of the endothelium; naturally occurring anticoagulant pathways; the fibrinolytic system, which degrades fibrin; and unimpeded blood flow, which serves to dilute activated clotting factors and limit contact of platelets and leukocytes with the vessel wall.

A. Nonthrombogenic Properties of Endothelium

Intact endothelium is thromboresistant (Fig. 1). It does not activate platelets or coagulation and it elaborates substances that inhibit coagulation, prevent platelet aggregation, and promote fibrinolysis. These properties can be lost if endothelial cells are activated or injured.

Endothelial cells influence platelets by synthesizing and releasing nitric oxide (NO) and prostacyclin, substances that inhibit platelet aggregation and induce vasodilatation (6–9). Endothelial cells also release tissue-type plasminogen activator (t-PA) and its major regulator, type 1 plasminogen activator inhibitor (PAI-1), two of the key components of the fibrinolytic system (10). By expressing annexin II, a coreceptor for t-PA and plasminogen, endothelial cells bind released t-PA and circulating plasminogen and provide a surface on which plasmin is generated (11,12).

Two of the natural anticoagulant pathways also depend on components of the endothelium. Heparan sulfate found on the abluminal surface of endothelial cells binds and activates antithrombin, a major inhibitor of thrombin and other clotting enzymes. The importance of antithrombin as a natural anticoagulant is underscored by the fact that patients deficient in this inhibitor are prone to thrombosis (13).

Endothelial cells also express thrombomodulin and endothelial cell protein C receptor (EPCR), key components of the protein C anticoagulant pathway (13,14). Thrombomodulin is a transmembrane protein that serves as a receptor for thrombin. Once bound to thrombomodulin, thrombin undergoes a conformational change at its active site that converts it from a procoagulant enzyme into a potent activator of protein C. Activated protein C (APC) serves as an anticoagulant by proteolytically degrading and inactivating two important cofactors of coagulation, activated factor V and activated factor VIII (factor Va and factor VIIIa, respectively). This

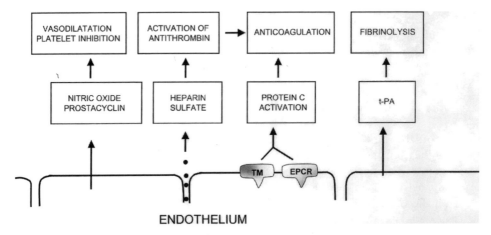

Figure 1 Nonthrombogenic properties of the vessel wall. Endothelial cells produce nitric oxide and prostacyclin, substances that cause vasodilatation and inhibit platelet aggregation. Heparan sulfate on the abluminal surface of endothelial cells activates circulating antithrombin, thereby promoting its anticoagulant activity. Thrombomodulin (TM) binds thrombin and converts it from a procoagulant enzyme into a potent activator of protein C. Activated protein C (APC) downregulates thrombin generation by inactivating factors Va and VIIIa. Endothelial cell protein C receptor (EPCR) binds protein C and localizes it on the cell surface where it can be activated by thrombomodulin-bound thrombin. Endothelial cells also synthesize and release tissue plasminogen activator (t-PA) and urinary plasminogen activator (u-PA), which initiate fibrinolysis by converting plasminogen to plasmin.

reaction, which occurs on negatively charged phospholipid surfaces, requires protein S as a cofactor (13,14).

The density of thrombomodulin expression is highest on small blood vessels, which present a greater surface area than larger vessels. To compensate for the reduced density of thrombomodulin, endothelial cells lining large blood vessels also express EPCR, a transmembrane protein that binds both protein C and APC. By concentrating protein C on the endothelial cell surface, EPCR promotes protein C activation by the thrombin/thrombomodulin complex (14).

The physiological importance of the protein C anticoagulant pathway is highlighted by the fact that patients deficient in protein C or protein S are prone to thromboembolism (15). More common than congenital protein C or protein S deficiency is the syndrome of activated protein C resistance, a disorder found in 2–6% of white populations (16,17). Over 90% of cases of activated protein C resistance are caused by a point mutation in the factor V gene that leads to the Arg residue at position 506 in factor V being replaced with a Gln residue. This mutant factor V is designated factor V Leiden. Although common in whites, the factor V Leiden mutation is not found in African blacks, Chinese, Japanese, or American Indian populations (18). This phenomenon has been explained by evidence that the factor V Leiden mutation arose through a founder effect about 30,000 years ago, a time after evolutionary divergence of white, African, and Asian populations (19). Persistence of the mutation through the centuries may reflect its potential evolutionary advantages. Women with the factor V Leiden mutation appear to have reduced menstrual bleeding (20), and premature infants carrying the mutation may be less prone to intraventricular hemorrhage (21).

The 506 bond in factor Va is the initial APC cleavage site on factor Va, and hydrolysis of this bond accelerates subsequent APC-mediated factor Va degradation (17). Because of the mutation at position 506, activated factor V Leiden is cleaved and inactivated by APC more slowly than wild-type factor Va, resulting in more persistent thrombin generation. This phenomenon may explain why patients with the factor V Leiden mutation are prone to venous thromboembolism (17).

B. Naturally Occurring Anticoagulant Pathways

In addition to antithrombin and the protein C pathway, tissue factor pathway inhibitor (TFPI) forms the basis of a third naturally occurring anticoagulant pathway. Because coagulation occurs at sites of vascular injury, all three anticoagulant pathways modulate clotting on the vessel wall. The antithrombin and protein C anticoagulant pathways are localized to the vessel wall, because, as described above, components of these pathways are found on the endothelium. The activity of TFPI is concentrated at sites of vascular injury where exposed tissue factor initiates coagulation by binding factor VIIa. A bivalent Kunitz-type inhibitor, TFPI inhibits the factor VIIa/tissue factor complex in a two-step fashion. TFPI first binds and inactivates factor Xa, and the TFPI/factor Xa complex then inactivates tissue factor–bound factor VIIa (22). Because formation of the TFPI/factor Xa complex is a prerequisite for efficient inhibition of the factor VIIa/tissue factor complex, the system ensures that some factor Xa generation occurs before the clotting mechanism is shut down.

C. Fibrinolytic System

Fibrinolysis is initiated by plasminogen activators that convert plasminogen, an inactive proenzyme, to plasmin. Plasmin then effects fibrinolysis by degrading fibrin into soluble fibrin degradation products (23). Two immunologically distinct plasminogen activators are found in blood; t-PA and urokinase plasminogen activator (u-PA). Both plasminogen activators are released from endothelial cells. Monocytes also synthesize and release u-PA and express annexin II on their surface (24). Released u-PA binds to u-PA receptors on the cell surface, whereas annexin II serves as a coreceptor for t-PA and plasminogen where it can locally convert plasminogen to plasmin. Cell surface plasmin likely represents one mechanism by which these cells degrade extracellular matrix proteins as they pass from the intravascular space into the tissues (23). The fibrinolytic system is regulated at two levels; plasminogen activators are inhibited by plasminogen activator inhibitors, the most important of which is PAI-1. Circulating plasmin is primarily inactivated by α_2-antiplasmin. Secondary plasmin inhibitors include α_2-macroglobulin and α_1-antitrypsin (23).

An association between congenital plasminogen deficiency and venous thromboembolism has been reported in several families (25,26). The abnormality appears to be inherited in an autosomal fashion with heterozygotes having plasminogen levels half those of normals. Increased PAI-1 levels or defective synthesis or release of t-PA are potential acquired causes of impaired fibrinolysis. Although there are reports of venous thromboembolism in association with these abnormalities (27), a causal relationship has yet to be established.

By serving as a binding site for t-PA and plasminogen, annexin II localizes fibrinolysis on the endothelial cell surface (11,12). The interaction of plasminogen with annexin II is mediated by its lysine-binding kringles. Lipoprotein(a) Lp(a) competes with plasminogen for annexin II binding. This phenomenon may explain why increased levels of Lp(a) are a risk factor for arterial thrombosis (28,29). However, there is little evidence for an association between elevated Lp(a) levels and venous thrombosis.

Increased levels of homocysteine also impair the binding of t-PA to annexin II (30). Although it is possible that reduced fibrinolytic activity may contribute to the increased risk of arterial and venous thromboses in patients with hyperhomocysteinemia, a causal relationship has yet to be established. Exposure of cultured endothelial cells to homocysteine induces an endoplasmic reticulum stress response characterized by overexpression of genes that influence cell proliferation and hemostatic balance. Homocysteine exposure reduces cell proliferation, promotes apoptosis, and induces mitochondrial damage (31,32). These phenomena also may contribute to the increased risk of thrombosis in patients with hyperhomocysteinemia (33,34).

D. Blood Flow

Venous return from the lower extremities is enhanced by contraction of the calf muscles, which propels blood upward from the legs. Valves in the deep veins of the legs maintain this upward blood flow. The avascular valve cusps depend on the ambient blood for their nutrient supply. With venous stasis, oxygen tension in the venous blood declines, thereby compromising oxygen supply to the valve cusps. Under hypoxic conditions, endothelial cells display a prothrombotic phenotype and express tissue factor and other activators of coagulation (34). With impaired blood flow there is accumulation of activated clotting factors, a process that can amplify clotting. These phenomena may explain the propensity of venous thrombi to arise in the venous sinuses of the calf or the valve cusp pockets of the deep calf veins. They also explain why immobility and venous obstruction, conditions that promote venous stasis, are risk factors for venous thromboembolism.

III. Thrombogenic Stimuli

Venous thromboembolism occurs when procoagulant stimuli overwhelm natural anticoagulant mechanisms and the capacity of the fibrinolytic system to degrade the resultant fibrin. Procoagulant stimuli can result from excessive activation of coagulation, vessel wall damage, or stasis, particularly when protective pathways are compromised by genetic abnormalities associated with excessive coagulation. Protective pathways include the nonthrombogenic properties of the vessel wall, natural anticoagulant pathways, and the fibrinolytic system.

A. Activation of Coagulation

Coagulation factors circulate as inactive zymogens. Each zymogen is converted to an active enzyme that activates the next zymogen in the coagulation pathway. Although the coagulation system can be initiated in vitro via intrinsic or extrinsic pathways, initiation in vivo is mediated by tissue factor and occurs through the extrinsic pathway.

Tissue factor is not normally expressed by blood-contacting cells. Inflammatory cytokines, such as interleukin-1 (IL-1) or tumor necrosis factor (TNF), can induce tissue factor expression by monocytes. Activated or damaged endothelial cells express receptors that tether leukocytes, platelets, and tissue factor–bearing monocytes or cell particles onto their surface (35–37). In addition to tissue factor expression, tethered leukocytes can amplify vascular damage by generating free radicals or releasing hydrolytic enzymes (35,36).

There are other links between inflammation and thrombosis. Inflammatory cytokines trigger the internalization of thrombomodulin, thereby reducing its density on the endothelial cell surface (13,14). This decreases the capacity for protein C activation. Shedding of EPCR contributes to the defect in the protein C anticoagulant pathway (14). Thrombin cleaves EPCR from the endothelial cell surface. By binding to circulating APC, soluble EPCR prevents it from degrading its substrates, a phenomenon that further compromises the protein C anticoagulant pathway.

Although a small fraction of circulating factor VII is activated, factor VIIa has little or no proteolytic activity until bound to tissue factor. Once the factor VIIa/tissue factor complex is formed, the catalytic efficiency of factor VIIa is increased (38) and it activates factors IX and X. Activation of factor X is more efficient, and the resultant factor Xa generates small amounts of thrombin that amplify the system by activating platelets and factors V and VIII. Factor VIIIa on the surface of activated platelets binds factor IXa to form intrinsic tenase. This complex is more efficient than the factor VIIa/ tissue factor complex (so-called extrinsic tenase) at activating factor X. Consequently, the bulk of factor X activation is effected by intrinsic tenase rather than extrinsic tenase (39). This phenomenon explains why patients with hemophilia A and B who lack factor VIII or factor IX, respectively, have a hemorrhagic diathesis despite intact initiation of coagulation via extrinsic tenase.

Factor Xa combines with factor Va on the activated platelet surface to form prothrombinase, the complex that activates prothrombin. The resultant thrombin then converts fibrinogen to fibrin. Fibrin monomers spontaneously polymerize to form fibrin polymer. The fibrin polymer is cross linked by activated factor XIII (factor XIIIa), a thrombin-activated transglutaminase. Cross linking stabilizes the fibrin mesh and renders it more resistant to lysis (38).

Thrombin generation is tightly regulated by TFPI, antithrombin, and the protein C anticoagulant pathway (13). By inhibiting factor VIIa in a factor Xa–dependent fashion, TFPI blocks the initiation of coagulation (13,22). In contrast, antithrombin and activated protein C block the propagation of coagulation (22). Antithrombin accomplishes this task by inhibiting factor Xa and thrombin, whereas activated protein C targets factors Va and VIIIa, the cofactors in prothrombinase and intrinsic tenase, respectively (14).

Using sensitive biochemical markers, healthy subjects exhibit low-level activation of coagulation which progressively increases with age (40,41). Levels of markers of activation of coagulation are elevated in some patients with congenital deficiencies of antithrombin, protein C, or protein S, and in those with antiphospholipid antibody syndrome, patients who also are at risk for thrombosis (42–44). Increased activation of coagulation in these states likely reflects defective regulatory mechanisms. Systemic impairment in the regulation of coagulation may explain why patients with unprovoked deep vein thrombosis are just as likely to develop recurrence in the opposite leg as they are in the leg in which the incident event occurred.

Patients with malignancy are at higher risk for thrombosis (45). Activation of coagulation in these subjects is likely to be multifactorial in origin (46–48). Some malignant cells express tissue factor, whereas others may expose tissue factor after chemotherapy or radiotherapy-induced cell death. Tissue factor also can be expressed by cytokine-activated monocytes. In addition to tissue factor–mediated activation of coagulation, some malignant cells elaborate a cysteine protease that can trigger coagulation by directly activating factor X (49).

B. Vessel Wall Damage

Although the normal vessel wall is nonthrombogenic, damage or injury to the endothelium can trigger the activation of platelets and coagulation. Direct vascular wall damage exposes tissue factor and subendothelial matrix proteins. Exposed tissue factor binds factor VIIa and initiates coagulation. Coincidentally, platelets adhere to exposed subendothelial matrix proteins where they become activated, thereby providing a surface on which clotting factors assemble (34). Activated platelets release thromboxane A_2 and adenosine diphosphate (ADP), substances that activate ambient platelets. Platelet activation also triggers conformational changes in glycoprotein (GP) IIb/IIIa, the most abundant receptor on the platelet surface. Once it is conformationally activated, GPIIb/IIIa binds fibrinogen and bridges adjacent platelets to form platelet aggregates (47).

Platelet aggregation and fibrin formation at sites of vascular injury explain, at least in part, the high incidence of venous thrombosis complicating major orthopedic surgery of the lower limbs. Local hypoxia caused by venous stasis is likely to be a contributing factor. Under hypoxic conditions, endothelial cells express receptors for leukocytes. Monocytes tethered to these receptors elaborate tissue factor that can trigger coagulation and express receptors for factor X and fibrinogen that can localize coagulation factors on their surface (35,36). Use of a thigh tourniquet in patients undergoing knee arthroplasty increases venous stasis and subsequent hypoxia in the calf. This may explain the high incidence of calf vein thrombosis in these patients (5).

In addition to direct trauma and hypoxia, endothelial cells also can be activated by exposure to endotoxin, inflammatory cytokines, such as IL-1 and TNF, and products of coagulation, particularly thrombin. Perturbed endothelial cells assume a procoagulant phenotype. They express tissue factor, attract tissue factor–bearing monocytes, and internalize thrombomodulin, which are alterations that promote coagulation. Under hypoxic conditions, endothelial cells may elaborate a protease that directly activates factor X (34), thereby augmenting thrombin generation. Concomitant synthesis and release of PAI-1 impairs local fibrinolysis. Perturbed endothelial cells also synthesize endothelins, substances that cause local vaso-constriction and promote platelet aggregation.

C. Venous Stasis

Venous stasis can be caused by systemic or local factors. Systemic factors include immobility and increased blood viscosity, whereas venous obstruction and venous dilatation are local factors that can contribute to stasis. With immobility, blood pools in the venous sinuses of the calf, which are dilated with recumbency (50). The importance of immobility in the pathogenesis of venous thrombosis is highlighted by the observation from autopsy studies that the prevalence of thrombosis is increased in patients confined to bed for more than a week before death (51). Furthermore, preoperative immobility is associated with a higher incidence of postoperative thrombosis (52–54), and after surgery, patients remain at risk for venous thromboembolism until they are fully mobile (55–57). The observations that thrombosis is more frequent in the paralyzed limb of stroke patients, whereas it occurs with equal frequency in both legs of paraplegics (58,59), provide additional evidence for the importance of immobility as a risk factor for venous thrombosis.

Venous stasis is likely to be the major factor predisposing patients to travel-related thrombosis (60). The risk of thrombosis increases exponentially with air travel times beyond 6 hrs, and there is a suggestion that the risk can be lowered by the use of graded compression stockings (61,62).

Increased blood viscosity causes venous stasis as does venous dilatation. Blood viscosity is increased with the elevated hematocrit that occurs in polycythemia. Hypergammaglobulinemia, dysproteinemia, and elevated levels of fibrinogen also can be associated with increased blood viscosity. This phenomenon could account for the increased risk of thrombosis in patients with these disorders. In addition to increased blood viscosity, acquired activated protein C resistance in patients with multiple myeloma also may render them prone to thrombosis (63). Stasis secondary to venous dilatation may explain why patients with varicose veins have an increased risk of thrombosis, particularly if they are bedridden. Estrogen causes venous dilatation (64). This could contribute to the increased risk of thrombosis during pregnancy and in women using estrogen-containing oral contraceptives or hormone replacement therapy (64).

As a local cause of venous stasis, venous obstruction may contribute to the risk of venous thrombosis in patients with pelvic tumors. Likewise, persistent venous obstruction after extensive proximal deep vein thrombosis may predispose patients to ipsilateral recurrence. Local venous stasis may also underlie the propensity for thrombosis in the left iliac vein during pregnancy (65). Thus, pressure from the enlarging uterus compresses the right common iliac artery which overlies the left common iliac vein. Raised central venous pressure produces venous stasis in the lower extremities. This phenomenon could explain why patients with heart failure are prone to thrombosis (66,67).

D. Impaired Compensatory Mechanisms

Venous thrombosis occurs when procoagulant stimuli overwhelm natural protective mechanisms. Patients with congenital deficiency of antithrombin, protein C, or protein S are prone to thrombosis, because naturally occurring anticoagulant pathways are compromised. Mutations in thrombomodulin or EPCR that limit protein C activation may also render patients prone to thrombosis (68,69).

A deficiency in heparin cofactor II, a secondary inhibitor of thrombin, has been associated with thrombosis. However, the risk of thrombosis in family members with heparin cofactor II deficiency appears similar to that in unaffected family members (70). Consequently, a causal relationship between heparin cofactor II deficiency and thrombosis has yet to be established.

Patients with activated protein C resistance are at increased risk of thrombosis because of excessive thrombin generation. Increased thrombin generation also may underlie the propensity to thrombosis in subjects with the prothrombin gene mutation. This G to A substitution at nucleotide 20210 in the 3'-untranslated region of the prothrombin gene is associated with elevated levels of prothrombin (71). With an allele frequency about half that of factor V Leiden, the prothrombin gene mutation is the second most common genetic risk factor for thrombosis, and occurs in about 2% of the white population.

Patients with elevated levels of factor VIII also have the potential for excessive thrombin generation. This could explain the observation that elevated factor VIII levels are associated with an increased risk of recurrent venous thromboembolism (72–74). Some studies also suggest an association between elevated levels of factor IX or factor X and venous thromboembolism (75,76). Elevated levels of these clotting factors appears to be an independent risk factor for thrombosis in patients who also have the factor V Leiden mutation (77,78).

Some dysfibrinogenemias have been associated with an increased risk of thrombosis, although most are asymptomatic or associated with a hemorrhagic diathesis (79,80). Potential mechanisms by which dysfibrinogenemia could lead to thrombosis include production of fibrin that is resistant to lysis because of reduced affinity for t-PA or defective thrombin binding to fibrin (79–81).

Impaired fibrinolysis can also predispose patients to thrombosis. Decreased fibrinolytic activity occurs in the early postoperative period (82–86), and has been reported in the last trimester of pregnancy (87,88), in women taking oral contraceptives (89) and in obese subjects (90,91). Fibrinolytic activity in the leg veins is less than that in arm veins (92), an observation that may partly explain why venous thrombi occur in the leg veins more frequently than in arm veins. The relative reduction in fibrinolytic activity in leg veins compared with arm veins is more pronounced in elderly people (93), which could account, at least in part, for the age-related increase in the risk of thrombosis.

There are isolated reports of familial abnormalities in fibrinolysis associated with thrombosis (94), but these appear to be rare. Impaired fibrinolysis in patients with established venous thromboembolism appears to be an acquired defect, mainly due to increased levels of PAI-1 (94). There is no evidence that defective fibrinolysis predicts recurrent thrombosis in this setting (94).

IV. Conclusions

The pathogenesis of venous thromboembolism is complex and often involves an interplay between genetic and acquired factors. Patients with genetic defects that predispose them to thrombosis have a lifelong risk of thrombosis, about half of which are triggered by environmental stimuli, such as surgery, cancer, or estrogen use. Because of the high background frequency of factor V Leiden and the prothrombin gene mutation in the general population, patients with more than one thrombophilic defect are being identified with increasing frequency. These individuals are more prone to thrombosis than those with a single abnormality. Thus, thrombosis can be viewed as a multigenic disorder in which susceptible individuals have one or more genetic mutations with clinical events occurring when superimposed environmental factors trigger thrombosis. In many cases, however, the inciting precipitant cannot be identified nor can an underlying genetic abnormality be detected. Such patients with unprovoked or idiopathic venous thromboembolism have an ongoing risk of recurrent thrombosis when anticoagulation therapy is stopped after 3, 6, 12, or 27 months (95–98). Further studies are needed to identify the underlying triggers to thrombosis in these patients.

References

1. Kakkar VV, Howe CT, Flance C, Clarke MB. Natural history of postoperative deep-vein thrombosis. Lancet 1969; 2:230–232.
2. Nicolaides AN, Kakkar VV, Field ES, Renney JTG. The origin of deep vein thrombosis: a venographic study. Br J Radiol 1971; 44:653–663.

3. Moser KM, LeMoine JR. Is embolic risk conditioned by location of deep venous thrombosis? Ann Intern Med 1981; 94:439-444.
4. Freiman DG. The structure of thrombi. In: Colman RW, Hirsh J, Marder V, Salzman EW, eds. Hemostasis and Thrombosis: Basic Principles and Clinical Practice. 2nd ed. Philadelphia: Lippincott, 1987:1123-1135.
5. Geerts WH, Heit JA, Clagett GP, Pineo GF, Colwell CW, Anderson FA Jr, Wheeler HB. Prevention of venous thromboembolism. Chest 2001; 119:132S-175S.
6. Griffith TM, Edwards DH, Lewis MJ, Newby AC, Henderson AH. The nature of endothelial-derived vascular relaxant factor. Nature 1984; 308:645-647.
7. Palmer RM, Ferrige AG, Moncada S. Nitric oxide release accounts for the biological activity of endothelium-derived relaxing factor. Nature 1987; 327:524-526.
8. Radomski MW, Palmer RM, Moncada S. Endogenous nitric oxide inhibits platelet adhesion to vascular endothelium. Lancet 1987; 2:1057-1058.
9. Moncada S, Gryglewski R, Bunting S, Vane JR. An enzyme isolated from arteries transforms prostaglandin endoperoxides to an unstable substance that inhibits platelet aggregation. Nature 1976; 263:663-665.
10. Loskutoff DJ, Edgington TE. Synthesis of a fibrinolytic activator and inhibitor by endothelial cells. Proc Natl Acad Sci USA 1977; 74:3903-3907.
11. Hajjar KA, Jacovina AT, Chacko J. An endothelial cell receptor for plasminogen/tissue plasminogen activator I. Identity with annexin II. J Biol Chem 1994; 269:21191-21197.
12. Cesarman GM, Guevara CA, Hajjar KA. An endothelial cell receptor for plasminogen/tissue plasminogen activator (t-PA). II. Annexin II-mediated enhancement of t-PA-dependent plasminogen activation. J Biol Chem 1994; 269:21198-21203.
13. Esmon CT. Protein C: The regulation of natural anticoagulant pathways. Science 1987; 235:1348-1352.
14. Esmon CT, Xu J, Gu JM, Qu D, Laszik Z, Ferrell G, Stearns-Kurosawa DJ, Kurosawa S, Taylor FB Jr, Esmon NL. Endothelial protein C receptor. Thromb Haemost 1999; 82:251-258.
15. Heijboer H, Brandjes DPM, Buller HR, Sturk A, tenCate JW. Deficiencies of coagulation-inhibiting and fibrinolytic proteins in outpatients with deep vein thrombosis. N Engl J Med 1990; 323:1512-1516.
16. Dahlback B. Inherited thrombophilia: resistance to activated protein C as a pathogenic factor of venous thromboembolism. Blood 1995; 85:607-614.
17. Nicolaes GA, Dahlback B. Factor V and thrombotic disease: description of a Janus-faced protein. Arterioscl Thromb Vasc Biol 2002; 22:530-538.
18. Rees DC, Cox M, Clegg JB. World distribution of factor V Leiden. Lancet 1995; 346:1133-1134.
19. Zivelin A, Griffin JH, Xu X, Pabinger I, Samama M, Conard J, Brenner B, Eldor A, Seligsohn U. A single genetic origin for a common Caucasian risk factor for venous thrombosis. Blood 1997; 89:397-402.
20. Lindqvist PG, Zoller B, Dahlback B. Improved hemoglobin status and reduced

menstrual blood loss among female carriers of factor V Leiden—an evolutionary advantage? Thromb Haemost 2001; 86:1122–1123.

21. Gopel W, Gortner L, Kohlmann T, Schultz C, Moller J. Low prevalence of large intraventricular haemorrhage in very low birth weight infants carrying the factor V Leiden or prothrombin G20210A mutation. Acta Paediatr 2001; 90:1021–1024.

22. Broze GJ Jr. Tissue factor pathway inhibitor. Thromb Haemost 1995; 74:90–93.

23. Collen D. The plasminogen (fibrinolytic) system. Thromb Haemost 1999; 82:259–270.

24. Kim J, Hajjar KA. Annexin II: a plasminogen-plasminogen activator co-receptor. Front Biosci 2002; 7:d341–d348.

25. Wille-Jorgensen M, Mortensen JZ, Madsen AG, Thorsen S. A family with reduced plasminogen activator activity in blood associated with recurrent venous thrombosis. Scand J Haematol 1982; 29:217–223.

26. Johansson L, Hedner U, Nilsson IM. A family with thromboembolic disease associated with deficient fibrinolytic activity in vessel wall. Acta Med Scand 1978; 203:477–480.

27. Prins MH, Hirsh J. A critical review of the evidence supporting a relationship between impaired fibrinolysis and venous thromboembolism. Arch Intern Med 1991; 151:1721–1731.

28. Miles LA, Fless GM, Levin EG, Scanu AM, Plow EF. A potential basis for the thrombotic risks associated with lipoprotein (a). Nature 1989; 339:301–333.

29. Hajjar KA, Gavish D, Breslow JL, Nachman RL. Lipoprotein(a) modulation of endothelial cell surface fibrinolysis and its potential role in atherosclerosis. Nature 1989; 339:303–305.

30. Hajjar KA, Mauri L, Jacovina AT, Zhong F, Mirza UA, Padovan JC, Chait BT. Tissue plasminogen activator binding to the annexin II tail domain. Direct modulation by homocysteine. J Biol Chem 1998; 273:9987–9993.

31. Austin RC, Sood SK, Dorward AM, Singh G, Shaughnessy SG, Pamidi S, Outinen PA, Weitz JI. Homocysteine-dependent alterations in mitochondrial gene expression, function and structure. Homocysteine and H202 act synergistically to enhance mitochondrial damage. J Biol Chem 1998; 273:30808–30817.

32. Outinen PA, Sood SK, Pfeifer SI, Pamidi S, Podor TJ, Li J, Weitz JI, Austin RC. Homocysteine-induced endoplasmic reticulum stress and growth arrest leads to specific changes in gene expression in human vascular endothelial cells. Blood 1999; 94:959–967.

33. den Heijer M, Koster T, Blom HJ, Bos GM, Briet E, Reitsma PH, Vandenbroucke JP, Rosendaal FR. Hyperhomocysteinemia as a risk factor for deep-vein thrombosis. N Engl J Med 1996; 334:759–762.

34. den Heijer M, Rosendaal FR, Blom HJ, Gerrits WB, Bos GM. Hyperhomocysteinemia and venous thrombosis: a meta-analysis. Thromb Haemost 1998; 80:874–877.

35. McEver RP. Adhesive interactions of leukocytes, platelets, and the vessel wall during hemostasis and inflammation. Thromb Haemost 2001; 86:746–756.

36. McEver RP. P-selectin and PSGL-1: exploiting connections between inflammation and venous thrombosis. Thromb Haemost 2002; 87:364–365.

37. Giesen PL, Rauch U, Bohrmann B, Kling D, Roque M, Fallon JT, Badimon JJ, Himber J, Riederer MA, Nemerson Y. Blood-borne tissue factor: another view of thrombosis. Proc Natl Acad Sci USA 1999; 96:2311–2315.

38. Colman RW, Marder VJ, Salzman EW, Hirsh J. Overview of hemostasis. In: Colman RW, Hirsh J, Marder VJ, Salzman EW, eds. Hemostasis and Thrombosis: Basic Principles and Clinical Practice. 3rd ed. Philadelphia: Lippincott, 1994:3–18.

39. Hockin MF, Jones KC, Everse SJ, Mann KG. A model for the stoichiometric regulation of blood coagulation. J Biol Chem 2002; 277:18322–18333.

40. Bauer KA, Weiss LM, Sparrow D, Vokonas PS, Rosenberg RD. Aging-associated changes in indices of thrombin generation and protein C activation in humans. Normatic Aging Study. J Clin Invest 1987; 80:1527–1534.

41. Mari D, Mannucci PM, Coppola R, Bottasso B, Bauer KA, Rosenberg RD. Hypercoagulability in centenarians: the paradox of successful aging. Blood 1995; 85:3144–3149.

42. Bauer KA, Goodman TL, Kass BL, Rosenberg RD. Elevated factor Xa activity in the blood of asymptomatic patients with congenital antithrombin deficiency. J Clin Invest 1985; 76:826–836.

43. Bauer KA, Broekmans AW, Bertina RM, Conard J, Horellou MH, Samama MM, Rosenberg RD. Hemostatic enzyme generation in the blood of patients with hereditary protein C deficiency. Blood 1988; 71:1418–1426.

44. Ginsberg JS, Demers C, Brill-Edwards P, Johnston M, Bona R, Burrows RF, Weitz J, Denburg JA. Increased thrombin generation and activity in patients with systemic lupus erythematosus and anticardiolipin antibodies: evidence for a prothrombotic state. Blood 1993; 81:2958–2963.

45. Rickles FR, Levine MN. Epidemiology of thrombosis in cancer. Acta Haematol 2001; 106:6–12.

46. Falanga A, Rickles FR. Pathophysiology of the thrombophilic state in the cancer patient. Semin Thromb Hemost 1999; 25:173–182.

47. Lee AY, Levine MN. The thrombophilic state induced by therapeutic agents in the cancer patient. Semin Thromb Haemost 1999; 25:137–145.

48. Rickles FR, Falanga A. Molecular basis for the relationship between thrombosis and cancer. Thromb Res 2001; 102:V215–V224.

49. Gordon SG, Franks C, Lewis B. Cancer procoagulation A: a factor X activating procoagulant from malignant tissue. Thromb Res 1975; 6:127–137.

50. Almen T, Bylander G. Serial phlebography of the normal leg during muscular contraction and relaxation. Acta Radiol 1962; 57:264.

51. Gibbs NM. Venous thrombosis of the lower limbs with particular reference to bed rest. Br J Surg 1957; 45:209.

52. Flordal PA, Bergqvist D, Burmark US, Ljungstrom KG, Torngren S. Risk factors for major thromboembolism and bleeding tendency after elective general surgical operations. Eur J Surg 1996; 162:783–789.

53. Heatley RV, Hughes LE, Morgan A, Okwonga W. Preoperative or postoperative deep vein thrombosis. Lancet 1976; 1:437–439.

54. Clarke-Pearson DL, DeLong Er, Synan IS, Coleman RE, Creasman WT. Variables associated with postoperative deep venous thrombosis: a prospective study of 411 gynecology patients and creation of a prognostic model. Obstet Gynecol 1987; 69:146–150.

55. Turpie AGG, Gallus AS, Beattie WS, Hirsh J. Prevention of venous thrombosis in patients with intracranial disease by intermittent pneumatic compression of the calf. Neurology 1977; 27:435–438.

56. Gallus AS, Hirsh J, O'Brien SE, McBride JA, Tuttle RJ, Gent M. Prevention of venous thrombosis with small subcutaneous doses of heparin. JAMA 1976; 235:1980–1982.

57. Gardlund B. Randomised, controlled trial of low-dose heparin for prevention of fatal pulmonary embolism in patients with infectious diseases. Lancet 1996; 347:1357–1361.

58. Warlow C, Ogston D, Douglas AS. Deep vein thrombosis of the legs after strokes. BMJ 1976; 1:1178–1181.

59. Bors E, Conrad CA, Massel TB. Venous occlusion of lower extremities in paraplegic patients. Surg Gynecol Obstet 1954; 99:451.

60. Gallus AS, Goghlan DC. Travel and venous thrombosis. Curr Opin Pulm Med 2002; 8:372–378.

61. Scurr JH, Machin SJ, Bailey-King S, Mackie IJ, McDonald S, Smith PD. Frequency and prevention of symptomless deep-vein thrombosis in long-haul flights: a randomised trial. Lancet 2001; 357:1485–1489.

62. Belaro G, Geroulakos G, Nicolaides AN, Myers KA, Winford M. Venous thromboembolism from air travel: the LONFLIT study. Angiology 2001; 52:369–374.

63. Zangari M, Saghafifar F, Anaissie E, Badros A, Desikan R, Fassas A, Mehta P, Morris C, Toor A, Whitfield D, Siegel E, Barlogie B, Fink L, Tricot G. Activated protein C resistance in the absence of factor V Leiden mutation is a common finding in multiple myeloma and is associated with an increased risk of thrombotic complications. Blood Coagul Fibrinolysis 2002; 13:187–192.

64. Goodrich SM, Wood JE. Peripheral venous distensibility and velocity of venous blood flow during pregnancy or during oral contraceptive therapy. Am J Obstet Gynecol 1964; 90:740.

65. Ginsberg JS. Thromboembolism and pregnancy. Thromb Haemost 1999; 82:620–625.

66. Simmons AV, Sheppard MA, Cox AF. Deep venous thrombosis after myocardial infarction: predisposing factors. Br Heart J 1973; 35:623–625.

67. Anderson GM, Hull E. The effect of dicumarol upon the mortality and incidence of thromboembolic complications in congestive heart failure. Am Heart J 1950; 39:697.

68. Kunz G, Ohlin AK, Adami A, Zoller B, Svensson P, Lane DA. Naturally occurring mutations in the thrombomodulin gene leading to impaired expression and function. Blood 2002; 99:3564–3653.

69. Biguzzi E, Merati G, Liaw PC, Pucciarelli P, Oganesyan N, Qu D, Gu JM, Fetiveau R, Esmon CT, Mannucci PM, Faioni EM. A 23bp insertion in the endothelial protein C receptor (EPCR) gene impairs EPCR function. Thromb Haemost 2001; 86:945–948.

70. Bertina RM, van der Linden IK, Engesser L, Muller HP, Brommer EJ. Hereditary heparin cofactor II deficiency and the risk of development of thrombosis. Thromb Haemost 1987; 47:196–200.

71. Poort SR, Rosendaal FR, Reitsma PH, Bertina RM. A common genetic variation of the 3′-untranslated region of the prothrombin gene is associated with elevated plasma prothrombin levels and an increase in venous thrombosis. Blood 1996; 88:3698–3703.

72. Kyrle PA, Minar E, Hirschl M, Bialonczyk C, Stain M, Schneider B, Weltermann A, Speiser W, Lechner K, Eichinger S. High plasma levels of factor VIII and the risk of recurrent venous thromboembolism. N Engl J Med 2000; 343:457–462.

73. Kraaijenhagen RA, in't Anker PS, Koopman MM, Reitsma PH, Prins MH, van den Ende A, Buller HR. High plasma concentration of factor VIIIc is a major risk factor for venous thromboembolism. Thromb Haemost 2000; 83:5–9.

74. Kamphuisen PW, Eikenboom JC, Bertina RM. Elevated factor VIII levels and the risk of thrombosis. Arterioscler Thromb Vasc Biol 2001; 21:731–738.

75. van Hylckama Vlieg A, van der Linden IK, Bertina RM, Rosendaal FR. High levels of factor IX increase the risk of venous thrombosis. Blood 2002; 95:3678–3682.

76. Meijers JC, Tekelenburg WL, Bouma BN, Bertina RM, Rosendaal FR. High levels of coagulation factor XI as a risk factor for venous thrombosis. N Engl J Med 2000; 342:696–701.

77. Folsom AR, Cushman M, Tsai MY, Aleksic N, Heckbert SR, Boland LL, Tsai AW, Yanez ND, Rosamond WD. A prospective study of venous thromboembolism in relation to factor V Leiden and related factors. Blood 2002; 99:2720–2725.

78. Lensen R, Bertina RM, Vandenbroucke JP, Rosendaal FR. High factor VIII levels contribute to the thrombotic risk in families with factor V Leiden. Br J Haematol 2001; 114:380–386.

79. Lijnen HR, Soria J, Soria C, Collen D, Caen JP. Dysfibrinogenemia (fibrinogen Dusard) associated with impaired fibrin-enhanced plasminogen activation. Thromb Haemost 1984; 51:108–109.

80. Liu CY, Koehn JA, Morgan FJ. Characterization of fibrinogen New York 1. A dysfunctional fibrinogen with a deletion of Bβ(9-72) corresponding exactly to exon 2 of the gene. J Biol Chem 1985; 260:4390–4396.

81. Meh DA, Mosesson MW, Siebenlist KR, Simpson-Haidaris PJ, Brennan SO, DiOrio JP, Thompson K, Di Minno G. Fibrinogen naples I (BβA68T) non-substrate thrombin-binding capacities. Thromb Res 2001; 103:63–73.

82. Comp PC, Jacocks RM, Taylor FB Jr. The dilute whole blood clot lysis assay: a screening method for identifying postoperative patients with a high incidence of deep venous thrombosis. J Lab Clin Med 1979; 93:120–127.

83. Crandon AJ, Peel KR, Anderson JA, Thompson V, McNicol GP. Post-operative deep vein thrombosis: identifying high-risk patients. BMJ 1980; 291:343–344.

84. Clayton JK, Anderson JA. GP McNicol GP. Preoperative prediction of post-operative deep vein thrombosis. BMJ 1976; 2:910–912.

85. Gallus AS, Hirsh J, Gent M. Relevance of preoperative and postoperative blood tests to postoperative leg-vein thrombosis. Lancet 1973; 2:805–809.

86. Gordon-Smith IC, Hickman JA, LeQuesne LP. Postoperative fibrinolytic activity and deep vein thrombosis. Br J Surg 1974; 61:213–218.

87. Menon IS, Peberdy M, Rannie RH, et al. A comparative study of blood fibrinolytic activity in normal women, pregnant women and women on oral contraceptives. J Obstet Gynaecol Br Commonw 1970; 77:752.

88. Bonnar J, McNicol GP, Douglas AS. Fibrinolytic enzyme system and pregnancy. BMJ 1969; 3:387–389.

89. Asted B, Isacson S, Nilssonetal IM, et al. Thrombosis and oral contraceptives: possible predisposition. BMJ 1973; 4:631.

90. Grace CS, Goldrick RD. Fibrinolysis and body fluid: interrelationships between blood fibrinolysis, body composition and parameters of lipid and carbohydrate metabolism. J Atheroscler Res 1968; 4:705.

91. Ogston D, McAndrew GM. Fibrinolysis in obesity. Lancet 1964; 2:1205.

92. Pandolfi M, Robertson B, Isacson S, Nilsson IM. Fibrinolytic activity of human veins in arms and legs. Thromb Diath Haemorrh 1968; 20:247.

93. Robertson BR, Pandolfi M, Nilsson IM. "Fibrinolytic capacity" in healthy volunteers at different ages as studied by standardized venous occlusions of arms and legs. Acta Med Scand 1972; 191:199–202.

94. Prins MH, Hirsh J. A critical review of the evidence supporting a relationship between impaired fibrinolytic activity and venous thromboembolism. Arch Intern Med 1991; 151:1721–1731.

95. Kearon C, Gent M, Hirsh J, Weitz J, Kovacs MJ, Anderson DR, Turpie AG, Green D, Ginsberg JS, Wells P, MacKinnon B, Julian JA. A comparison of three months of anticoagulation with extended anticoagulation for a first episode of idiopathic venous thromboembolism. N Engl J Med 1999; 341:901–907.

96. Pinede L, Ninet J, Duhaut P, Chabaud S, Demolombe-Rague S, Durieu I, Nony P, Sanson C, Boissel JP. Investigators of the "Duree Optimale du Traitement AntiVitamines K" (DOTAVK) Study. Comparison of 3 and 6 months of oral anticoagulant therapy after a first episode of proximal deep vein thrombosis or pulmonary embolism and comparison of 6 and 12 weeks of therapy after isolated calf deep vein thrombosis. Circulation 2001; 103:2453–2460.

97. Agnelli G, Prandoni P, Santamaria MG, Bagatella P, Iorio A, Bazzan M, Moia M, Guazzaloca G, Bertoldi A, Tomasi C, Scannapieco G, Ageno W. Warfarin Optimal Duration Italian Trial Investigators. Three months versus one year of oral anticoagulant therapy for idiopathic deep venous thrombosis. Warfarin Optimal Duration Italian Trial Investigators. N Engl J Med 2001; 345:165–169.

98. Kearon C. Duration of anticoagulation for venous thromboembolism. J Thromb Thrombolysis 2001; 12:59–65.

4

Prophylaxis of Venous Thromboembolism

RUSSELL D. HULL and GRAHAM F. PINEO

University of Calgary
Calgary, Alberta, Canada

I. Introduction

Deep vein thrombosis most commonly arises in the deep veins of the calf muscles or, less commonly, in the proximal deep veins of the leg. Deep vein thrombosis confined to the calf veins is associated with a low risk of clinically important pulmonary embolism (1–3). However, without treatment, approximately 20% of calf vein thrombi extend into the proximal venous system where they may pose a serious and potentially life-threatening disorder (3–5). Untreated proximal venous thrombosis is associated with a 10% risk of fatal pulmonary embolism and at least a 50% risk of pulmonary embolism or recurrent venous thrombosis (1–3). Furthermore, the post-phlebitic syndrome is associated with extensive proximal venous thrombosis and carries its own long-term morbidity.

It is now well established that clinically important pulmonary emboli arise from thrombi in the proximal deep veins of the legs (3,6–9). Other less common sources of pulmonary embolism include the deep pelvic veins, renal veins, the inferior vena cava, the right heart, and occasionally axillary veins. The clinical significance of pulmonary embolism depends on the size of the embolus and the cardiorespiratory reserve of the patient.

Various risk factors predispose to development of venous thromboembolism (see Chap. 3).

II. Prevention of Venous Thromboembolism

There are two approaches to the prevention of fatal pulmonary embolism: (1) primary prophylaxis is carried out using either drugs or physical methods that are effective for preventing deep vein thrombosis and (2) secondary prevention involves the early detection and treatment of subclinical venous thrombosis by screening postoperative patients with objective tests that are sensitive for venous thrombosis. Primary prophylaxis is preferred in most clinical circumstances. Furthermore, prevention of deep vein thrombosis and pulmonary embolism is more cost effective than treatment of the complications when they occur (10–14). Secondary prevention by case-finding studies should never replace primary prophylaxis. It should be reserved for patients in whom primary prophylaxis is either contraindicated or ineffective.

The prevention of thrombosis can be directed toward three components of Virchow's triad: blood flow, factors within the blood itself, and the vascular endothelium. Some methods act on all three components, resulting in a reduction of venous stasis, prevention of the hypercoagulable state induced by tissue trauma and other factors, and protection of the endothelium. Whichever method is used, where possible, prophylaxis should be initiated prior to induction of anesthesia, as it has been demonstrated that the thrombotic process commences intraoperatively (15) and may persist for days or weeks following surgery.

For patients undergoing general surgical procedures, the pattern of practice based on numerous clinical trials has been to start prophylaxis 2 hr preoperatively with either unfractionated heparin or low molecular weight heparin (16–21). This approach has been shown to be both effective and safe, and indeed it has resulted in a significant decrease in the incidence of fatal pulmonary embolism in surgical patients (16, 17). For patients undergoing high-risk orthopedic surgical procedures such as total hip or total knee replacement or surgery for hip fracture because of concern about excess bleeding, commencement of prophylaxis has been delayed. Thus, in Europe, prophylaxis is commenced 10–12 hr preoperatively (22–29), whereas in North America, prophylaxis is usually started 12–24 hr postoperatively (30–37). This difference in patterns of practice may account for the difference in the rates of postoperative venous thrombosis and bleeding in Europe and North America (38).

There is now good evidence that the timing of the initial administration of a prophylactic agent has a significant impact on the incidence of postoperative venous thrombosis. Starting low molecular weight heparin (dalteparin) at half the daily dose within 2 hr of hip replacement surgery followed by a further half dose 6–8 hr later and then using the usual daily dose once a day significantly decreased the incidence of venous thrombosis when compared with placebo or warfarin (39,40). Compared with warfarin started the evening before surgery, the incidence of venographically proven deep vein thrombosis was 25.8% versus 14.6% with low molecular weight heparin ($P = .006$). The incidence of proximal venous thrombosis was similar in the two groups. Although there was no difference in the incidence of major bleeding, patients on low molecular weight heparin had more bleeding complications involving the operative site and a greater percentage required postoperative transfusions (40). In the North American Fragmin Trial, starting low molecular weight heparin (dalteparin) within 2 hr before surgery or within 4–6 hr after surgery for total hip replacement significantly decreased the incidence of deep vein thrombosis demonstrated by venography when compared with warfarin started the night of surgery (41). The incidence of deep vein thrombosis detected by venography was 10.7% for low molecular weight heparin started preoperatively, 13.1% for low molecular weight heparin started postoperatively, and 24% for patients on warfarin ($P < .001$). The incidence of proximal deep vein thrombosis in the three groups was 0.8% for the two low molecular weight heparin groups versus 3.0% for the warfarin group ($P = .04$). The initial dose was half the usual high-risk dose. There was no difference in the incidence of major bleeding reported by the principal investigators; however, assessment of major bleeding from time 0 to day 8 by the Central Adjudication Committee identified an increased incidence of major bleeding in the patients with low molecular weight heparin started preoperatively compared with either the postoperative low molecular weight heparin group or the warfarin group. The results of the two studies comparing the early initiation of low molecular weight heparin with warfarin were compared with two previous studies where warfarin prophylaxis was compared with low molecular weight heparin started 12 hr preoperatively or 12–24 hr postoperatively (42). In this systematic review, it was shown that the incidence of post-operative venous thrombosis was significantly lower in the two clinical trials starting prophylaxis in close proximity to surgery compared with the studies where low molecular weight heparin was started either 12 hr preoperatively or 12–24 hr postoperatively (42) (Figs. 1–3). There was no increase in the incidence of major bleeding. Starting low molecular weight heparin (enoxaparin) no more than 8 hr postoperatively also led to a significant decrease in the incidence of venous thrombosis in patients undergoing total knee replacement when compared with warfarin started on the night of surgery, although there was an increase in the incidence of total bleeding rates (43).

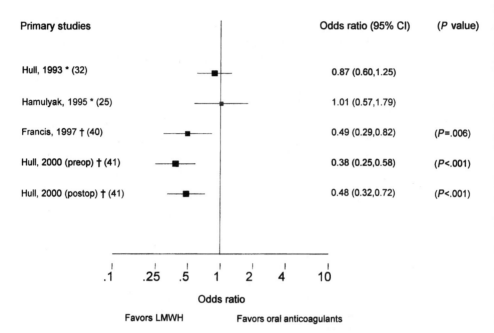

Figure 1 Primary study odds ratios for all deep vein thromboses. Odds ratios are indicated by boxes. Horizontal lines represent 95% confidence intervals. Odds ratios less than 1 favor low molecular weight heparins (LMWH); odds ratios greater than 1 favor oral anticoagulants. *Study using remote timing prophylaxis. †Study using close proximity timing prophylaxis. (Adapted from Ref. 42.)

The regimen of low molecular weight heparin started 4–6 hr after surgery at half the usual high-risk dose and then continuing with the usual high-risk dose the following day was included in the most recent American College of Chest Physicians (ACCP) recommendations for patients under-going elective hip replacement (20). As discussed later, there has been concern about the associated use of neuraxial anesthesia and low molecular weight heparin prophylaxis because of a cluster of spinal hematomas (44). This intriguing difference between the incidence of bleeding complications in Europe and the United States may arise from local practice patterns with a predominant tendency toward once daily low molecular weight prophylaxis in Europe and twice daily prophylaxis using a higher total daily dose in the United States. Since half the usual high-risk dose of the low molecular weight heparin is administered using the close proximity postoperative regimen, and the average time of initiation after spinal anesthesia was 9

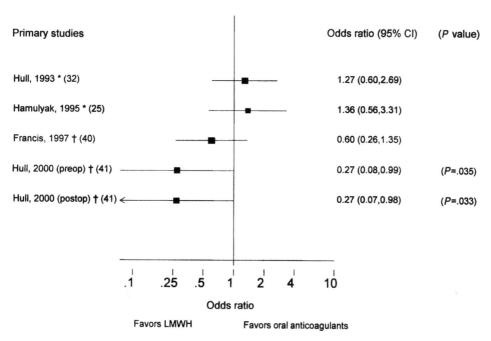

Figure 2 Primary study odds ratios for proximal deep vein thrombosis. Odds ratios are indicated by boxes. Horizontal lines represent 95% confidence intervals. Odds ratios less than 1 favor low molecular weight heparins (LMWH); odds ratios greater than 1 favor oral anticoagulants. *Study using remote timing prophylaxis. †Study using close proximity timing prophylaxis. (Adapted from Ref. 42.)

hr, the close proximity postoperative regimen may be a safe approach in conjunction with spinal anesthesia.

Evidence from a number of other recent randomized clinical trials using newer antithrombotic agents started in close proximity to surgery suggest that the early commencement of prophylaxis plays a role in the improved efficacy of these agents when compared with accepted standards for prophylaxis. The antithrombin, recombinant hirudin, started 2 hr preoperatively was superior to the low molecular weight heparin (enoxaparin) started the night before surgery for both total and proximal deep vein thrombosis (45). Studies with the direct thrombin inhibitor, melagatran (subcutaneous form) and ximelagatran (oral form), produced interesting results. When melagatran by subcutaneous injection twice daily was started immediately before surgery and continued for 2–3 days, followed by ximelagatran in different doses twice daily, the deep vein thrombosis rates

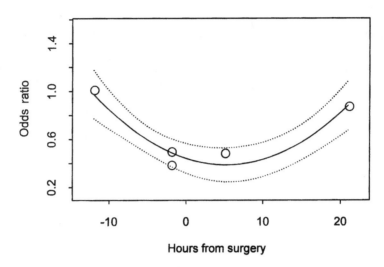

Figure 3 Quadratic fit for study odds ratio for deep vein thrombosis versus the number of hours from surgery for the first dose of low molecular weight heparin. The upper and lower dashed lines indicate the 95% confidence intervals for the true odds ratio. (Adapted from Ref. 42.)

were either equivalent to or significantly lower than those seen with low molecular weight heparin (dalteparin) started the night before surgery in patients undergoing total hip or total knee replacement (46,47). When ximelagatran and low molecular weight heparin (enoxaparin) were started the morning after surgery, the venous thromboembolism rates were significantly lower with enoxaparin treatment, with no difference in major bleeding rates (48).

Studies with the synthetic pentasaccharide, fondaparinux (Arixtra), suggest that the timing of commencement of this agent may in part account for the superior efficacy when compared with low molecular weight heparin (enoxaparin). In a dose-finding study, fondaparinux was started 6 hr following surgery in five different doses and compared with enoxaparin started 12–24 hr after the end of surgery. Depending on the dose of fondaparinux, the deep vein thrombosis rates were either equivalent to or significantly lower than those with enoxaparin (49). In four Phase III clinical trials, fondaparinux was started 6 hr following the end of surgery and given once daily and compared with enoxaparin either started the night before surgery or 12–24 hr after the finish of surgery in patients undergoing total hip or total knee replacement or surgery for hip fracture (50–54).These studies all showed fondaparinux to be superior to enoxaparin for the reduction of deep vein thrombosis, although the decrease in the North American hip replacement study was not statistically significant. Other clinical trials, most of which are currently ongoing, have used a similar approach with the new agents starting 6–8 hr postoperatively and compared with low molecular weight heparin started 12–24 hr postoperatively.

Without prophylaxis, the frequency of fatal pulmonary embolism ranges from 0.1 to 0.8% in patients undergoing elective general surgery (55–57), 2 to 3% in patients undergoing elective hip replacement (58), and 4 to 7% in patients undergoing surgery for a fractured hip, (59). The need for prophylaxis after elective hip replacement has been questioned because of the low incidence of fatal pulmonary embolism in patients participating in clinical trials (60). However, review of data from the National Confidential Enquiry into Peri-Operative Deaths (NCEPOD) indicates that pulmonary embolism continues to be the commonest cause of death following total hip replacement surgery; 35% of patients who died had pulmonary embolism confirmed at autopsy (61). Factors increasing the risk of postoperative venous thrombosis include advanced age, malignancy, previous venous thromboembolism, obesity, heart failure, or paralysis.

The ideal prophylactic agents for venous thromboembolism are described in Table 1. Prophylactic measures most commonly used are low-dose or adjusted-dose unfractionated heparin, low molecular weight heparin, oral anticoagulant (international normalized ratio [INR] 2–3), and intermittent pneumatic compression. Recently, the pentasaccharide fonda-parinux (Arixtra) has been approved for use in the United States for patients undergoing surgery for total hip or total knee replacement or for hip fracture.

There has been recent concern regarding the use of regional anesthesia in the form of intraspinal or epidural anesthesia and/or analgesia and the use of prophylactic anticoagulants. Spinal hematomas have been reported with the use of intravenous or subcutaneous heparin and warfarin treatment, but most of these complications occurred in patients with complex

Table 1 Features of an Ideal Prophylactic Method for Venous Thromboembolism

Effective compared with placebo or active approaches
Safe
Good compliance with patient, nurses, and physicians
Ease of administration
No need for laboratory monitoring
Cost effective

clinical problems (62). With the advent of low molecular weight heparin and the increased use of regional anesthesia, concern was raised regarding the potential risk of neuraxial damage due to bleeding when both procedures are used together. Surveys among anesthetists in Europe suggested that the likelihood of spinal hematoma in this setting was remote (63,64). However, recent experience in the United States with the use of neuraxial anesthesia and analgesia and the postoperative administration of low molecular weight heparin has resulted in a number of case reports of spinal hematoma, many of which caused permanent neurological damage (44). Many of these occurred with continued epidural analgesia, many of the procedures were traumatic, and several patients have been on nonsteroidal anti-inflammatory drugs (44). Other risk factors appear to be age over 75 years and female gender. At this stage, the U.S. Food and Drug Administration (USFDA) has recommended caution when neuraxial anesthesia is used in the presence of low molecular weight heparin prophylaxis. The American Association of Regional Anesthesia Committee has recently reviewed these issues and new guidelines are expected.

III. Extended Out-of-Hospital Prophylaxis

It is widely recognized that the risk of developing deep vein thrombosis increases after total hip arthroplasty (65). The need for in-hospital prophylaxis has been firmly established. The Sixth ACCP Consensus Conference recommends anticoagulant prophylaxis for at least 7–10 days following elective total hip replacement surgery (20). Although thromboprophylaxis is routinely administered for total hip replacement patients, it is commonly stopped at the time of discharge from hospital. In a recent epidemiological study by White and colleagues (66), a large linked hospital discharge database revealed the mean length of hospital stay after primary and revision total hip arthroplasty was 6.9 and 8.0 days, respectively. The period of risk for the development of venous thromboembolism was shown to extend well beyond this initial hospital stay (66). In this study of hip arthroplasty patients, White et al. reported that 76% of thromboembolic cases were diagnosed after hospital discharge. The median time for diagnosing these thromboembolic events was 17 days after hip arthroplasty. The median time for diagnosing venous thromboembolism following total knee arthroplasty was 7 days; suggesting that extended prophylaxis may not be required in such knee patients.

For major orthopedic surgery, the current recommendations from the Sixth ACCP Consensus Conference indicate that the use of extended out-of-hospital prophylaxis in patients undergoing total hip arthroplasty with low molecular weight heparin may reduce the incidence of clinically important venous thromboembolism, and this approach is recommended at least for high-risk patients. Because of uncertainty regarding cost effectiveness, this is currently a grade 2A recommendation (20).

There have been six randomized clinical trials comparing extended prophylaxis with low molecular weight heparin to placebo in patients undergoing total hip replacement who have received either low molecular weight heparin (enoxaparin or dalteparin) or warfarin for in-hospital prophylaxis (26–29,36,67). All of these trials indicated that deep vein thrombosis rates were decreased with extended prophylaxis. A systematic review of all six clinical trials demonstrated a significant decrease in both total and proximal deep vein thrombosis as demonstrated by bilateral venography, but this also demonstrated a significant decrease in symptomatic venous thromboembolism occurring during the treatment period (68). There was no major bleeding in the out-of-hospital phase of any of these trials; indicating that the risk/benefit ratio strongly favored extended prophylaxis (Figs. 4–6).

The NNT_B (number needed to be treated) provides a useful public health overview (67). Only 24–28 patients required out-of-hospital low molecular weight heparin prophylaxis to prevent one new episode of out-of-hospital proximal venous thrombosis compared with out-of-hospital

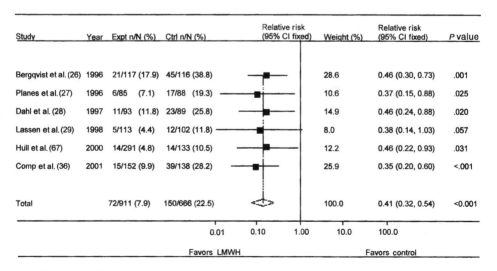

Study	Year	Expt n/N (%)	Ctrl n/N (%)	Relative risk (95% CI fixed)	Weight (%)	Relative risk (95% CI fixed)	P value
Bergqvist et al. (26)	1996	21/117 (17.9)	45/116 (38.8)		28.6	0.46 (0.30, 0.73)	.001
Planes et al. (27)	1996	6/85 (7.1)	17/88 (19.3)		10.6	0.37 (0.15, 0.88)	.025
Dahl et al. (28)	1997	11/93 (11.8)	23/89 (25.8)		14.9	0.46 (0.24, 0.88)	.020
Lassen et al. (29)	1998	5/113 (4.4)	12/102 (11.8)		8.0	0.38 (0.14, 1.03)	.057
Hull et al. (67)	2000	14/291 (4.8)	14/133 (10.5)		12.2	0.46 (0.22, 0.93)	.031
Comp et al. (36)	2001	15/152 (9.9)	39/138 (28.2)		25.9	0.35 (0.20, 0.60)	<.001
Total		72/911 (7.9)	150/666 (22.5)		100.0	0.41 (0.32, 0.54)	<0.001

0.01   0.10   1.00   10.0   100.0

Favors LMWH   Favors control

Figure 4 The relative risk for all deep vein thrombosis during the out-of-hospital time interval; summary and individual study results. (Adapted from Ref. 68.)

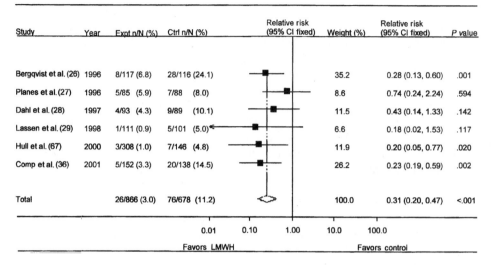

Figure 5 The relative risk for proximal deep vein thrombisis during the out-of-hospital time interval; summary and individual study results. (Adapted from Ref. 68.)

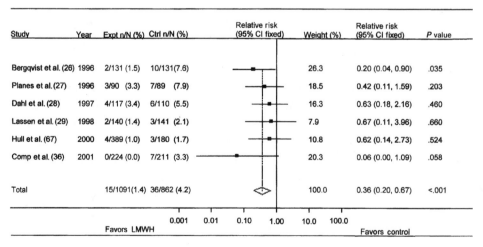

Figure 6 The relative risk for symptomatic venous thromboembolism during the out-of-hospital time interval; summary and individual study results. (Adapted from Ref. 68.)

placebo in patients having elective hip arthroplasty in the United States and Canada (67).

From a population perspective, extended prophylaxis will prevent 41 cases of proximal deep vein thrombosis for every 1000 patients having elective hip surgery. Even if the death rate is as low as 8% of these 41 cases, extended prophylaxis will allow the saving of about 3.5 lives per 1000 patients undergoing elective hip surgery by preventing fatal pulmonary embolism. Although a 0.35% mortality rate is low, it would be recognized that these deaths are preventable; for every 500,000 patents undergoing elective hip surgery in North America, extended prophylaxis would save 1750 lives. Even if the death rate is as low as 0.1%, this still reflects 500 lives saved (67).

Based on the findings of these studies, extended prophylaxis with low molecular weight heparin has been shown to be effective and safe in the prevention of deep vein thrombosis after total hip arthroplasty. The use of low molecular weight heparin prophylaxis was associated with substantive risk reductions. Thus, the recommended 7- to 10-day prophylaxis regimen following total hip arthroplasty is suboptimal.

The optimal duration of extended prophylaxis remains uncertain. The intervals of extended out-of-hospital prophylaxis that were evaluated in the randomized clinical trials by using venographic endpoints ranged from 19 to 28 days. This interval is in harmony with the finding that patients with venographically confirmed symptomatic deep vein thrombosis after hip surgery in whom prophylaxis was stopped at hospital discharge were readmitted on average 17 days after surgery (66). Thus, in all patients undergoing elective hip surgery, 19–28 days would seem a reasonable duration for use of extended low molecular weight heparin prophylaxis. Two economic analyses have indicated that out-of-hospital antithrombotic prophylaxis after total hip replacement with the use of low molecular weight heparin is cost effective (69,70).

Extended prophylaxis with acecoumarol was compared with low molecular weight heparin for extended prophylaxis to 30 days following total hip replacement. Deep vein thrombosis rates were similar, but there was significantly more bleeding with acecoumarol (71). Extended prophylaxis to day 28 in patients undergoing total knee replacement did not significantly lower the rates of venous thrombosis when compared with 7–10 days of prophylaxis with low molecular weight heparin (36).

In patients undergoing cancer surgery, extended prophylaxis to 25–31 days with low molecular weight heparin was superior to prophylaxis for 6–10 days (72). Extended prophylaxis is currently being studied in patients undergoing surgery for hip fracture and in high-risk medical patients. The advent of effective oral agents will simplify the approach to extended prophylaxis, but concerns about cost will remain a problem.

Patterns of clinical practice with the respect of the prevention of venous thromboembolism and the appropriate use of anticoagulants for the treatment of thrombotic disease have been influenced very strongly by recent consensus conferences (20,73). Recommendations from the Sixth ACCP Consensus Conference on Antithrombotic Therapy (20) and the International Consensus Statement on the Prevention of Venous Thromboembolism (73) have recently been published. Rules of evidence for assessing the literature were applied to all recommendations regarding prevention and treatment of venous thrombosis, thereby indicating which recommendations were based on rigorous randomized trials, which were based on extrapolation of evidence from related clinical disorders, and which were based only on nonrandomized clinical trials or case series (74).

IV. Specific Prophylactic Measures

A.   Low Molecular Weight Heparin

A number of low molecular weight heparins have been evaluated by randomized clinical trials in moderate-risk general surgical patients including many who underwent cancer surgery (18,19,21,75–78). In randomized clinical trials comparing low molecular weight heparin with unfractionated heparin, the low molecular weight heparins given once or twice daily have been shown to be as effective or more effective in preventing thrombosis (18,19,21,76–78). In most of the trials, similarly low frequencies of bleeding for low molecular weight heparin and low-dose unfractionated heparin were documented, although the incidence of bleeding was significantly lower in the low molecular weight heparin group as evidenced by a reduction in the incidence of wound hematoma, severe bleeding, and the number of patients requiring reoperation for bleeding (18,19).

A number of randomized control trials have been performed with low molecular weight heparin comparing it with either unfractionated heparin or warfarin for the prevention of venous thrombosis following total hip replacement. The most recent trials using bilateral venography are shown in Table 2 (22–32,41). The drugs under investigation and their dosage schedules vary from one clinical trial to another, making comparisons across trials difficult. Furthermore, it has been shown that even within the same clinical trial there can be considerable intercenter variability (32). Major bleeding rates and definitions of major bleeding vary across trials as well, making comparisons difficult.

Although the number of patients undergoing total knee replacement now equals those undergoing total hip replacements, there have been fewer trials in this patient population. Recent clinical trials comparing low molec-

Table 2 Recent Randomized Trials of Low Molecular Weight Heparin Versus Heparin or Warfarin Prophylaxis for Deep Vein Thrombosis Following Hip Replacement Surgery: Total Deep Vein Thrombosis and Major Bleeding

Reference no.	Treatment	No. of patients	Total deep vein thrombosis (%)	Major bleeding (%)
30	Enoxaparin	258	19.4	3.3
	Unfractionated heparin	263	23.3	5.7
22	Nadroparin	198	12.6	0.5
	Unfractionated heparin	199	16.0	1.5
23	Dalteparin	67	30.2	1.4[a]
	Unfractionated heparin	68	42.4	7.4
24	Enoxaparin	120	12.5	1.6
	Heparin	108	25.0	0
31	Enoxaparin	136	21.0	4.0
	Enoxaparin	136	6.0	1.0
	Heparin	142	1.5	6.0
32	Tinzaparin	332	21.0	2.8
	Warfarin	340	23.0	1.5
25	Nadroparin	195	13.8	1.5[b]
	Warfarin	196	13.8	2.3
40	Dalteparin	192	15.0	2.0
	Warfarin	190	26.0	1.0
41	Dalteparin	496	10.7	2.8
	Dalteparin	487	13.1	1.8
	Warfarin	489	24.0	2.0

[a] Serious bleeding.
[b] Clinically important plus minor bleeding for combined hip and knee replacement patients.

ular weight heparin with warfarin are shown in Table 3 (25,32,34,35,43). Although the rates of deep vein thrombosis with low molecular weight heparin are significantly lower than those with warfarin, the rates continue to be high.

Multiple meta-analyses have shown that low molecular weight heparin and low-dose heparin are equally effective in preventing venous thrombosis in general surgery (79–82), but low molecular weight heparin is more effective in orthopedic surgery (79–82). Bleeding rates were higher with low-dose heparin in patients undergoing general surgery.

Two recent decision analyses compared the cost effectiveness of enoxaparin with warfarin in patients undergoing hip replacement (83,84).

Table 3 Randomized Control Trials of Low Molecular Weight Heparin Prophylaxis Versus Warfarin for Deep Vein Thrombosis Following Total Knee Replacement: Total Deep Vein Thrombosis and Major Bleeding

Reference no.	Treatment	No. of patients	Total deep vein thrombosis (%)	Major bleeding (%)
32	Tinzaparin	317	45.0	0.9
	Warfarin	324	54.0	2.0
34	Enoxaparin	206	37.0	2.1
	Warfarin	211	52.0	1.8
35	Ardeparin	232	27.0[a]	7.9[b]
	Warfarin	222	38.0	4.4
25	Nadroparin	65	24.6	1.5[c]
	Warfarin	61	37.7	2.3
43	Enoxaparin	173	38.0	5.2
	Warfarin	176	59.0	2.3

[a] Venogram on operated leg only.
[b] Overt bleeding—total.
[c] Clinically important and minor bleeding for combined hip and knee replacement patients.

Although enoxaparin was more expensive than low-dose warfarin, its cost effectiveness compared favorably with other medical interventions. A recent economic evaluation of low molecular weight heparin versus warfarin prophylaxis after total hip or knee replacement identified that low molecular weight heparin was cost effective (85).

Recent studies have shown that low molecular weight heparin is superior to low-dose unfractionated heparin in patients suffering multiple trauma (86) and equally effective in medical patients (87,88).

B. Low-Dose Heparin

The effectiveness of low-dose unfractionated heparin for preventing deep vein thrombosis following general surgery has been established by multiple randomized clinical trials (17–19). Low-dose subcutaneous heparin is usually given in a dose of 5000 units 2 hr preoperatively, and postoperatively every 8 or 12 hr. Most of the patients in these trials underwent abdominothoracic surgery, particularly for gastrointestinal disease, but patients having gynecological and urological surgery as well as mastectomies or vascular procedures were also included. Pooled data from meta-analyses confirm that low-dose heparin significantly reduces the incidence of all deep vein thrombosis, proximal deep vein thrombosis, and all pulmonary emboli including fatal pulmonary emboli (17,79–82). The International Multicentre Trial also established the effectiveness of low-dose heparin for preventing fatal pulmonary embolism, a clinically and significantly striking reduction from 0.7 to 0.1% ($P < .005$) (16).

The incidence of major bleeding complications is not increased by low-dose heparin, but there is an increase in minor wound hematomas. The platelet count should be monitored regularly in all patients on low-dose heparin to detect the rare, but significant, development of heparin-induced thrombocytopenia.

C. Intermittent Leg Compression

The use of intermittent pneumatic leg compression prevents venous thrombosis by enhancing blood flow in the deep veins of the legs, thereby preventing venous stasis. It also increases blood fibrinolytic activity, which may contribute to its antithrombotic properties. Intermittent pneumatic leg compression is effective for preventing venous thrombosis following cardiac surgery (89) and in patients undergoing neurosurgery (90–92). In patients undergoing hip surgery, intermittent pneumatic compression of the calf is effective for preventing calf vein thrombosis, but it is less effective against proximal vein thrombosis than warfarin sodium (93,94). Intermittent pneumatic compression of the calf decreased venous thrombosis following knee replacement (95,96).

Intermittent pneumatic compression is virtually free of clinically important side effects and offers a valuable alternative in patients who have a high risk of bleeding. It may produce discomfort in the occasional patient, and it should not be used in patients with an overt incidence of leg ischemia caused by peripheral vascular disease. A variety of well-accepted, comfortable, and effective intermittent pneumatic devices are currently available which may be applied preoperatively, at the time of operation, or in the early postoperative period. These devices should be used for the entire period until the patient is fully ambulatory with only temporary removal for nursing care or physiotherapy.

With a shortened hospital stay, use of intermittent pneumatic compression becomes of limited value. A greater problem, however, is one of compliance (97,98). In addition to poor compliance, a recent study documented the fact that key outcome-related parameters such as the rate of pressure rise and the maximum pressure applied to various parts of the leg were less than anticipated most of the time in patients having intermittent pneumatic compression following elective hip surgery (98). Disappointingly, an intensive nursing training program did not improve these outcomes.

D. Graduated Compression Stockings

Graduated compression stocks are a simple, safe, and moderately effective form of thromboprophylaxis. It is by no means clear how graduated compression stockings achieve a thromboprophylactic effect. It has been shown that they increase the velocity of venous blood flow, and thus graduated compression stockings are recommended in low-risk patients and as an adjunct in those at medium and high risk (99–101). The only major contra-indication is peripheral vascular disease. The majority of studies in patients undergoing general abdominal and gynecological procedures have shown a reduction in the incidence of deep vein thrombosis. A comprehensive meta-analysis concluded that, in studies using objective methods, there was a highly significant risk reduction of 68% in patients at moderate risk of postoperative thromboembolism (101). However, there is no conclusive evidence that graduated compression stockings are effective in reducing the incidence of fatal and nonfatal pulmonary embolism. It is not known whether wearing graduated compression stockings following discharge from hospital is efficacious. Graduated compression stockings may be useful in preventing the postphlebitic syndrome following an episode of proximal deep vein thrombosis (102) and in reducing the likelihood of thrombosis during prolonged airline travel (103).

E. Oral Anticoagulants

For prophylaxis, oral anticoagulants (coumarin derivatives) can be commenced preoperatively, at the time of surgery, or in the early postoperative period (104). Oral anticoagulants commenced at the time of surgery or in the early postoperative period may not prevent small venous thrombi from forming during surgery or soon after surgery, because the antithrombotic effect is not achieved until the third or fourth postoperative day. However, oral anticoagulants are effective in inhibiting the extension of these thrombi, thereby preventing clinically important venous thromboembolism.

The postoperative use of warfarin following total hip or total knee replacement surgery has been compared with low molecular weight heparin (25,32,40,41,43,105) or intermittent pneumatic compression (94,106) with little or no difference in the incidence of postoperative venous thrombosis or bleeding. However, more recent studies using earlier intervention with low molecular weight heparin have demonstrated superior efficacy when compared with warfarin, started the night of surgery and closely controlled using a warfarin nomogram (41). Another clinical trial using clinical endpoints for venous thromboembolism demonstrated superior efficacy of low molecular weight heparin although the majority of patients on warfarin had an INR of less than 2 (105).

When warfarin was initiated 7–10 days preoperatively to prolong prothrombin time (PT) 1.5–3.0 sec and then less intense warfarin was started the night of surgery, the results were similar to those when warfarin was started the night before surgery (104).

In patients with hip fractures, warfarin was more effective than either aspirin or placebo (107). Compared with placebo, very low doses of oral anticoagulants (warfarin 1 mg per day) decreased the postoperative thrombosis rate in patients undergoing gynecological surgery or major general surgery (108) and decreased the thrombosis rate in indwelling central line catheters in one study (109) but not another (110). Very low-dose warfarin, however, did not provide protection against deep vein thrombosis following hip or knee replacement (111).

F. Other Agents

Although meta-analyses indicate that aspirin decreases the frequency of venous thrombosis following general or orthopedic surgery, this reduction is significantly less than that obtained using other agents (112). Interest in the use of aspirin in hip fracture patients was fueled by the awareness that this agent significantly reduces the incidence of stroke and myocardial infarction in this patient population. The Pulmonary Embolism Prevention (PEP) Trial compared the use of aspirin versus placebo in a large number of patients undergoing surgery for hip fracture (113). Although there was extensive contamination with other prophylactic measures, there was a significant decrease in fatal pulmonary embolism with the use of aspirin, whereas the fatal and nonfatal cardiovascular events and all-cause mortality were no different. Wound-related and gastrointestinal bleeding and the need for blood transfusions were all significantly more frequent in the aspirin-treated patients. Aspirin cannot be recommended for the prevention of venous thrombosis in high-risk patients (20). Also, although intravenous dextran has been shown to be effective in the prevention of venous thrombosis following major orthopedic surgery, it is cumbersome, expensive, and associated with significant side effects. It has, therefore, been replaced by other agents.

V. New Antithrombotic Agents

For many years, unfractionated heparin and warfarin were the only agents available for the prevention and treatment of thrombotic disorders. Over the past 15 years, the low molecular weight heparins have found their place in the physicians' armamentarium. More recently, a plethora of new specific antithrombotic agents have been described and a number have been used in Phase II and Phase III clinical trials. The most advanced of these agents are inhibitors of factor X, factor II (thrombin), or the factor VIIa tissue factor complex. Heparin and low molecular weight heparin can be made available for absorption by the oral route, and a large Phase III study has been completed comparing the efficacy and safety of oral heparin with low molecular weight heparin in patients undergoing total hip replacement. Only the pentasaccharide fondaparinux (Arixtra) has been approved for clinical use by the USFDA. These agents and a number of other innovative antithrombotic agents are under extensive study for the prevention and treatment of both venous and arterial thrombotic disorders, and more information will become available in the coming years.

The pentasaccharide fondaparinux is a highly selective factor X inhibitor with a high affinity for antithrombin. When fondaparinux binds to antithrombin, it induces a confirmational change which markedly increases the rate of factor Xa inhibition. When antithrombin then binds to activated factor X, the fondaparinux is released and thus continues the process. Inhibition of factor Xa leads to less generation of thrombin, but unlike other antithrombotic agents, fondaparinux does not inhibit other coagulation proteins or affect platelet function or aggregation. Fondaparinux has a long half-life (17 hr), permitting once daily dosing. Fondaparinux has the further advantage of being a wholly synthetic molecule, which is not dependant on animal sources as are the heparins, and it does not produce heparin-associated antibodies. Of some concern is the fact that the antithrombotic activity cannot be blocked by any of the known agents, and the FDA has mandated that caution be used in elderly patients who may have decreased renal function because of a concern that there may be accumulation of the drug. It was also stated that "differences in efficacy and safety between Arixtra and the comparator may have been influenced by factors such as the timing of the first dose of the drug after surgery," an observation which had previously been made (114).

In a dose-finding study, fondaparinux was shown to have a highly reproducible and linear dose-dependent inhibition of thrombosis, as well as a dose-dependent increase in major bleeding (49). Fondaparinux has been compared with the low molecular weight heparin enoxaparin in more than 7000 patients undergoing orthopedic procedures in Phase III clinical trials (50–53). The fondaparinux protocol was the same in all four studies (i.e., 2.5 mg sc started 6 hr after the operation with the second injection 12 hr or longer after the first). In the hip fracture study, enoxaparin, 40 mg, was started an average of 18 hr postoperatively; in the knee replacement study, enoxaparin, 30 mg, twice daily an average of 21 hr postoperatively; in the European hip replacement study, enoxaparin, 40 mg, was started 12 hr preoperatively; and in the North American hip replacement study, enoxaparin, 30 mg, twice daily was started a mean of 13 hr postoperatively. In the hip fracture study, there was a significant decrease in both total and proximal deep vein thrombosis rates with fondaparinux with no difference in the major bleeding rates, although minor bleeding was increased with fondaparinux (50). In the knee replacement study, there was a significant decrease in the total deep vein thrombosis rates with fondaparinux but proximal rates were similar; however, there was a significant increase in major bleeding as indicated by the bleeding index in the fondaparinux group (51). In the European total hip replacement study, there was a significant decrease in both total and proximal deep vein thrombosis rates in the fondaparinux group (52), whereas in the North American study, there was a significant difference in venographically proven distal deep vein thrombosis but not for proximal deep vein thrombosis (53). In both studies, the bleeding index was similar in both groups. When all studies were pooled, there was a significant decrease in both total and proximal deep vein thrombosis rates with fondaparinux but no difference in the incidence of symptomatic events (54). The incidence of major bleeding was increased in the fondaparinux group (54).

The specific direct thrombin inhibitor melagatran (subcutaneous form) or ximelagatran (oral form) has undergone extensive study. In the first study, subcutaneous melagatran in three doses was given twice daily for 2 days beginning immediately before surgery with the second dose being given on the evening of surgery, and on day 3 oral ximelagatran in three different doses was started in a twice daily fashion for 6–9 days (46). The control was dalteparin, 5000 units, started the evening before surgery and continued daily. Bilateral venography showed there was no difference in total or proximal deep vein thrombosis rates within the various groups. In the second study (METHRO II), a combination of subcutaneous melagatran starting immediately before surgery and continued twice daily for 2–3 days in four dose levels was followed by ximelagatran in four different doses orally twice daily and compared with dalteparin, 5000 units, started the evening before surgery (47). A highly significant dose-dependent decrease in deep vein thrombosis rates was seen for both total hip and total knee replacement patients. Also, a dose-dependent decrease in proximal deep vein thrombosis and pulmonary embolism was found in the total population. Total bleeding was not significantly different between the treatment groups. In a Phase III study in patients undergoing total hip replacement surgery, ximelagatran, 24 mg twice daily, was compared with enoxaparin, 30 mg twice daily, both being initiated the morning after surgery (48). Enoxaparin-treated patients had significantly fewer events of venous thromboembolism (venographic and symptomatic venous thromboembolism) compared with ximelagatran-treated patients. Bleeding rates were low and comparable between the groups. A study with a similar design in patients undergoing total knee replacement surgery has not yet been reported.

When unfractionated heparin or low molecular weight heparin are given orally, there is little evidence of absorption in that there is little, if any, change in the levels of various coagulation tests including factor Xa levels. However, if an agent such as sodium N-[8-(2-hydroxy-benzoyl)amino] caprylate (SNAC) is combined with unfractionated heparin, there is significant absorption when compared with unfractionated heparin without the carrier (115,116). In a Phase II study, SNAC heparin has been shown to have a significant antithrombotic effect when compared with subcutaneous low molecular weight heparin (116). A large international clinical trial comparing two doses of SNAC heparin started 6 hr postoperatively and given three times daily by mouth was compared with enoxaparin, 30 mg twice daily, started 12–24 hr postoperatively. The results of this clinical trial will become available in the near future. The technology is also available for delivering low molecular weight heparin by the oral route in either the liquid or the dry form. Therefore, in spite of the development of a host of new oral antithrombotic agents, there may well be a role for oral heparin and oral low molecular weight heparin in both the prevention and treatment of thrombotic disorders, particularly in the out-of-hospital setting.

VI. Specific Recommendations

The recommended primary prophylactic approach depends on the patient's risk category and, in surgical patients, the type of surgery.

In assessing the literature relating to the prevention of venous thromboembolism, the rules of evidence as defined by Guyatt et al. have been used (74). They are summarized as follows:

> Level I: Randomized trials with low false-positive (1) and low false-negative (2) errors
> Level II: Randomized trials with high false-positive (1) and high false-negative (2) errors
> Level III: Nonrandomized concurrent cohort studies
> Level IV: Nonrandomized historical cohort studies
> Level V: Case series

Unless indicated, all recommendations in the following section are based on Level I evidence (24,73).

A. High-Risk Patients

Elective Hip Replacement

Several approaches are effective. Subcutaneous low molecular weight heparin given once or twice daily is effective and safe (20,73). Several such agents are approved for use in Europe and North America. At present, in North America, these agents are approved for postoperative use only. Prophylaxis with oral anticoagulants adjusted to maintain an INR of 2.0–3.0 is effective and is associated with a low risk of bleeding (20). Other effective approaches include adjusted-dose subcutaneous unfractionated heparin and intermittent pneumatic compression (20,73). However, rates of proximal venous thrombosis are higher with intermittent pneumatic compression than high risk doses of pharmacological prophylaxis.

Elective Knee Replacement

The current prophylaxis of choice is low molecular weight heparin given once or twice daily postoperatively (20,73). Oral anticoagulants are less effective than low molecular weight heparin, and intermittent pneumatic compression was shown in earlier studies to be effective and to be a useful alternative.

Hip Fractures

Two approaches to prophylaxis are available: oral anticoagulation (INR = 2–3) (20) or fixed-dose subcutaneous low molecular weight heparin started preoperatively (20,73). The combined use of intermittent pneumatic compression with low molecular weight heparin or warfarin may provide additional benefit in certain patients (not Level I).

Multiple Trauma

Multiple trauma represents a high risk for thrombosis. Low molecular weight heparin is the prophylaxis of choice (20,86). Intermittent pneumatic compression has been recommended, where feasible, because it does not cause any risk for bleeding (20). Other alternatives include low-dose unfractionated heparin or warfarin based on extrapolation from other high-risk situations such as hip fracture and hip replacement surgery. Insertion of an inferior vena cava filter has been recommended for very high-risk situations where anticoagulants may be contraindicated, but this recommendation is based on Level V data.

Acute Spinal Cord Injury Associated with Paralysis

Low molecular weight heparin is the most effective prophylaxis (20,73). Adjusted-dose heparin has also been shown to be effective. Low-dose heparin and intermittent pneumatic compression are less effective. Combining intermittent pneumatic compression with low molecular weight heparin or adjusted-dose heparin may provide additional benefit, but this is not supported by clinical trial data.

B. Moderate-Risk Patients

Neurosurgery

These patients should receive intermittent pneumatic compression. This approach may be used in conjunction with graduated compression stockings. Low-dose heparin is an acceptable alternative (20,73).

General Abdominal, Thoracic, or Gynecological Surgery

In moderate-risk patients, the use of subcutaneous low-dose unfractionated heparin (5000 units every 8 or 12 hr) or subcutaneous low molecular weight heparin is recommended (20,73). Subcutaneous low molecular weight heparin is as effective as subcutaneous heparin prophylaxis, and it has the advantage of a once-daily injection. An alternative recommendation is the use of intermittent pneumatic compression until the patient is ambulatory. This method is indicated in patients at high risk for bleeding. Pharmacological methods may be combined with graduated compression stockings in selected patients.

C. Low-Risk Patients

Apart from early ambulation, specific prophylaxis is usually not recommended (20,73). However, prophylaxis for low-risk patients is recommended in certain circumstances. It is the clinical custom in some countries to use graduated compression stockings, but this is not based on evidence from clinical trials.

D. Other Conditions

Medical Patients

Medical patients should be classified as low, moderate, or high risk for venous thromboembolism, depending on their underlying medical condition and other comorbid factors, such as immobility, previous deep vein thrombosis, or cancer. Low-risk patients should be considered for graduated compression stockings. For patients following myocardial infarction who have no other significant risk factors, anticoagulation with heparin/warfarin is recommended (20,73). In the presence of congestive heart failure and/or pulmonary infections/pneumonia, either low-dose heparin or low molecular weight heparin is recommended (20,73,117). For patients with ischemic strokes and lower limb paralysis, low-dose heparin or low molecular weight heparin is recommended (20,73). Intermittent pneumatic compression may be used for high-risk patients who are at high risk of bleeding, although this is not based on clinical trial data.

In a recent multicenter study in acutely ill medical patients (including congestive heart failure, acute respiratory failure, or medical conditions associated with at least one additional risk factor for venous thromboembolism), low molecular weight heparin (enoxaparin), 40 mg daily, was shown significantly to decrease the incidence of venographically demonstrated deep vein thrombosis when compared with enoxaparin, 20 mg, or a placebo (118). Prophylaxis was continued for 6–14 days. The observed benefit with the 40-mg dose was maintained at 3 months. There was no difference in death rates nor in the incidence of major bleeding. Recently, a clinical trial has been launched in high-risk medical patients to determine if extended prophylaxis with enoxaparin out to day 38 is superior to initial prophylaxis for 9–14 days with an ultrasound endpoint. Similarly, a study has recently been completed but not yet reported comparing low molecular weight heparin (dalteparin) for 14 days with a placebo in high-risk medical patients also using an ultrasound endpoint. At this time, there have been no studies which are adequately powered to show a difference in efficacy between unfractionated heparin and low molecular weight heparin in high-risk medical patients (117).

Pregnancy

Although low molecular weight heparin has not been approved for use in pregnancy, it has been widely used for both prevention and treatment of venous thromboembolism. Review of safety data on the use of low molecular weight heparin for prevention or treatment of venous thromboembolism in pregnancy have been published (119,120). These studies indicate that low molecular weight heparin has an acceptable incidence of adverse events, even in this relatively high-risk population. There have been a number of reports of thrombosis of mechanical prosthetic heart valves in pregnant patients treated with different doses of low molecular weight heparin including full therapeutic doses (121–123) and including three recent deaths reported from South Africa. In a clinical study of pregnant women with prosthetic heart valves given low molecular weight heparin (1 mg/kg bid) to reduce the risk of thromboembolism, two of seven women developed clots resulting in blockage of the valve and leading to maternal and fetal death. There are postmarketing reports of prosthetic valve thrombosis in pregnant women with prosthetic heart valves while receiving low molecular weight heparin for thromboprophylaxis. These events resulted in maternal death or surgical interventions. The use of low molecular weight heparin injection is not recommended for thromboprophylaxis in pregnant women with prosthetic heart valves (124). This has led to a warning from the FDA regarding the use of low molecular weight in such patients (124). In a randomized clinical trial, low molecular weight heparin (dalteparin) (average 4631 factor Xa units per day) or subcutaneous unfractionated heparin (mean 20,569 units per day) for either prevention or treatment of venous thromboembolism (125). Treatment lasted for approximately 32 weeks (125). There were no thromboembolic complications in either group, but there was significantly more bleeding with unfractionated heparin. Two patients in the unfractionated heparin group suffered lumbosacral compression fractures, whereas none was seen in the dalteparin group. In a follow-up to this study, bone density measurements were carried out in 46 patients from the previous group at 1 week, 6 weeks, 16 weeks, and 52 weeks (126). Bone density measurements were normal in the dalteparin group but significantly decreased in the unfractionated heparin group up to 52 weeks, and a few patients who were followed up to 3 years continued to show decreased bone density. This study clearly favors the use of low molecular weight heparin for the management of venous thromboembolism in pregnancy (126).

There have been reports of congenital anomalies in infants born to women who received low molecular weight heparin during pregnancy including cerebral anomalies, limb anomalies, hypospadias, peripheral vascular malformation, fibrotic dysplasia, and cardiac defects. A cause and effect relationship has not been established nor has the incidence been shown to be higher than in the general population (124).

Numerous studies have indicated that patients with hereditary thrombophilia have an increased incidence of complications of pregnancy including first-trimester abortion, intrauterine growth retardation, stillbirths, preeclampsia, and abruptio placentae (127,128). Studies are currently underway to determine if the administration of low molecular weight heparin through pregnancy can prevent these events.

At the present time, either unfractionated heparin or low molecular weight heparin are recommended for the prevention or treatment of venous thromboembolism in pregnancy (129). Most recommendations include the use of factor Xa levels periodically to monitor treatment with low molecular weight heparin. Patients with mechanical heart valves and the antiphospholipid antibody syndrome require special attention (124,129). Clearly, further randomized clinical trials in the management of thrombotic problems in pregnancy are required.

VII. Conclusions

There are now effective measures for the prevention of venous thromboembolism in most medical and surgical conditions. Based on information from Level 1 clinical trials and systematic reviews, recommendations for the prevention of venous thromboembolism can be made for most circumstances encountered by the physician or surgeon. Where such information is not available, recommendations must be based on extrapolation from similar circumstances in which the risk reduction is known. Unfortunately, even when effective prophylactic agents are available, they are commonly not applied, particularly in medical patients at risk of venous thromboembolism. Death from pulmonary embolism is one of the most preventable causes of death in hospital practice. The ultimate goal of prophylaxis should be the elimination of fatal pulmonary embolism in medical and surgical patients, a goal that at the present time is still unfulfilled.

References

1. Hull RD, Hirsh J, Carter CJ, Jay RM, Ockelford PA, Buller HR, Turpie AG, Powers P, Kinch D, Dodd PE. Diagnostic efficacy of impedance plethysmography for clinically suspected deep vein thrombosis: a randomized trial. Ann Intern Med 1985; 102:21–28.
2. Huisman MV, Buller HR, ten Cate JW, Vreeken J. Serial impedance plethysmography for suspected deep venous thrombosis in outpatients. The Amsterdam General Practitioner Study. N Engl J Med 1986; 314:823–828.
3. Kakkar VV, Howe CT, Flanc C, Clarke MB. Natural history of postoperative deep vein thrombosis. Lancet 1969; 2:230–233.
4. Lagerstedt CI, Olsson CG, Fagher BO, Oqvist BW, Albrechtsson U. Need for long term anticoagulant treatment in symptomatic calf vein thrombosis. Lancet 1985; 2:515–518.
5. Lohr JM, James KV, Deshmukh RM, Hasselfeld KA. Calf vein thrombi are not a benign finding. Am J Surg 1995; 170:86–90.
6. Moser KM, Le Moine JR. Is embolic risk conditioned by location of deep venous thrombosis? Ann Intern Med 1981; 94:439–444.
7. Sevitt S, Gallagher N. Venous thrombosis and pulmonary embolism. A clinicopathological study in injured and burned patients. Br J Surg 1961; 48:475–489.
8. Mavor GE, Galloway JMD. The iliofemoral venous segment as a source of pulmonary emboli. Lancet 1967; 1:871–874.
9. Hull RD, Hirsh J, Carter CJ, Raskob GE, Gill GJ, Jay RM, Leclerc JR, David M, Coates G. Diagnostic value of ventilation-perfusion lung scanning in patients with suspected pulmonary embolism. Chest 1985; 88:819–828.
10. Salzman EW, Davies GC. Prophylaxis of venous thromboembolism. Analysis of cost-effectiveness. Ann Surg 1980; 191:207–218.
11. Hull R, Hirsh J, Sackett DL, Stoddart GL. Cost-effectiveness of primary and secondary prevention of fatal pulmonary embolism in high risk surgical patients. Can Med Assoc J 1982; 127:990–995.

12. Oster G, Tuden RL, Colditz GA. A cost-effectiveness analysis of prophylaxis against deep vein thrombosis in major orthopedic surgery. JAMA 1987; 257: 203–208.

13. Bergqvist D, Matzsch T, Jendteg S, Lindgren B, Persson U. The cost-effectiveness of prevention of post-operative thromboembolism. Acta Chir Scand Suppl 1990; 556:36–41.

14. Hauch O, Khattar SC, Jorensen LN. Cost-benefit analysis of prophylaxis against deep vein thrombosis in major orthopaedic surgery. Semin Thromb Hemost 1991; 17(Suppl 3):280–283.

15. Sharnoff JG, DeBlasio G. Prevention of fatal postoperative thromboembolism by heparin prophylaxis. Lancet 1970; 2:1006–1007.

16. International Multicentre Trial. Prevention of fatal postoperative pulmonary embolism by low doses of heparin. Lancet 1975; 2:45–51.

17. Collins R, Scrimgeour A, Yusef S, Peto R. Reduction in fatal pulmonary embolism and venous thrombosis by perioperative administration of sub-cutaneous heparin. N Engl J Med 1988; 318:1162–1173.

18. Kakkar VV, Cohen AT, Edmonson RA, Phillips MJ, Cooper DJ, Das SK, Maher KT, Sanderson RM, Ward VP, Kakkar S. Low molecular weight versus standard heparin for prevention of venous thromboembolism after major abdominal surgery. Lancet 1993; 341:259–265.

19. Kakkar VV, Boeckl O, Boneau B, Bordenave L, Brehm OA, Brucke P, Cocceri S, Cohen AT, Galland F, Haas S, Jarrige J, Koppenhagen K, LeQuerrec A, Parraguette E, Prandoni P, Roder JD, Roos M, Ruschemeyer C, Siewert JR, Vinazzer H, Wenzel E. Efficacy and safety of a low molecu-lar weight heparin and standard unfractionated heparin for prophylaxis of postoperative venous thromboembolism: European multicenter trial. World J Surg 1997; 21:2–9.

20. Geerts WH, Heit JA, Clagett GP, Pineo GF, Colwell CW, Anderson FA Jr, Wheeler HB. Prevention of venous thromboembolism. Chest 2001; 119(Suppl): 132S–175S.

21. Bergqvist D, Burmark US, Flordal PA, Frisell J, Hallbook T, Hedberg M, Horn A, Kelty E, Kvitting P, Lindhagen A. Low molecular weight heparin started before surgery as prophylaxis against deep vein thrombosis: 2500 versus 5000 Xal units in 2070 patients. Br J Surg 1995; 82:496–501.

22. Leyvraz PF, Bachmann F, Hoek J, Buller HR, Postel M, Samama M, Vandenbrook MD. Prevention of deep vein thrombosis after hip replacement: randomised comparison between unfractionated heparin and low molecular weight heparin. BMJ 1991; 303:543–548.

23. Eriksson BI, Kälebo P, Anthymyr BA, Wadenvik H, Tengborn L, Risberg B. Prevention of deep vein thrombosis and pulmonary embolism after total hip replacement. J Bone Joint Surg Am 1991; 73-A(4):484–493.

24. Planes A, Vochelle N, Fagola M, Feret J, Bellaud M. Prevention of deep vein thrombosis after total hip replacement: the effect of low molecular weight heparin with spinal and general anaesthesia. J Bone Joint Surg Br 1991; 73-B:418–422.

25. Hamulyak K, Lensing AW, van der Meer J, Smid WM, van Ooy A, Hoek JA.

Subcutaneous low-molecular-weight heparin or oral anticoagulants for the prevention of deep-vein thrombosis in elective hip and knee replacement? Thromb Haemost 1995; 74(6):1428–1431.

26. Bergqvist D, Benoni G, Bjorgell O, Fredin H, Hedlundh U, Nicolas S, Nilsson P, Nylander G. Low molecular weight heparin (enoxaparin) as prophylaxis against venous thromboembolism after total hip replacement. N Engl J Med 1996; 335(10):696–700.

27. Planes A, Vochelle N, Darmon JY, Fagola M, Bellaud M, Huet Y. Risk of deep-venous thrombosis after hospital discharge in patients having undergone total hip replacement: double-blind randomized comparison of enoxaparin versus placebo. Lancet 1996; 348:224–228.

28. Dahl OE, Andreassen G, Aspelin T, Muller C, Mathiesen P, Nyhus S, Abdelnoor M, Solhaug JH, Arnesen H. Prolonged thromboprophylaxis following hip replacement surgery—results of a double-blind, prospective, randomized, placebo-controlled study with dalteparin (Fragmin). Thromb Haemost 1997; 77(1):26–31.

29. Lassen MR, Borris LC, Anderson BS, Jensen HP, Skejo Bro HP, Andersen G, Petersen AO, Siem P, Horlyck E, Jensen BV, Thomsen PB, Hansen BR, Erin-Madsen J, Moller JC, Rotwitt L, Christensen F, Nielsen AB, Appelquist E, Tjalve E, et al. Efficacy and safety of prolonged thromboprophylaxis with a low-molecular-weight heparin (dalteparin) after total hip arthroplasty—the Danish prolonged prophylaxis (DaPP) study. Thromb Res 1998; 89:281–287.

30. Levine MN, Hirsh J, Gent M, Turpie AG, Leclerc J, Powers PJ, Jay RM, Neemeh J. Prevention of deep vein thrombosis after elective hip surgery: a randomized trial comparing low molecular weight heparin with standard unfractionated heparin. Ann Intern Med 1991; 114(7):545–551.

31. Colwell CW Jr, Spiro TE, Trowbridge AA, Morris BA, Kwaan HC, Blaha JD, Comerota AJ, Skoutakis VA. Use of enoxaparin, a low molecular weight heparin and unfractionated heparin for the prevention of deep venous thrombosis after elective hip replacement. J Bone Joint Surg Am 1994; 76-A(1):3–14.

32. Hull RD, Raskob G, Pineo G, Rosenbloom D, Evans W, Mallory T, Anquist K, Smith F, Hughes G, Green D. A comparison of subcutaneous low-molecular-weight heparin with warfarin sodium for prophylaxis against deep-vein thrombosis after hip or knee implantation. N Engl J Med 1993; 329(19):1370–1376.

33. Leclerc JR, Geerts WH, Desjardins L, Jobin F, Laroche F, Delorme F, Haviernick S, Atkinson S, Bourgouin J. Prevention of deep vein thrombosis after major knee surgery—a randomised, double-blind trial comparing a low molecular weight heparin fragment (enoxaparin) to placebo. Thromb Haemost 1992; 67(4):417–423.

34. Leclerc JR, Geerts WH, Desjardins L, Laflamme GH, L'Esperance B, Demers C, Kassis J, Cruikshank M, Whitmen L, Delorme F. Prevention of venous thromboembolism after knee arthroplasty—a randomized, double-blind trial comparing enoxaparin with warfarin. Ann Intern Med 1996; 124:619–626.

35. Heit JA, Berkowitz SD, Bona R, Cabanas V, Corson JD, Elliott CG, Lyons

R. Efficacy and safety of low molecular weight heparin (ardeparin sodium) compared to warfarin for the prevention of venous thromboembolism after total knee replacement surgery: A double blind, dose ranging study. Thromb Haemost 1997; 77(1):32–38.

36. Comp PC, Spiro TE, Friedman RJ, Whitsett TL, Johnson GJ, Gardiner GA, Landon GC, Jové Mfor the enoxaparin Clinical Trial Group. Prolonged enoxaparin therapy to prevent venous thromboembolism after primary hip or knee replacement. J Bone Joint Surg Am 2001; 83-A:336–345.

37. Kearon C, Hirsh J. Starting prophylaxis for venous thromboembolism postoperatively. Arch Intern Med 1995; 155:366–372.

38. Hull RD, Brant RF, Pineo GF, Stein PD, Raskob GE, Valentine KA. Preoperative vs postoperative initiation so low-molecular-weight heparin prophylaxis against venous thromboembolism in patients undergoing elective hip replacement. Arch Intern Med 1999; 159:137–141.

39. Torholm C, Broeng L, Jorgensen PS, Bjerregaard P, Josephsen L, Jorgensen PK, Hagen K, Knudsen JB. Thromboprophylaxis by low-molecular-weight heparin in elective hip surgery. A placebo controlled study. J Bone Joint Surg Br 1991; 73-B:434–438.

40. Francis CW, Pellegrini VD Jr, Totterman S, Boyd AD, Marder VJ, Liebert KM, Stulberg BN, Ayers DC, Rosenberg A, Kessler C, Johanson NA. Prevention of deep vein thrombosis after total hip arthroplasty: comparison of warfarin and dalteparin. J Bone Joint Surg Am 1997; 79-A(9):1365–1372.

41. Hull RD, Pineo GF, Francis C, Bergqvist D, Fellenius C, Soderberg K, Holmqvist A, Mant M, Dear R, Baylis B, Mah A, Brant R. Low-molecular-weight heparin prophylaxis using dalteparin in close proximity to surgery vs. warfarin in hip arthroplasty patients. Arch Intern Med 2000; 160:2199–2207.

42. Hull RD, Pineo GF, Stein PD, Mah AF, MacIsaac SM, Dahl OE, Ghali WA, Butcher MS, Brant RF, Bergqvist D, Hamulyák K, Francis CW, Marder VJ, Raskob GE. Timing of initial administration of low-molecular-weight heparin prophylaxis against deep vein thrombosis in patients following elective hip arthroplasty. Arch Intern Med 2001; 161:1952–1960.

43. Fitzgerald RH Jr, Spiro TE, Trowbridge AA, Gardiner GA, Whitsett TL, O'Connell MB, Ohar JA, Young TR, Enoxaparin Clinical Trial Group. Prevention of venous thromboembolic disease following primary total knee arthroplasty. A randomized, multicenter, open-label, parallel-group comparison of enoxaparin and warfarin. J Bone Joint Surg Am 2001; 83-A(6):900–906.

44. Horlocker TT, Heit JA. Low molecular weight heparin: Biochemistry, pharmacology, perioperative prophylaxis regimens, and guidelines for regional anesthetic management. Anesth Analg 1997; 85:874–885.

45. Eriksson BI, Ekman S, Kalebo P, Zachrisson B, Bach D, Close P. Prevention of deep vein thrombosis after total hip replacement: direct thrombin inhibition with recombinant hirudin, CGP 39393. Lancet 1996; 347:635–639.

46. Eriksson BI, Arfwidsson AC, Frison L, Eriksson UG, Bylock A, Kälebo P, Fager G, Gustafsson D. A dose-ranging study of the oral direct thrombin

inhibitor, ximelagatran, and its subcutaneous form, melagatran, compared with dalteparin in the prophylaxis of thromboembolism after hip or knee replacement: METHRO 1. Thromb Haemost 2002; 87:231–237.

47. Eriksson BI, Lindbratt S, Kalebo P, Bylock A, Frison L, Welin L, Dahl O, Gustafsson D. METHRO II: dose-response study of the novel oral, direct thrombin inhibitor, H 376/95 and its subcutaneous formulation melagatran, compared with dalteparin as thromboembolic prophylaxis after total hip or total knee replacement. Haemostasis 2000; 30(Suppl 1):20.

48. Colwell CW, Berkowitz SD, Davidson BL, Lotke PA, Ginsberg JS, Lieberman JR, Neubauer J, Whipple JP, Peters GR, Francis CW. Randomized, double-blind, comparison of ximelagatran, an oral direct thrombin inhibitor, and enoxaparin to prevent venous thromboembolism (VTE) after total hip arthroplasty (THA). Blood 2001; 98:706a.

49. Turpie AGG, Gallus AS, Hoek JA, for the Pentasaccharide Investigators. A synthetic pentasaccharide for the prevention of deep-vein thrombosis after total hip replacement. N Engl J Med 2001; 344:619–625.

50. Eriksson BI, Bauer KA, Lassen MR, Turpie AGG. Fondaparinux compared with enoxaparin for the prevention of venous thromboembolism after hip-fracture surgery. N Engl J Med 2001; 345:1298–1304.

51. Bauer KA, Eriksson BI, Lassen MR, Turpie AGG. Fondaparinux compared with enoxaparin for the prevention of venous thromboembolism after elective knee surgery. N Engl J Med 2001; 345:1305–1310.

52. Lassen MR, Bauer KA, Eriksson BI, Turpie AGG, for the European Pentasaccharide Hip Elective Surgery Study (EPHESUS) Steering Committee. Postoperative fondaparinux versus preoperative enoxaparin for prevention of venous thromboembolism in elective hip-replacement surgery: a randomised double-blind comparison. Lancet 2002; 359:1715–1720.

53. Turpie AGG, Bauer KA, Eriksson BI, Lassen MR, for the PENTATHLON 2000 Study Steering Committee. Postoperative fondaparinux versus postoperative enoxaparin for prevention of venous thromboembolism after elective hip-replacement surgery: a randomised double-blind trial. Lancet 2002; 359:1721–1726.

54. Bounameaux H, Perneger T. Fondaparinux: a new synthetic pentasaccharide for thrombosis prevention. Lancet 2002; 359:1710–1711.

55. Kakkar VV, Adams PC. Preventive and therapeutic approach to thromboembolic disease and pulmonary embolism: can death from pulmonary embolism be prevented? J Am Coll Cardiol 1986; 8(6 Suppl B):146B–158B.

56. Skinner DB, Salzman EW. Anticoagulant prophylaxis in surgical patients. Surg Gynecol Obstet 1967; 125:741–746.

57. Shephard RM Jr, White HA, Shirkey AL. Anticoagulant prophylaxis of thromboembolism in post-surgical patients. Am J Surg 1966; 112:698–702.

58. Coventry MB, Nolan DR, Beckenbaugh RD. "Delayed" prophylactic anticoagulation: a study of results and complications in 2,012 total hip arthoplasties. J Bone Joint Surg Am 1973; 55-A:1487–1492.

59. Eskeland G, Solheim K, Skjorten F. Anticoagulant prophylaxis, throm-

boembolism and mortality in elderly patients with hip fracture: a controlled clinical trial. Acta Chir Scand 1966; 131:16–29.

60. Murray DW, Britton AR, Bulstrode CJK. Thromboprophylaxis and death after total hip replacement. J Bone Joint Surg Br 1996; 78-B(6):863–870.

61. Campling EA, Devlin HB, Hoile RW, Lunn JN. The report of the national confidential enquiry into perioperative deaths (NCEPOD) 1991/92, London HM30.

62. Vandermeulen EP, Van Aken H, Vermylen J. Anticoagulants and spinal-epidural anesthesia. Anesth Analg 1994; 79:1165–1177.

63. Bergqvist D, Lindblad B, Matzsch T. Risk of combining low molecular weight heparin for thromboprophylaxis and epidural or spinal anesthesia. Semin Thromb Hemost 1993; 19(Suppl 1):147–151.

64. Dahlgren N, Tornebrandt K. Neurological complications after anaesthesia; a follow-up of 18,000 spinal and epidural anaesthetics performed over three years. Acta Anaesthesiol Scand 1995; 39:872–880.

65. Dahl OE, Aspelin T, Arnesen H, Seljeflot I, Kierulf P, Ruyter R, Lyberg T. Increased activation of coagulation and formation of late deep venous thrombosis following discontinuation of thromboprophylaxis after hip replacement surgery. Thromb Res 1995; 80:299–306.

66. White RH, Romano PS, Zhou H, Rodrigo J, Bargar W. Incidence and time course of thromboembolic outcomes following total hip or knee arthroplasty. Arch Intern Med 1998; 158:1525–1531.

67. Hull RD, Pineo GF, Francis C, Bergqvist D, Fellenius C, Soderberg K, Holmqvist A, Mant M, Dear R, Baylis B, Mah A, Brant R, for the North American Fragmin Trial Investigators. Low-molecular-weight heparin prophylaxis using dalteparin extended out-of-hospital vs in-hospital warfarin/out-of-hospital placebo in hip arthroplasty patients. A double-blind, randomized comparison. Arch Intern Med 2000; 160:2208–2215.

68. Hull RD, Pineo GF, Stein PD, Mah AF, MacIsaac SM, Dahl OE, Butcher M, Brant RF, Ghali WA, Bergqvist D, Raskob GE. Extended out-of-hospital low-molecular-weight heparin prophylaxis against deep venous thrombosis in patients after elective hip arthroplasty: a systematic review. Ann Intern Med 2001; 135:858–869.

69. Bergqvist D, Jonsson B. Cost-effectiveness of prolonged out-of-hospital prophylaxis with low-molecular-weight heparin following total hip replacement. Haemostasis 2000; 30(Suppl 2):130–135.

70. Sarasin FP, Bounameaux H. Out of hospital antithrombotic prophylaxis after total hip replacement: Low-molecular-weight heparin, warfarin, aspirin or nothing? A cost-effectiveness analysis. Thromb Haemost 2002; 87:586–592.

71. Samama ChM, Barré J, Fiessenger JN, Rosencher N. Long term venous thromboembolism prophylaxis after total hip replacement: a comparison of low molecular weight heparin with oral anticoagulant. Thromb Haemost Suppl 2001; OC2343 (abstr).

72. Bergqvist D, Agnelli G, Cohen AT, Eldor A, Nilsson PE, Le Moigne-Amrani A,

Dietrich-Neto F. Duration of prophylaxis against venous thromboembolism with enoxaparin after surgery for cancer. N Engl J Med 2002; 346:975–980.

73. Nicolaides AN, Breddin HK, Fareed J, Goldhaber S, Haas S, Hull R, Kalodiki E, Myers K, Samama M, Sasahara A. Prevention of venous thromboembolism. International Consensus Statement. Guidelines compiled in accordance with the scientific evidence. Int Angiol 2001; 20:1–37.

74. Guyatt G, Schunëmann H, Cook D, Jaeschke R, Pauker S, Bucher H. Grades of recommendation for antithrombotic agents. Chest 2001; 119(1 Suppl):3S–7S.

75. Bergqvist D, Matzsch T, Burmark U, Frisell J, Guilbaud O, Hallbook T, Horn A, Lindhagen A, Ljungner H, Ljungstrom KG. Low molecular weight heparin given the evening before surgery compared with conventional low dose heparin in prevention of thrombosis. Br J Surg 1988; 75:888–891.

76. Caen JP. A randomized double-blind study between a low molecular weight heparin Kabi 2165 and standard heparin in the prevention of deep vein thrombosis in general surgery. A French multicenter trial. Thromb Haemost 1988; 59:216–220.

77. Nurmohamed MT, Verhaeghe R, Haas S, Iriarte JA, Vogel G, van Rij AM, Prentice CR, ten Cate JW. A comparative trial of a low molecular weight heparin (enoxaparin) versus standard heparin for the prophylaxis of postoperative deep vein thrombosis in general surgery. Am J Surg 1995; 169:567–571.

78. ENOXACAN Study Group. Efficacy and safety of enoxaparin versus unfractionated heparin for prevention of deep vein thrombosis in elective cancer surgery: a double-blind randomized multicentre trial with venographic assessment. Br J Surg 1997; 84:1099–1103.

79. Leizorovicz A, Haugh MC, Chapuis FR, Samama MM, Boissel JP. Low molecular weight heparin in prevention of perioperative thrombosis. BMJ 1992; 305:913–920.

80. Nurmohamed MT, Rosendaal FR, Buller HR, Dekker E, Hommes DW, Vandenbroucke JP, Briet E. Low-molecular-weight heparin versus standard heparin in general and orthopaedic surgery: a meta-analysis. Lancet 1992; 340:152–156.

81. Koch A, Bouges S, Ziegler S, Dinkel H, Daures JP, Victor N. Low molecular weight heparin and unfractionated heparin in thrombosis prophylaxis after major surgical intervention: update of previous meta-analyses. Br J Surg 1997; 84:750–759.

82. Palmer AJ, Koppenhagen K, Kirchhof B, Weber U, Bergemann R. Efficacy and safety of low molecular weight heparin, unfractionated heparin and warfarin for thrombo-embolism prophylaxis in orthopaedic surgery: a meta-analysis of randomised clinical trials. Haemostasis 1997; 27:75–84.

83. O'Brien BJ, Anderson DR, Goeree R. Cost-effectiveness of enoxaparin versus warfarin prophylaxis against deep vein thrombosis after total hip replacement. Can Med Assoc J 1994; 150(7):1083–1089.

84. Menzin J, Colditz GA, Regan MM, Richner RE, Oster G. Cost-effectiveness

of enoxaparin vs. low dose warfarin in the prevention of deep vein thrombosis after total hip replacement surgery. Arch Intern Med 1995; 155:757–764.

85. Hull RD, Raskob GE, Pineo GF, Feldstein W, Rosenbloom D, Gafni A, Green D, Feinglass J, Trowbidge AA, Elliott CG. Subcutaneous low-molecular-weight heparin vs warfarin for prophylaxis of deep vein thrombosis after hip or knee implantation: an economic perspective. Arch Intern Med 1997; 157:298–303.

86. Geerts WH, Jay RM, Code KI, Chen E, Szalai JP, Saibil EA, Hamilton PA. A comparison of low dose heparin with low molecular weight heparin as prophylaxis against venous thromboembolism after major trauma. N Engl J Med 1996; 335(10):701–707.

87. Harenberg J, Roebruck P, Heene DL, on behalf of the Heparin Study in Internal Medicine Group. Subcutaneous low molecular weight heparin versus standard heparin and the prevention of thromboembolism in medical inpatients. Haemostasis 1996; 26:127–139.

88. Bergmann JF, Neuhart E. A multicenter randomized double-blind study of enoxaparin compared with unfractionated heparin in the prevention of venous thromboembolic disease in elderly inpatients bedridden for an acute medical illness. Thromb Haemost 1996; 76:529–534.

89. Ramos R, Salem BI, De Pawlikowski MP, Coordes C, Eisenberg S, Leidenfrost R. The efficacy of pneumatic compression stockings in the prevention of pulmonary embolism after cardiac surgery. Chest 1996; 109(1):82–85.

90. Turpie AG, Gallus A, Beattie WS, Hirsh J. Prevention of venous thrombosis in patients with intracranial disease by intermittent pneumatic compression of the calf. Neurology 1977; 27:435–438.

91. Turpie AG, Delmore T, Hirsh J, Hull R, Genton E, Hiscoe C, Gent M. Prevention of venous thrombosis by intermittent sequential calf compression in patients with intracranial disease. Thromb Res Suppl 1979; 15:611–616.

92. Skillman JJ, Collins RE, Coe NP, Goldstein BS, Shapiro RM, Zervas NT, Bettmann MA, Salzman EW. Prevention of deep vein thrombosis in neurosurgical patients: a controlled, randomized trial of external pneumatic compression boots. Surgery 1978; 83:354–358.

93. Hull RD, Raskob GE, Gent M, McLoughlin D, Julian D, Smith FC, Dale NI, Reed-Davis R, Lofthouse RN, Anderson C. Effectiveness of intermittent pneumatic leg compression for preventing deep vein thrombosis after total hip replacement. JAMA 1990; 263:2313–2317.

94. Francis CW, Pellegrini VD Jr, Marder VJ, Totterman S, Harris CM, Gabriel KR, Azodo MV, Liebert KM. Comparison of warfarin and external pneumatic compression in prevention of venous thrombosis after total hip replacement. JAMA 1992; 267(21):2911–2915.

95. Hull RD, Delmore TJ, Hirsh J, Gent M, Armstrong P, Lofthouse R, MacMillan A, Blackstone I, Reed-Davis R, Detwiler RC. Effectiveness of intermittent pulsatile elastic stockings for the prevention of calf and thigh vein thrombosis in patients undergoing elective knee surgery. Thromb Res 1979; 16:37–45.

96. McKenna R, Galante J, Bachmann F, Wallace DL, Kaushal PS, Meredith P. Prevention of venous thromboembolism after total knee replacement by high-dose aspirin or intermittent calf and thigh compression. Br Med J 1980; 280:514–517.

97. Comerota AJ, Katz ML, White JV. Why does prophylaxis with external pneumatic compression for deep vein thrombosis fail? Am J Surg 1992; 164:265–268.

98. Haddad FS, Kerry RM, McEwan JA, Appleton L, Garbuz DS, Masri BA, Duncan CP. Unanticipated variations between expected and delivered pneumatic compression therapy after elective hip surgery: a possible source of variation in reported patient outcomes. J Arthroplasty 2001; 16:37–46.

99. Meyerowitz BR, Nelson R. Measurement of the velocity of blood in lower limb veins with and without compression surgery. Surgery 1964; 56:481–486.

100. Sigel B, Edelstein AL, Felix WR Jr, Memhardt CR. Compression of the deep venous system of the lower leg during inactive recumbency. Arch Surg 1973; 106:38–43.

101. Wells PS, Lensing AWA, Hirsh J. Graduated compression stockings in the prevention of postoperative venous thromboembolism. A meta-analysis. Arch Intern Med 1994; 154:67–72.

102. Brandjes DPM, Buller HR, Heijboer H, Huisman MV, de Rijk M, Jagt H, ten Cate JW. Randomised trial of effect of compression stockings in patients with symptomatic proximal vein thrombosis. Lancet 1997; 349:759–762.

103. Scurr JH, Machin SJ, Bailey-King S, Mackie IJ, McDonald S, Smith PD. Frequency and prevention of symptomless deep-vein thrombosis in long-haul flights: a randomised trial. Lancet 2001; 357:1485–1489.

104. Francis CW, Pellegrini VD Jr, Leibert KM, Totterman S, Azodo MV, Harris CM, Cox C, Marder VJ. Comparison of two warfarin regimens in the prevention of venous thrombosis following total knee replacement. Thromb Haemost 1996; 75:706–711.

105. Colwell CW Jr, Collis DK, Paulson R, McCutchen JW, Bigler GT, Lutz S, Hardwick ME. Comparison of enoxaparin and warfarin for the prevention of venous thromboembolic disease after total hip arthroplasty. J Bone Joint Surg Am 1999; 81-A:932–940.

106. Paiement GD, Wessinger SJ, Waltman WC, Harris WH. Low dose warfarin versus external pneumatic compression for prophylaxis against venous thromboembolism following total hip replacement. J Arthroplasty 1987; 2:23–26.

107. Powers PJ, Gent M, Jay RM, Julian DH, Turpie AG, Levine M, Hirsh J. A randomized trial of less intense postoperative warfarin or aspirin therapy in the prevention of venous thromboembolism after surgery for fractured hip. Arch Intern Med 1989; 149:771–774.

108. Poller L, McKernan A, Thomson JM, Elstein M, Hirsch PJ, Jones JB. Fixed minidose warfarin: a new approach to prophylaxis against venous thrombosis after major surgery. BMJ 1987; 295:1309–1312.

109. Bern MM, Lokich JJ, Wallach SR, Bothe A Jr, Benotti PN, Arkin CF, Greco FA, Huberman M, Moore C. Very low doses of warfarin can prevent thrombosis in central venous catheters. Ann Intern Med 1990; 112:423–428.

110. Heaton DC, Han DY, Inder A. Minidose (1 mg) warfarin as prophylaxis for central vein catheter thrombosis. Intern Med J 2002; 32:84–88.

111. Dale C, Gallus A, Wycherley A, Langlois S, Howie D. Prevention of venous thrombosis with minidose warfarin after joint replacement. BMJ 1991; 303: 224.

112. Antiplatelet Trialists' Collaboration. Collaborative overview of randomized trials of antiplatelet therapy. III: Reduction in venous thrombosis and pulmonary embolism by antiplatelet prophylaxis among surgical and medical patients. BMJ 1994; 308:235–246.

113. Pulmonary Embolism Prevention (PEP) Trial collaborative Group. Prevention of pulmonary embolism and deep vein thrombosis with low dose aspirin: Pulmonary Embolism Prevention (PEP) trial. Lancet 2000; 355:1295–1302.

114. Hull RD, Pineo GF. A synthetic pentasaccharide for the prevention of deep-vein thrombosis. N Engl J Med 2001; 345:291.

115. Rivera TM, Leone-Bay A, Paton D, Leipold HR, Baughman RA. Oral delivery of heparin in combination with Sodium N-[8-(2-Hydroxybenzoyl)-amino]caprylate: pharmacological considerations. Pharm Res 1997; 14:1830–1834.

116. Baughman RA, Kapoor SC, Agarwal RK, Kisicki J, Catella-Lawson F, Fitzgerald GA. Oral delivery of anticoagulant doses of heparin: a randomized, double-blind, controlled study in humans. Circulation 1998; 98:1610–1615.

117. Mismetti P, Laporte-Simitsidis S, Tardy B, Cucherat M, Buchmuller A, Juillard-Delsart D, Decousus H. Prevention of venous thromboembolism in internal medicine with unfractionated or low-molecular-weight heparins: a meta-analysis of randomised clinical trials. Thromb Haemost 2000; 83:14–19.

118. Samama MM, Cohen AT, Darmon JY, Desjardins L, Eldor A, Janbon C, Leizorovicz A, Nguyen H, Olsson CG, Turpie AG, Weisslinger N. A comparison of enoxaparin with placebo for the prevention of venous thromboembolism in acutely ill medical patients. Prophylaxis in Medical Patients with Enoxaparin Study Group. N Engl J Med 1999; 341:793–800.

119. Sanson BJ, Lensing AWA, Prins MH, Ginsberg JS, Barkagan ZS, Lavenne-Pardonge E, Brenner B, Dulitzky M, Nielsen JD, Boda Z, Turi S, MacGillavry MR, Hamulyak K, Theunissen IM, Hunt BJ, Buller HR. Safety of low-molecular-weight heparin in pregnancy: a systematic review. Thromb Haemost 1999; 81:668–672.

120. Lepercq J, Conard J, Borel-Derlon A, Darmon JY, Boudignat O, Francoual C, Priollet P, Cohen C, Yvelin N, Schved JF, Tournaire M, Borg JY. Venous thromboembolism during pregnancy: a retrospective study of enoxaparin safety in 624 pregnancies. Br J Obstet Gynaecol 2001; 108:1134–1140.

121. Roberts N, Ross D, Flint SK, Arya R, Blott M. Thromboembolism in pregnant women with mechanical prosthetic heart valves anticoagulated with low molecular weight heparin. Br J Obstet Gynaecol 2001; 108:327–329.

122. Leyh RG, Fischer S, Ruhparwar A, Haverich A. Anticoagulation for prosthetic heart valves during pregnancy: is low-molecular-weight heparin an alternative? Eur J Cadiothorac Surg 2002; 21:577–579.

123. Lev-Ran O, Kramer A, Gurevitch J, Shapira I, Mohr R. Low-molecular-weight heparin for prosthetic heart valves: treatment failure. Ann Thorac Surg 2000; 69:264–266.

124. MedWatch Website at www.fda.gov/medwatch, Bulletin 2002.

125. Pettilä V, Kaaja R, Leinonen P, Ekblad U, Kataja M, Ikkala E. Thrombo-prophylaxis with low molecular weight heparin (dalteparin) in pregnancy. Thromb Res 1999; 96:275–282.

126. Pettilä V, Leinonen P, Markkola A, Hiilesmaa V, Kaaja R. Postpartum bone mineral density in women treated for thromboprophylaxis with unfractionated heparin or LMW heparin. Thromb Haemost 2002; 87:182–186.

127. Sanson BJ, Friederich PW, Simioni P, Zanardi S, Hilsman MV, Girolami A, ten Cate JW, Prins MH. The risk of abortion and stillbirth in antithrombin III, protein C and protein S deficient women. Thromb Haemost 1996; 75:387–388.

128. Kupferminc MJ, Eldor A, Steinman N, Many A, Bar-am A, Jaffa A, Fait A, Lessing JB. Increased frequency of genetic thrombophilia in women with complications of pregnancy. N Engl J Med 1999; 340:9–13.

129. Ginsberg JS, Greer I, Hirsh J. Use of antithrombotic agents during pregnancy. Chest 2001; 119(1 Suppl):122S–131S.

5

Investigation of Suspected Deep Vein Thrombosis

WILLIAM H. GEERTS and RITA SELBY

University of Toronto
and Sunnybrook & Women's College Health Sciences Centre
Toronto, Ontario, Canada

I. Introduction

Deep vein thrombosis (DVT) is a common and hazardous clinical condition encountered by virtually all types of physicians. The observed prevalence of DVT is approximately 1 per 1000 persons in the general population per year (1–4). It is important to make or exclude the diagnosis of DVT accurately, since failure to treat DVT is associated with substantial morbidity and mortality, whereas overdiagnosis exposes patients to the dangers and inconvenience of anticoagulants.

Information derived primarily from postoperative patients demonstrates that the majority of deep venous thrombi arise in, and remain confined to, the small veins of the calf where they are generally asymptomatic and undergo spontaneous thrombolysis (5–7). Calf vein thrombi are unlikely to result in pulmonary embolism (5,8,9). However, approximately 10–30% of calf thrombi will extend into the popliteal and other more proximal veins (8,10,11); at this point, leg symptoms are more common and there is a substantial short-term risk of pulmonary embolism (10) and a long-term risk of chronic postthrombotic symptoms (12–14). Clinicians should also be

Table 1   Components of the Investigation of Suspected DVT

A. Determination of pretest probability
  1. Risk factors for venous thromboembolism
  2. History of the presentation
  3. Physical examination
  4. Consideration of alternate diagnoses
B. Laboratory testing
  1. Sensitive D-dimer
C. Imaging test
  1. Older tests—impedance plethysmography, contrast venography
  2. Doppler ultrasonography
  3. Newer tests—CT, MRV
D. Application of a formal diagnostic algorithm
  1. Incorporating clinical probability
  2. Incorporating a sensitive D-dimer
  3. Without formal clinical probability or D-dimer

DVT, deep vein thrombosis; CT, computed tomography; MRV, magnetic resonance venography.

aware that, among outpatients with leg swelling or pain, only 15–30% actually have the diagnosis of DVT confirmed on objective testing (15,16).

The investigative approach to a patient with suspected DVT has four important components (Table 1): (1) determination of the pretest probability based on the presence of risk factors for thrombosis, the history and physical examination, and consideration of alternate diagnoses; (2) the possible role of laboratory testing; (3) an objective imaging test of the venous system; and (4) application of a formal diagnostic/management algorithm.

II.   Risk Factors for DVT

The majority of patients with DVT have one or more risk factors for thrombosis that produce venous stasis, activate the coagulation system, and/ or result in venous endothelial injury (Table 2) (4,17–22). Recent surgery, trauma, lower extremity paresis, and immobility are relatively common precipitating factors for thrombosis (19,22). Increasing age and previous venous thromboembolism are also independent risk factors (3). Certain malignancies (particularly brain tumors and adenocarcinomas of the lung and gastrointestinal and genitourinary systems) and the treatment of cancer predispose to the development of DVT (17,23–26). Pregnancy and the use of exogenous estrogens as well as cardiorespiratory failure and some chronic

Table 2   Risk Factors for DVT[a]

Epidemiological and Clinical Risk Factors
   Increasing age
   Previous venous thromboembolism
   Certain cancers
   Cancer therapy (surgery, radiotherapy, chemotherapy, hormonal)
   Recent surgery
   Trauma (especially lower extremity)
   Immobility—bedrest, long-distance travel, plaster cast
   Lower extremity paresis—stroke, other neuromuscular disease, spinal cord injury
   Heart failure
   Respiratory failure
   Pregnancy and the postpartum period
   Estrogens—oral contraceptives, perimenopausal hormone replacement,
      raloxifene
   Inflammatory bowel disease
   Nephrotic syndrome
   Collagen vascular diseases—systemic lupus erythematosus, Behçet's syndrome
Molecular Hypercoagulability
   Factor V Leiden/activated protein C resistance
   Prothrombin 20210A variant
   Antiphospholipid antibody syndrome including lupus anticoagulant and
      anticardiolipin antibody
   Deficiency or abnormal function of antithrombin, protein C, protein S
   Elevated levels of clotting factor VIII, IX, or XI
   Hyperhomocysteinemia
   Myeloproliferative disorders including polycythemia rubra vera and essential
      thrombocytosis
   Dysfibrinogenemia
   Paroxysmal nocturnal hemoglobinuria
   Heparin-induced thrombocytopenia
   Disseminated intravascular coagulation

DVT, deep vein thrombosis.
[a] See also Chapter 4.

inflammatory diseases are additional clinical risk factors. An increasing number of inherited or acquired abnormalities of coagulation and its control mechanisms produce a hypercoagulable state that predisposes to the development of venous thrombi (27–30). Finally, there is accumulating evidence that clinical venous thromboembolism (VTE) often requires the concomitant occurrence of multiple risk factors, some genetic and others "environmental" (31).

III. Clinical Aspects of the Diagnosis of DVT

Leg swelling and/or pain are the cardinal symptoms experienced by patients
with proven DVT. The physical examination may include one or more of the
following signs: leg swelling, tenderness, warmth, erythema, or distended
superficial veins (32–34). Although it is well known that the history or
physical examination alone is an unreliable method to confirm or exclude a
diagnosis of DVT, there is now substantial evidence that a formal assessment of the key aspects of the clinical presentation (including risk factors for
thrombosis and consideration of alternate diagnoses) may assist in decision
making about further diagnostic testing (33–39). A clinical model that

Table 3 Clinical Model for Predicting Pretest Probability
of DVT

Clinical feature	Score
History	
Active cancer (ongoing treatment or within previous 6 months or palliative)	1
Paralysis, paresis, or recent plaster cast immobilization of the lower extremity	1
Recent bedrest >3 days or major surgery past 4 weeks	1
Physical Examination	
Localized tenderness along deep venous distribution	1
Entire leg swollen	1
Calf swelling 3 cm > contralateral side (measured 10 cm below tibial tuberosity)	1
Pitting edema confined to symptomatic leg	1
Dilated superficial vein(s)	1
Alternative Diagnosis	
Alternative diagnosis as likely or more likely than DVT	−2
Pretest Probability	
1. Sum of scores → ≤0 low probability	
1 or 2 moderate probability	
≥ 3 high probability	
2. Sum of scores → ≤ 1 DVT unlikely	
> 1 DVT possible	

DVT, deep vein thrombosis.
Source: Adapted from Refs. 35, 39, and 128.

separates patients with suspected DVT into low, moderate, and high risk has been validated (Table 3) (33,35). The primary components of this clinical predictive model are risk factors for thrombosis, physical signs, and the presence of a possible alternate diagnosis (Table 4) (16,40). The model has recently been simplified to categorize patients into those unlikely to have DVT and those with possible DVT (39,41).

Although a clinical probability model alone cannot be used to exclude the diagnosis of DVT (42,43), the appropriate use of a formal clinical

Table 4   Differential Diagnosis for Suspected DVT

Musculoskeletal
   Lower extremity injury
   Muscle strain or tear
   Arthritis of the knee or ankle including gout
   Heterotopic ossification
   Sarcoma
Vascular
   Acute postthrombotic syndrome
   Chronic venous insufficiency
   Superficial venous thrombosis
   Varicose veins
   Peripheral arterial disease
   May-Thurner syndrome
   Femoral or popliteal artery aneurysm
Dermatological
   Cellulitis
   Dermatitis
   Erythema nodosum
Focal Collections
   Popliteal (Baker's) cyst (intact, leaking, or ruptured)
   Hematoma
   Abscess
   Pelvic mass resulting in venous compression
Neurological
   Leg swelling due to lower extremity paralysis
   Nerve root irritation
   Reflex sympathetic dystrophy
Drug-induced
   Calcium channel blockers
   Corticosteroids
Lymphedema

DVT, deep vein thrombosis.

predictive model can significantly reduce the need for more costly diagnostic tests (42–45). Informal clinical assessment of pretest probability has recently been shown to be almost as useful as the application of a formal predictive model (46,47). However, caution must be used with all clinical predictive models for DVT, since there is substantial interobserver variability in the assignment of risk score (37,48,49). In centers that incorporate clinical probability into diagnostic protocols for DVT, efforts should be made to standardize this process through education, wall charts, preprinted assessment sheets, or computer-generated algorithms.

IV. Laboratory Tests in the Investigation of Suspected DVT

The role of D-dimer testing and the important precautions related to its use are discussed in detail in Chapter 8 (50–53). Among patients with suspected DVT, there is now considerable evidence that the combination of low clinical probability and a negative sensitive D-dimer result can end the investigation process without the need to perform any venous imaging (38,41–45,54–59). Furthermore, a negative D-dimer combined with a negative Doppler ultrasound examination may avoid the need for serial imaging (38,42,55–57,59–61). Some physicians are prepared to exclude VTE based on a negative sensitive D-dimer alone (42,62), whereas others caution against this (59). In either case, users of D-dimer must be aware that the predictive value of D-dimer is affected not only by the specific test used (63–66) and the patient population in which the test is applied (67) but also by the handling of the blood sample, by who performs the test (68), by the presence of cancer (69), the extent and age of the thrombus (70), and the use of anticoagulation (70). More data on the impact of D-dimer testing on usual practice in a broad spectrum of clinical settings are required to determine its effect on routine practice and cost effectiveness (71).

V. Older Imaging Tests for DVT

Fibrinogen leg scanning, impedance plethysmography, radionuclear thrombus scans, and contrast venography have largely or entirely been replaced by venous Doppler ultrasonography because of major limitations of each of the older tests (72).

A. Ascending Contrast Venography

Contrast venography has long been considered to be the "gold standard" diagnostic test for DVT (40,72–74). A technically complete, normal venogram excludes proximal and calf DVT (40), and an intraluminal filling defect seen on multiple views confirms this diagnosis. However, ascending contrast venography is now infrequently performed for a number of reasons, including the following: difficulty obtaining venous access on the patient's foot, pain associated with the procedure, contraindications and complications related to the use of intravenous contrast, the considerable technical skill (no longer widely available) required to perform high-quality venography, frequent nondiagnostic studies, considerable interobserver variability in its evaluation, high costs, and the widespread availability and acceptance of noninvasive imaging (75–79). Contrast venography is currently considered when noninvasive tests cannot be performed or are nondiagnostic, and it is still utilized as the primary efficacy outcome in some clinical trials (9,73).

B. Impedance Plethysmography

In the 1970s, there was interest in developing a noninvasive test that could reliably diagnose DVT. Impedance plethysmography (IPG) was shown to identify which symptomatic patients required anticoagulation (9,72,77,80–82). Although the accuracy of IPG was subsequently shown to be inferior to Doppler ultrasonography (9,83–86), the prospective outcome studies using serial IPG generally demonstrated the safety of withholding anticoagulant therapy if proximal DVT was ruled out (15,81,84). Because of limitations associated with this test, IPG has appropriately been replaced by venous Doppler ultrasound imaging (9,72,83,84,87,88).

VI. Venous Doppler Ultrasonography

Compression Doppler ultrasonography (DUS) has emerged as the diagnostic test of choice for patients with suspected DVT, since it is accurate for proximal DVT, noninvasive, widely available, relatively inexpensive, and repeatable (52,72,79,89). The procedure is generally performed quickly and is potentially portable. An additional advantage of DUS is the ability of this test to identify the alternate diagnosis in a proportion of patients who have acute DVT excluded (e.g., superficial venous thrombosis, popliteal cyst, muscle hematoma) (90).

Duplex scanning combines B-mode or two-dimensional ultrasound cross-sectional imaging of the veins with Doppler assessment of blood flow (79,91). The addition of color flow features facilitates the identification of vessels and determination of flow patterns (92). The most reliable DUS criterion for DVT is abnormal compressibility of a deep venous segment

(79,93,94). Veins containing thrombi do not collapse completely with gentle compression by the ultrasound probe. Other supplemental criteria include the absence of flow, increased intraluminal echogenicity, and venous distension. Using contrast venography as the reference standard, the sensitivity and specificity of DUS for proximal DVT both exceed 95% (84,89,93,95,96). There is controversy as to whether the study could be restricted to the common femoral and popliteal veins only (7,9,93,97) or whether the entire proximal deep venous system should be imaged (79,98,99). Noncompressibility restricted to the common femoral vein alone is associated with a high false-positive rate; primarily due to iliac vein compression by pelvic masses (100). We prefer to attempt to image the deep veins from the inferior vena cava down to the origin of the popliteal vein. For the deep veins of the calf, both the sensitivity and specificity of DUS are reduced (to 60–70% or less) (89,101).

Among patients with a negative DUS at presentation, repeating the study 5–7 days later will detect DVT in only 1–2% (16,89,102). For this reason, some physicians believe that repeat testing is not justified (103).

Diagnostic strategies based on the detection of proximal DVT by DUS and the withholding of anticoagulation in patients without evidence of proximal DVT have been shown to be safe (16,84,89,93,102,105,105). Calf DVT has less clinical importance than proximal DVT, and therefore most of the published studies of DUS have not attempted to assess patients for calf DVT (8,9,15,16,81,84,89,100,102). In a cohort study of 1290 patients with negative proximal DUS that remained negative 1 week later, the rate of proven VTE at 6 months was only 0.7%; strongly supporting the safety of this approach (102). Another prospective study randomized 985 consecutive out-patients with suspected DVT to an approach based on either serial DUS or IPG (84). The safety of both approaches was demonstrated with no fatal pulmonary emboli and with low rates of VTE over the subsequent 6 months (1.5 vs 2.6%, respectively).

Clinicians must also be aware of the limitations of Doppler ultrasonography, which include the following: DUS studies may be nondiagnostic because of poor patient cooperation, morbid obesity, marked edema or tenderness, venous anatomical variability or lower extremity injuries, casts or immobilization devices, false-positive and false-negative rates of approximately 5% for proximal DVT, the requirement for an experienced, highly skilled operator as well as expensive equipment, and reduced accuracy for calf DVT (100,106). DUS often does not directly visualize the iliac veins or the femoral vein as it passes through the adductor canal and nonoccluding thrombi may be missed in these and other locations. The accuracy of DUS for asymptomatic DVT in high-risk patients is also reduced (to about 60% for proximal DVT) (89,107,108).

VII.   Other Imaging Tests for DVT

A.   Computed Tomographic Venography

Contrast computed tomographic venography (CTV) can be utilized to investigate patients suspected of having DVT. Unsuspected DVT is sometimes detected on CT scans performed for other reasons, especially in patients with pelvic malignancy. Currently, CTV is used in patients who have an inadequate proximal DUS, as a means to investigate for iliac vein thrombosis, and as part of an algorithm for suspected pulmonary embolism (PE) along with CT pulmonary angiography (109–112). Indirect CTV, using the same bolus of intravenous contrast given for CT pulmonary angiography, may be used to image the deep veins from the iliac crest to the proximal calf 2–4 min after the intravenous injection for the pulmonary study (110,111,113,114). Some of the limitations of this technique, including flow artifacts, poor opacification of the deep veins, difficulties distinguishing acute from chronic DVT, and interobserver variability, may lead to misinterpretation of CTV (110,115). Although this modality is being used routinely in some centers, it has not yet been adequately evaluated and is associated with moderate additional radiation (115).

B.   Magnetic Resonance Venography

Magnetic resonance techniques are very promising in the investigation of patients with suspected DVT. Magnetic resonance venography (MRV) appears to be as accurate as contrast venography for the diagnosis of acute DVT (72,116–119) and may be more accurate than DUS, especially for pelvic and calf DVT (120,121). A central, low-signal filling defect surrounded by a hyperintense signal associated with the absence of flow is considered to be positive. One type of MRV, known as magnetic resonance direct thrombus imaging, can directly visualize a thrombus against a suppressed background and was recently shown to be accurate for symptomatic DVT (119). MRV involves no radiation and does not require the injection of contrast. Apart from the noninvasive nature of the study, other potential advantages of MRV include the ability to image pelvic veins, the capacity to confirm alternate diagnoses, and the potential to distinguish acute from chronic DVT (122,123). Furthermore, MRV may be used as a noninvasive adjunct to MR angiography of the pulmonary arteries in the investigation of suspected PE (124,125). MRV may have special roles in suspected DVT or PE in pregnancy, in situations where the limb is not accessible to other imaging (e.g., with long-leg casts), and in the investigation of possible recurrent thrombosis. However, a greater number of studies including a broad spectrum of patients and with larger samples are still required. Clinical management studies using MRV are also necessary. MRV requires prolonged patient cooperation, it remains very expensive, access to routine MRV is restricted in most centers, and experience in the interpretation of this test is limited.

VIII. Algorithms in the Investigation of Suspected DVT

Figures 1 and 2 outline two variations of diagnostic algorithms for the investigation of suspected DVT based primarily on DUS (42,59,72). If an initial proximal DUS is negative, repeating the study in 5–7 days will detect thrombi that have extended into the popliteal vein since the first test. If a repeat test is also negative, anticoagulants can be withheld and no further testing is required (16,102). The main problems with the serial DUS approach are the low rates of conversion (1–2%) from negative to positive on repeat testing (16,35,55,77,89,102) and the inconvenience and cost of multiple tests (77,103,126). A number of strategies have been proposed to improve the efficiency of a DUS-based approach. In some centers, including the deep calf veins in the DUS assessment (if the proximal veins have no

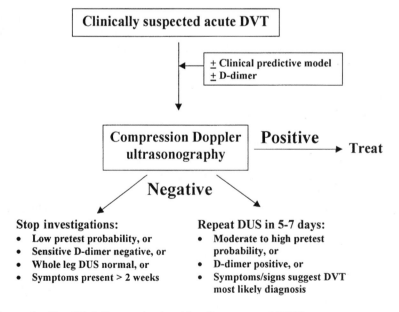

Figure 1 Simplified diagnostic algorithm for suspected DVT.

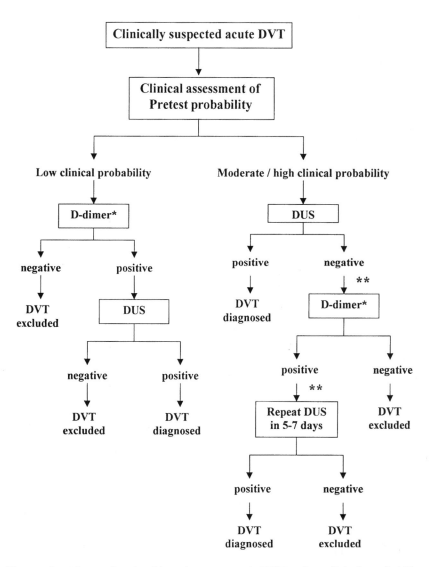

Figure 2 Diagnostic algorithm for suspected DVT using clinical probability assessment, D-dimer testing, and DUS. *, This applies to a sensitive D-dimer assay that has been well validated in the diagnosis of DVT. **, An alternative option would be to obtain a contrast venogram if clinical probability is high.

evidence of thrombus), is a strategy to avoid serial ultrasound testing. This is not desirable for several reasons: (1) the sensitivity of DUS for calf vein thrombosis is less than for proximal DVT and the false-positive rate is higher (89), (2) calf vein imaging is much more likely to be technically inadequate, (3) examining the deep calf veins substantially increases the time required to perform the study, and (4) if the study is felt to demonstrate calf DVT, this poses a clinical dilemma about the subsequent management; that is, to treat with anticoagulants or to obtain serial ultrasounds and only treat if there is progression of the calf thrombus into the popliteal vein (127).

Alternate strategies to reduce the need for serial DUS testing include determination of clinical probability and/or D-dimer levels (41,59). Studies have demonstrated that anticoagulation may be withheld from patients with a low clinical probability of DVT and negative D-dimer (41,42,45,56,128). Serial DUS imaging can also be avoided if the initial DUS is negative and there is either a low pretest probability (35,42,59) or a negative D-dimer result (38,42,55–57,59,61). These approaches are just as safe as and may be more cost effective than serial imaging (42,61).

If the DUS result is discordant with the clinical impression (DUS positive with a low pretest probability or DUS negative in a patient with a high clinical probability), further testing should be considered because of a substantial reduction in the predictive values in these settings (33,89). Among patients with higher prevalence of VTE, for example, those with cancer or others with a high clinical probability, the D-dimer has demonstrated sensitivities of only 80 and 65% and should either not be used or should be accompanied by at least a single DUS (69,129,130).

For hospitalized patients in whom DVT is suspected after regular hours, there is rarely a need to obtain a DUS urgently. Most of these patients can receive a single, therapeutic dose of subcutaneous low molecular weight heparin and the DUS obtained the following day. For outpatients with suspected DVT who present after regular hours, the DUS can also generally be delayed until the following day by administration of a therapeutic dose of low molecular weight heparin, discharging the patient home, and arranging for imaging the following day during regular working hours (129,131). In both groups, the only patients who require urgent diagnosis are those in whom the risk of bleeding is so high that even brief anticoagulation is considered to be unsafe.

IX. Calf DVT

As discussed earlier, there is strong evidence that a diagnostic approach to suspected DVT based on proving or excluding proximal DVT is safe and efficient (15,16,35,52,55,81,84,102). Therefore, the safety of not searching for symptomatic calf DVT has been established in a number of large studies in which impedance plethysmography or proximal venous Doppler ultrasonography was used to investigate patients with leg symptoms—among these patients, a proportion had calf DVT as the cause of their presentation (7,9). Furthermore, DUS is less accurate for calf DVT than for proximal DVT, because the calf veins are smaller, flow is slower, and there is a greater likelihood of anatomical variability. Whether or not it is beneficial to detect and then treat symptomatic calf DVT remains controversial (127,132–134). Calf DVT rarely results in clinically important PE (5,8,9,15,81,84,135). Only about 5–20% of calf DVT will extend proximally if untreated—this is most likely to occur in the first week or two after the initial presentation (7,8,10,84,136,137). This observation is the basis for repeating the DUS 5–7 days after an initial negative study in patients who present with suspected DVT. However, since the majority of those with possible DVT do not have this condition, only 1–2% of symptomatic patients will convert the DUS from negative to positive.

In the overwhelming majority of symptomatic patients, we restrict DUS imaging to the proximal veins for the following reasons: (1) DUS of the calf veins is less accurate than of the proximal veins and, therefore, imaging of the calf veins will result in false-positive results, (2) we are uncertain about whether or not calf DVT requires treatment, and (3) imaging the calf and proximal veins substantially prolongs the time required to perform the DUS reliably compared with imaging the proximal veins only. However, we generally do obtain DUS of the calf and proximal veins for patients in whom serial testing will be very difficult, for those with higher than usual risk of extension (e.g., patients who are immobile or have plaster casts), and for those with persistent calf symptoms on follow-up to help resolve this diagnostic dilemma.

X. Approach to Suspected Recurrent DVT

After an episode of DVT, chronic or recurrent leg swelling and/or discomfort are very common (14,138,139). Although such patients are at risk for recurrent DVT once anticoagulation has been discontinued, postthrombotic syndrome is at least as common as true recurrence (12,140,141). The diagnosis of recurrent DVT is more difficult than the initial presentation, because many patients have residual imaging abnormalities (142). Every effort should be made to avoid overcalling a diagnosis of recurrent DVT, since, in the majority of patients, this condition is not confirmed by objective testing and because this diagnosis usually results in anticoagulation for life. Predictors of recurrent thrombosis include location of the initial DVT (proximal > distal; iliofemoral > popliteal; an idiopathic event; the presence of thrombophilia or cancer; persistent thrombosis on repeat imaging; and positivity of plasma D-dimer at the end of the treatment phase (143–147). The primary predictor of postthrombotic syndrome is recurrent DVT in the same leg (12).

If patients with suspected recurrent DVT have a normal DUS, further management can proceed as outlined for the initial presentations above (148,149). If the DUS is normal over the proximal deep venous system, repeating the study in 5–7 days should be considered unless the D-dimer result is also negative. Similarly, if the DUS demonstrates a noncompressible deep venous segment that was previously normal, a diagnosis of recurrence can be made (150,151). However, in a high proportion of patients, the DUS will be abnormal, and it is often difficult to ascertain whether this represents new disease or residual thrombosis from the original episode. In this case, contrast venography may be useful—if the venogram demonstrates an intraluminal filling defect or extension of thrombosis compared with previous imaging, a diagnosis of recurrence can be made (142,152). A negative D-dimer may also help resolve the uncertainty of possible recurrent DVT, although more data are required before this can be advocated as a routine strategy in suspected recurrence when there is residual disease (153). Finally, demonstration of an increase in the diameter of the common femoral or popliteal vein compared with a previous measurement also corresponds to venographic confirmation of recurrence (151). Conversely, it appears to be safe to withhold anticoagulation from patients with improved or stable venous diameters if there is no other evidence of recurrence (148). Again, further evidence of the safety of this approach is necessary.

It has been shown that 1 year after an acute proximal DVT, the Doppler ultrasound is still abnormal in 30–50% of patients (150,151,154, 155). The ultrasound appearance of thrombi of different ages changes over time (79). Older thrombi are more echogenic ("hyperechoic") than more recent thrombi, the vein diameter decreases with time, and collateral veins are often present (139,154,156). However, the role of the ultrasound appearance of thrombi in the investigation of suspected recurrent DVT has not been subjected to prospective trials. Patients who are still receiving oral anticoagulants and the international normalized ratio (INR) is in the therapeutic range have a very low risk of recurrent DVT—in this circumstance, we will often not do further testing (unless there is underlying malignancy) (157–159).

Magnetic resonance imaging may have a future role in the evaluation of suspected recurrent DVT, since the signal characteristics of thrombi change with time (118).

XI. Conclusions

Deep vein thrombosis is an important diagnosis to consider in patients with leg symptoms. At the same time, the majority of patients with suspected DVT do not have this diagnosis confirmed using objective testing. Consideration of risk factors for thrombosis is a key initial step followed, in the majority of patients, by Doppler ultrasonography. Strategies based on the detection or exclusion of proximal DVT have repeatedly been shown to be safe. A positive DUS in patients with a first episode of suspected DVT is usually sufficient evidence to commence anticoagulant therapy unless the clinical features make DVT unlikely. The formal assessment of clinical probability and D-dimer testing, if used properly, enhance the efficiency of diagnostic algorithms for suspected DVT. A low clinical probability combined with a negative sensitive D-dimer or a negative proximal DUS essentially excludes the diagnosis of DVT. Patients with moderate or high clinical suspicion of DVT should have DUS testing and, if the initial test is negative, a repeat study should be obtained 5–7 days later (unless a sensitive D-dimer result is also negative).

References

1. Anderson FA, Wheeler HB, Goldberg RJ, Hosmer DW, Patwardhan NA, Jovanovic B, Forcier A, Dalen JE. A population-based perspective of the hospital incidence and case-fatality rates of deep vein thrombosis and pulmonary embolism: The Worchester DVT Study. Arch Intern Med 1991; 151:933–938.
2. Hansson P-O, Welin L, Tibblin G, Eriksson H. Deep vein thrombosis and pulmonary embolism in the general population: 'the study of men born in 1913.' Arch Intern Med 1997; 157:1665–1670.
3. Silverstein MD, Heit JA, Mohr DN, Petterson TM, O'Fallon WM, Melton LJ. Trends in the incidence of deep vein thrombosis and pulmonary embolism: a 25-year population-based study. Arch Intern Med 1998; 158:585–593.
4. Heit JA. Venous thromboembolism epidemiology: implications for prevention and management. Semin Thromb Hemost 2002; 28(Suppl 2):3–13.
5. Kakkar VV, Howe CT, Flanc C, Clarke MB. Natural history of postoperative deep-vein thrombosis. Lancet 1969; 2:230–233.
6. Nicolaides AN, Kakkar VV, Fields ES, Renney JT. The origin of deep vein thrombosis: a venographic study. Br J Radiol 1971; 44:653–663.
7. Cogo A, Lensing AWA, Prandoni P, Hirsh J. Distribution of thrombosis in patients with symptomatic deep vein thrombosis. Implications for simplifying the diagnostic process with compression ultrasound. Arch Intern Med 1993; 153:2777–2780.

8. Moser KM, LeMoine JR. Is embolic risk conditioned by location of deep venous thrombosis? Ann Intern Med 1981; 94:439–444.

9. Kearon C, Julian JA, Newman TE, Ginsberg JS, for the McMaster Diagnostic Imaging Practice Guidelines Initiative. Noninvasive diagnosis of deep venous thrombosis. Ann Intern Med 1998; 128:663–677.

10. Huisman MV, Buller HR, ten Cate JW, van Royen EA, Vreeken J, Kersten M-J, Bakx R. Unexpected high prevalence of silent pulmonary embolism in patients with deep venous thrombosis. Chest 1989; 95:498–502.

11. Lagerstedt CI, Olsson C-G, Fagher BO, Oqvist BW, Albrechtsson U. Need for long-term anticoagulant treatment in symptomatic calf-vein thrombosis. Lancet 1985; 2:515–518.

12. Prandoni P, Lensing AWA, Cogo A, Cuppini S, Villalta S, Carta M, Cattelan AM, Polistena P, Bernardi E, Prins MH. The long-term clinical course of acute deep venous thrombosis. Ann Intern Med 1996; 125:1–7.

13. Brandjes DPM, Buller HR, Heijboer H, Huisman MV, de Rijk M, Jagt H, ten Cate J.W. Randomised trial of effect of compression stockings in patients with symptomatic proximal-vein thrombosis. Lancet 1997; 349:759–762.

14. Mohr DN, Silverstein MD, Heit JA, Petterson TM, O'Fallon WM, Melton LJ. The venous stasis syndrome after deep venous thromboembolism or pulmonary embolism: a population-based study. Mayo Clin Proc 2000; 75:1249–1256.

15. Huisman MV, Buller HR, ten Cate JW, Vreeken J. Serial impedance plethysmography for suspected deep venous thrombosis in outpatients: the Amsterdam General Practitioner Study. N Engl J Med 1986; 314:823–828.

16. Birdwell BG, Raskob GE, Whitsett TL, Durica SS, Comp PC, George JN, Tytle TL, McKee PA. The clinical validity of normal compression ultrasonography in outpatients suspected of having deep venous thrombosis. Ann Intern Med 1998; 128:1–7.

17. Cogo A, Bernardi E, Prandoni P, Girolami B, Noventa F, Simioni P, Girolami A. Acquired risk factors for deep-vein thrombosis in symptomatic outpatients. Arch Intern Med 1994; 151:164–168.

18. Rosendaal FR. Risk factors for venous thrombotic disease. Thromb Haemost 1999; 82:610–619.

19. Selby R, Geerts WH. Venous thromboembolism: risk factors and prophylaxis. Semin Respir Crit Care Med 2000; 21:493–501.

20. Heit JA, O'Fallon M, Petterson TM, Lohse CM, Silverstein MD, Mohr DN, Melton LJ. Relative impact of risk factors for deep vein thrombosis and pulmonary embolism, A population-based study. Arch Intern Med 2001; 162:1245–1248.

21. Kearon C. Epidemiology of venous thromboembolism. Semin Vasc Med 2001; 1:7–25.

22. Martinelli I. Risk factors in venous thromboembolism. Thromb Haemost 2001; 86:395–403.

23. Levitan N, Dowlati A, Remick SC, Tahsildar HI, Sivinski LD, Beyth R, Rimm AA. Rates of initial and recurrent thromboembolic disease among

patients with malignancy versus those without malignancy: risk analysis among Medicare claims data. Medicine 1999; 78:285–291.

24. Arkel YS. Thrombosis and cancer. Semin Oncol 2000; 27:362–374.

25. Lee AYY, Levin MN. Cancer and Thrombosis. Current Concepts in Patient Care. Wilton, CT: Chase Medical Communications, 2002:1–14.

26. Thodiyil PA, Kakkar AK. Variation in relative risk of venous thromboembolism in different cancers. Thromb Haemost 2002; 87:1076–1977.

27. Bertina RM. Molecular risk factors for thrombosis. Thromb Haemost 1999; 82:601–609.

28. Federman DG, Kirsner RS. An update on hypercoagulable disorders. Arch Intern Med 2001; 161:1051–1056.

29. Seligsohn U, Lubetsky A. Genetic predisposition to venous thrombosis. N Engl J Med 2001; 344:1222–1231.

30. Thomas RH. Hypercoagulability syndromes. Arch Intern Med 2001; 161:2433–2439.

31. Rosendaal FR. Venous thrombosis: a multicausal disease. Lancet 1999; 353:1167–1173.

32. Hirsh J, Hull RD, Raskob GE. Clinical features and diagnosis of venous thrombosis. J Am Coll Cardiol 1986; 8:114B–127B.

33. Wells PS, Hirsh J, Anderson DR, Lensing AWA, Foster G, Kearon C, Weitz J, D'Ovidio R, Cogo A, Prandoni P, Girolami A, Ginsberg JS. Accuracy of clinical assessment of deep-vein thrombosis. Lancet 1995; 345:1326–1330 [Erratum, Lancet 1995;346:516].

34. Kahn SR, Joseph L, Abenhaim L, Leclerc JR. Clinical prediction of deep vein thrombosis in patients with leg symptoms. Thromb Haemost 1999; 81:353–357.

35. Wells PS, Anderson DR, Bormanis J, Guy F, Mitchell M, Gray L, Clement C, Robinson KS, Lewandowski B. Value of assessment of pretest probability of deep-vein thrombosis in clinical management. Lancet 1997; 350:1795–1798.

36. Anand SS, Wells PS, Hunt D, Brill-Edwards P, Cook D, Ginsberg JS. Does this patient have deep vein thrombosis? JAMA 1998; 279:1094–1099.

37. Wells PS, Hirsh J, Anderson DR, Lensing AWA, Foster G, Kearon C, Weitz J, D'Ovidio R, Cogo A, Prandoni P, Girolami A, Ginsberg JS. A simple clinical model for the diagnosis of deep-vein thrombosis combined with impedance plethysmography: potential for an improvement in the diagnostic process. J Intern Med 1998; 243:15–23.

38. Wells PS, Anderson DR, Bormanis J, Guy F, Mitchell M, Gray L, Clement C, Robinson KS, Lewandowski B. Application of a diagnostic clinical model for the management of hospitalized patients with suspected deep-vein thrombosis. Thromb Haemost 1999; 81:493–497.

39. Wells PS, Rodger M, Forgie M, Anderson D, Kovacs M, Florack P, Waddell P, Kearon C, Dreyer J, Dubey N. A randomised trial in patients with suspected DVT comparing a D-dimer/clinical probability strategy to clinical probability, prior to ultrasound imaging. D-dimer safely reduces the need for diagnostic imaging (abst). Thromb Haemost 2001; (Suppl):OC41.

40. Hull RD, Hirsh J, Sackett DL, Taylor DW, Carter C, Turpie AGG, Powers P, Gent M. Clinical validity of a negative venogram in patients with clinically suspected venous thrombosis. Circulation 1981; 64:622–625.

41. Anderson DR, Wells PS, Kovacs MJ, Kearon C, Dreyer J, Forgie MA. A randomized trial in patients with suspected deep vein thrombosis comparing a D-dimer/clinical probability strategy to clinical probability, prior to ultrasound imaging. D-dimer safely reduces the need for diagnostic testing (abst). Blood 2001; 98:447.

42. Perrier A, Bounameaux H. Cost-effective diagnosis of deep vein thrombosis and pulmonary embolism. Thromb Haemost 2001; 86:475–487.

43. Tick LW, van Voorthuizen T, Hovens MMC, Leeuwenburgh I, Lobatto S, Stijnen PJ, van der Heul C, Huisman PM, Kramer MHH, Huisman MV. Effective and safe practical diagnosis of deep vein thrombosis in 811 patients referred to non-academic teaching hospitals; the PRADIA Study (abst). Thromb Haemost 2001; 38(Suppl).

44. Janes S, Ashford N. Use of a simplified clinical scoring system and D-dimer testing can reduce the requirement for radiology in the exclusion of deep vein thrombosis by over 20%. Br J Haematol 2001; 112:1079–1082.

45. Kearon C, Ginsberg JS, Douketis J, Crowther M, Brill-Edwards P, Weitz JI, Hirsh J. Management of suspected deep venous thrombosis in outpatients by using clinical assessment and D-dimer testing. Ann Intern Med 2001; 135:108–111.

46. Miron M-J, Perrier A, Bounameaux H. Clinical assessment of suspected deep vein thrombosis: comparison between a score and empirical assessment. J Intern Med 2000; 247:249–254.

47. Cornuz J, Ghali WA, Hayoz D, Stoianov R, Depairon M, Yersin B. Clinical prediction of deep venous thrombosis using two risk assessment methods in combination with rapid quantitative D-dimer testing. Am J Med 2002; 112:198–203.

48. Bigaroni A, Perrier A, Bounameaux H. Is clinical probability assessment of deep vein thrombosis by a score really standardized? [letter]. Thromb Haemost 2000; 83:788–789 [Erratum 2000;84:576].

49. Sanson B-J, Lijmer JG, MacGillavry MR, Turkstra F, Prins MH, Buller HR, on behalf of the ANTELOPE-Study Group. Comparison of a clinical probability estimate and two clinical models in patients with suspected pulmonary embolism. Thromb Haemost 2000; 83:199–203.

50. Bounameaux H, de Moerloose P, Perrier A, Reber G. Plasma measurement of D-dimer as diagnostic aid in suspected venous thromboembolism: an overview. Thromb Haemost 1994; 71:1–6.

51. Becker DM, Philbrick JT, Bachhuber TL, Humphries JE. D-dimer testing and acute venous thromboembolism. A shortcut to accurate diagnosis? Arch Intern Med 1996; 156:939–946.

52. Perrier A, Desmarais S, Miron M-J, de Moerloose P, Lepage R, Slosman D, Didier D, Unger P-F, Patenaude J-V, Bounameaux H. Non-invasive diagnosis of venous thromboembolism in outpatients. Lancet 1999; 353:190–195.

53. Kelly J, Rudd A, Lewis RR, Hunt BJ. Plasma D-dimers in the diagnosis of venous thromboembolism. Arch Intern Med 2002; 162:747–756.

54. Ginsberg JS, Kearon C, Douketis J, Turpie AGG, Brill-Edwards P, Stevens P, Panju A, Patel A, Crowther M, Andrew M, Massicotte MP, Hirsh J, Weitz JI. The use of D-dimer testing and impedance plethysmographic examination in patients with clinical indications of deep vein thrombosis. Arch Intern Med 1997; 157:1077–1081.

55. Bernardi E, Prandoni P, Lensing AWA, Agnelli G, Guazzaloca G, Scanna-pieco G, Piovella F, Verlato F, Tomasi C, Moia M, Scarano L, Girolami A. D-dimer testing as an adjunct to ultrasonography in patients with clini-cally suspected deep vein thrombosis: prospective cohort study. BMJ 1998; 317:1037–1040.

56. Aschwanden M, Labs K-H, Jeanneret C, Gehrig A, Jaeger KA. The value of rapid D-dimer testing combined with structural clinical evaluation for the diagnosis of deep vein thrombosis. J Vasc Surg 1999; 30:929–935.

57. Lennox AF, Delis KT, Serunkuma S, Zarka ZA, Daskalopoulou SE, Nicolaides AN. Combination of a clinical risk assessment score and rapid whole-blood D-dimer testing in the diagnosis of deep vein thrombosis in symptomatic patients. J Vasc Surg 1999; 30:794–804.

58. Kraaijenhagen RA, Piovella F, Bernardi E, Veralto F, Beckers EAM, Koopman MMW, Barone M, Camporese G, van Loon BJP, Prins MH, Prandoni P, Buller HR. The optimal diagnostic management strategy in patients with suspected deep vein thrombosis (abst). Thromb Haemost 2002; abstract OC40.

59. Kraaijenhagen RA, Piovella F, Bernardi E, Verlato F, Beckers EAM, Koopman MMW, Barone M, Camporese G, van Loon BJP, Prins MH, Prandoni P, Buller HR. Simplification of the diagnostic management of suspected deep vein thrombosis. Arch Intern Med 2002; 162:907–911.

60. Heijboer H, Ginsberg JS, Buller HR, Lensing AWA, Colly LP, ten Cate JW. The use of the D-dimer test in combination with non-invasive testing versus serial non-invasive testing alone for the diagnosis of deep-vein thrombosis. Thromb Haemost 1992; 67:510–513.

61. Perone N, Bounaneaux H, Perrier A. Comparison of four strategies for diagnosing deep vein thrombosis: a cost-effectiveness analysis. Am J Med 2001; 110:33–40.

62. Bates SM, Grand'maison A, Johnston M, Naguit I, Kovacs MJ, Ginsberg JS. A latex D-dimer reliably excludes venous thromboembolism. Arch Intern Med 2001; 161:447–453.

63. Freyburger G, Trillaud H, Labrouche S, Gauthier P, Javorschi S, Bernard P, Grenier N. D-dimer strategy in thrombosis exclusion. A gold standard study in 100 patients suspected of deep venous thrombosis or pulmonary embolism: 8 DD methods compared. Thromb Haemost 1998; 79:32–37.

64. van der Graaf F, van den Borne H, van der Kolk M, de Wild PJ, Janssen GWT, van Uum SHM. Exclusion of deep venous thrombosis with D-dimer testing. Comparison of 13 D-dimer methods in 99 outpatients suspected of

deep venous thrombosis using venography as reference standard. Thromb Haemost 2000; 83:191–198.

65. Dempfle C-E, Zips S, Ergul H, Heene DL, and the FACT study group. The fibrin assay comparison test (FACT). Evaluation of 23 quantitative D-dimer assays as basis for the development of D-dimer calibrators. Thromb Haemost 2001; 85:671–678.

66. Harper P, Marson M, Grimmer A, Monahan K, Humm G, Baker B. The rapid whole blood agglutination d-dimer assay has poor sensitivity for use as an exclusion test in suspected deep vein thrombosis. NZ Med J 2001; 114:61–64.

67. Righini M, Goehring C, Bounameaux H, Perrier A. Effects of age on the performance of common diagnostic tests for pulmonary embolism. Am J Med 2000; 109:357–361.

68. Chunilal SD, Brill-Edwards PA, Stevens PB, Joval JP, McGinnis JA, Rupwate M, Ginsberg JS. The sensitivity and specificity of a red blood cell agglutination D-dimer assay for venous thromboembolism when performed on venous blood. Arch Intern Med 2002; 162:217–220.

69. Lee AYY, Julian JA, Levine MN, Weitz JI, Kearon C, Wells PS, Ginsberg JS. Clinical utility of a rapid whole-blood D-dimer assay in patients with cancer who present with suspected acute deep venous thrombosis. Ann Intern Med 1999; 131:417–423.

70. Siragusa S, Terulla V, Pirrelli S, Porta C, Falaschi F, Anastasio R, Guarone R, Scarabelli M, Odero A, Bressan MA. A rapid D dimer assay in patients presenting at an emergency room with suspected acute venous thrombosis: accuracy and relation to clinical variables. Haematologica 2001; 86:856–861.

71. Goldstein NM, Kollef MH, Ward S, Gage BF. The impact of the introduction of a rapid D-dimer assay on the diagnostic evaluation of suspected pulmonary embolism. Arch Intern Med 2001; 161:567–571.

72. Tapson VF, Carroll BA, Davidson BL, Elliott CG, Fedullo PF, Hales CA, Hull RD, Hyers TM, Leeper KV, Morris TA, Moser KM, Raskob GE, Shure D, Sostman HD, Thompson BT. The diagnostic approach to acute venous thromboembolism. Clinical Practice Guideline. Am J Respir Crit Care Med 1999; 160:1043–1066.

73. de Valois JC, van Schalk CC, Verzijlbergen F, van Ramshorst B, Eikelboom BC, Meuwissen OJA. Contrast venography: from gold standard to "golden backup" in clinically suspected deep vein thrombosis. Eur J Radiol 1990; 11:131–137.

74. Lensing AWA, Buller HR, Prandoni P, Batchelor D, Molenaar AHM, Cogo A, Vigo M, Huisman PM, ten Cate JW. Contrast venography, the gold standard for the diagnosis of deep-vein thrombosis: improvement in observer agreement. Thromb Haemost 1992; 67:8–12.

75. Redman HC. Deep venous thrombosis: is contrast venography still the diagnostic "gold standard"? Radiology 1988; 168:277–278.

76. Bounameaux H, Prins M, Schmitt HE, Schneider PA. Venography of the lower limbs: pitfalls of the diagnostic standard. Invest Radiol 1992; 27:1009–1011.

77. Heijboer H, Cogo A, Buller HR, Prandoni P, ten Cate JW. Detection of deep vein thrombosis with impedance plethysmography and real-time compression ultrasonography in hospitalized patients. Arch Intern Med 1992; 152:1901–1903.

78. Couson F, Bounameaux C, Didier D, Geiser D, Meyerovitz MF, Schmitt H-E, Schneider P-A, Bounameaux H. Influence of variability of interpretation of contrast venography for screening of postoperative deep venous thrombosis on the results of a thromboprophylactic study. Thromb Haemost 1993; 70:573–575.

79. Fraser JD, Anderson DR. Deep venous thrombosis: recent advances and optimal investigation with US. Radiology 1999; 211:9–24.

80. Hull R, van Aken WG, Hirsh J, Gallus AS, Hoicka G, Turpie AGG, Walker I, Gent M. Impedance plethysmography using the occlusive cuff technique in the diagnosis of venous thrombosis. Circulation 1976; 53:696–700.

81. Hull RD, Hirsh J, Carter CJ, Jay RM, Ockelford PA, Buller HR, Turpie AG, Powers P, Kinch D, Dodd PE, Gill GJ, Leclerc JR, Gent M. Diagnostic efficacy of impedance plethysmography for clinically suspected deep-vein thrombosis: a randomized trial. Ann Intern Med 1985; 102:21–28.

82. Prandoni P, Vigo M, Huisman MV, Jonker J, Buller HR, ten Cate JW. Computerized impedance plethysmography, a new plethysmographic method to detect deep vein thrombosis (abst). Thromb Haemost 1987; 58(Suppl):24.

83. Anderson DR, Lensing AWA, Wells PS, Levine MN, Weitz JI, Hirsh J. Limitations of impedance plethysmography in the diagnosis of clinically suspected deep-vein thrombosis. Ann Intern Med 1993; 118:25–30.

84. Heijboer H, Buller HR, Lensing AWA, Turpie AGG, Colly LP, ten Cate JW. A comparison of real-time compression ultrasonography with impedance plethysmography for the diagnosis of deep-vein thrombosis in symptomatic outpatients. N Engl J Med 1993; 329:1365–1369.

85. Ginsberg JS, Wells PS, Hirsh J, Panju AA, Patel MA, Malone DE, McGinnis J, Stevens P, Brill-Edwards P. Reevaluation of the sensitivity of impedance plethysmography for the detection of proximal deep vein thrombosis. Arch Intern Med 1994; 154:1930–1933.

86. Wells PS, Hirsh J, Anderson DR, Lensing AWA, Foster G, Kearon C, Weitz J, Cogo A, Prandoni P, Minuk T, Thomson G, Benedetti L, Girolami A. Comparison of the accuracy of impedance plethysmography and compression ultrasonography in outpatients with clinically suspected deep vein thrombosis. A two centre paired-design prospective trial. Thromb Haemost 1995; 74:1423–1427.

87. Prandoni P, Lensing AWA, Buller HR, Carta M, Vigo M, Cogo A, Cuppini S, ten Cate JW. Failure of computerized impedance plethysmography in the diagnostic management of patients with clinically-suspected deep-vein thrombosis. Thromb Haemost 1991; 65:233–236.

88. Kahn SR, Joseph L, Grover SA, Leclerc JR. A randomized management study of impedance plethysmography vs. contrast venography in patients with

a first episode of clinically suspected deep vein thrombosis. Thromb Res 2001; 102:15–24.

89. Kearon C, Ginsberg JS, Hirsh J. The role of venous ultrasonography in the diagnosis of suspected deep venous thrombosis and pulmonary embolism. Ann Intern Med 1998; 129:1044–1049.

90. Borgstede JP, Clagett GE. Types, frequency, and significance of alternative diagnoses found during duplex Doppler venous examinations of the lower extremities of the lower extremities. J Ultrasound Med 1992; 11:85–89.

91. Vogel P, Laing FC, Jeffrey RB, Wing VW. Deep venous thrombosis of the lower extremity: US evaluation. Radiology 1987; 163:747–751.

92. Lewis BD, James EM, Welch TJ, Joyce JW, Hallett JW, Weaver AL. Diagnosis of acute deep venous thrombosis of the lower extremities: prospective evaluation of color Doppler flow imaging versus venography. Radiology 1994; 192:651–655.

93. Lensing AWA, Prandoni P, Brandjes D, Huisman PM, Vigo M, Tomasella G, Krekt J, ten Cate JW, Huisman MV, Buller HR. Detection of deep-vein thrombosis by real-time B-mode ultrasonography. N Engl J Med 1989; 320:342–345.

94. Cronan JJ. Venous thromboembolic disease: the role of US. Radiology 1993; 186:619–630.

95. Monreal M, Montserrat E, Salvador R, Bechini J, Donoso L, MaCallejas J, Foz M. Real-time ultrasound for diagnosis of symptomatic venous thrombosis and for screening of patients at risk: correlation with ascending conventional venography. Angiology 1989; 40:527–533.

96. Mattos MA, Londrey GL, Leutz DW, Hodgson KJ, Ramsey DE, Barkmeier LD, Stauffer ES, Spadone DP, Sumner DS. Color-flow duplex scanning for the surveillance and diagnosis of acute deep venous thrombosis. J Vasc Surg 1992; 15:366–376.

97. Pezzullo JA, Perkins AB, Cronan JJ. Symptomatic deep vein thrombosis: diagnosis with limited compression US. Radiology 1996; 198:67–70.

98. Frederick MG, Hertzberg BS, Kliewer MA, Paulson EK, Bowie JD, Lalouche KJ, DeLong DM, Carroll BA. Can the US examination for lower extremity deep venous thrombosis be abbreviated? A prospective study of 755 examinations. Radiology 1996; 199:45–47.

99. Maki DD, Kumar N, Nguyen B, Langer JE, Miller WT, Gefter WB. Distribution of thrombi in acute lower extremity deep venous thrombosis: implications for sonography and CT and MR venography. AJR 2000; 175:1299–1301.

100. Birdwell BG, Raskob GE, Whitsett TL, Durica SS, Comp PC, George JN, Tytle TL, Owen WL, McKee PA. Predictive value of compression ultra-sonography for deep vein thrombosis in symptomatic outpatients: clinical implications of the site of vein noncompressibility. Arch Intern Med 2000; 160:309–313.

101. Eskandari MK, Sugimoto H, Richardson T, Webster MW, Makaroun MS. Is color flow duplex a good diagnostic test for detection of isolated calf vein thrombosis in high risk patients? Angiology 2000; 51:705–710.

102. Cogo A, Lensing AWA, Koopman MMW, Piovella F, Siragusa S, Wells PS, Villalta S, Buller HR, Turpie AGG, Prandoni P. Compression ultrasonography for diagnostic management of patients with clinically suspected deep vein thrombosis: prospective cohort study. BMJ 1998; 316:17–20.

103. Bounameaux H, Perrier A. Compression ultrasonography for diagnosing deep vein thrombosis. Repeat testing is unjustified. BMJ 1998; 316:1534–1535.

104. O'Leary DH, Kane RA, Chase BM. A prospective study of the efficacy of B-scan sonography in the detection of deep venous thrombosis in the lower extremities. J Clin Ultrasound 1988; 16:1–8.

105. Vaccaro JP, Cronan JJ, Dorfman GS. Outcome analysis of patients with normal compression US examinations. Radiology 1990; 175:645–649.

106. Zwiebel WJ. Sources of error in duplex venography and an algorithmic approach to the diagnosis of deep venous thrombosis. Semin Ultrasound CT MR 1988; 9:286–294.

107. Wells PS, Lensing AWA, Davidson BL, Prins MH, Hirsh J. Accuracy of ultrasound for the diagnosis of deep venous thrombosis in asymptomatic patients after orthopedic surgery: a meta-analysis. Ann Intern Med 1995; 122:47–53.

108. Lensing AWA, Doris CI, McGrath FP, Cogo A, Sabine MJ, Ginsberg J, Prandoni P, Turpie AGG, Hirsh J. A comparison of compression ultrasound with color Doppler ultrasound for the diagnosis of symptomless postoperative deep vein thrombosis. Arch Intern Med 1997; 157:765–768.

109. Duwe KM, Shiau M, Budorick NE, Austin JHM, Berkmen YM. Evaluation of the lower extremity veins in patients with suspected pulmonary embolism: A retrospective comparison of helical CT venography and sonography. Am J Roentgenol 2000; 175:1525–1531.

110. Garg K, Kemp JL, Wojcik D, Hoehn S, Johnston RJ, Macey LC, Baron AE. Thromboembolic disease: comparison of combined CT pulmonary angiography and venography with bilateral leg sonography in 70 patients. Am J Roentgenol 2000; 175:997–1001.

111. Loud PA, Katz DS, Klippenstein DL, Shah RD, Grossman ZD. Combined CT venography and pulmonary angiography in suspected thromboembolic disease: Diagnostic accuracy for deep venous evaluation. Am J Roentgenol 2000; 174:61–65.

112. Yankelevitz DF, Gamsu G, Shah A, Rademaker J, Shaham D, Buckshee M, Cham MD, Henschke CI. Optimization of combined CT pulmonary angiography with lower extremity CT venography. Am J Roentgenol 2000; 174:67–69.

113. Cham MD, Yankelevitz DF, Shaham D, Shah AA, Sherman L, Lewis A, Rademaker J, Pearson G, Choi J, Wolff W, Prabhu PM, Galanski M, Clark RA, Sostman HD, Henschke CI. Deep venous thrombosis: detection by using indirect CT venography. Radiology 2000; 216:744–751.

114. Coche EE, Hamoir XL, Hammer FD, Hainaut P, Goffette PP. Using dual-detector helical CT angiography to detect deep venous thrombosis in patients with suspicion of pulmonary embolism: diagnostic value and additional findings. Am J Roentgenol 2001; 176:1035–1039.

115. Garg K, Mao J. Deep venous thrombosis: spectrum of findings and pitfalls in interpretation on CT venography. Am J Roentgenol 2001; 177:319–323.

116. Evans AJ, Sostman HD, Knelson MH, Spritzer CE, Newman GE, Paine SS, Beam CA. Detection of deep venous thrombosis: prospective comparison of MR imaging with contrast venography. Am J Roentgenol 1993; 161:131–139.

117. Carpenter JP, Holland GA, Baum RA, Owen RS, Carpenter JT, Cope C. Magnetic resonance venography for the detection of deep venous thrombosis: Comparison with contrast venography and duplex Doppler ultrasonography. J Vasc Surg 1993; 18:734–741.

118. Moody AR, Pollock JG, O'Connor AR, Bagnall M. Lower-limb deep venous thrombosis: direct MR imaging of the thrombus. Radiology 1998; 209:349–355.

119. Fraser DGW, Moody AR, Morgan PS, Martel AL, Davidson I. Diagnosis of lower-limb deep venous thrombosis: a prospective blinded study of magnetic resonance direct thrombus imaging. Ann Intern Med 2002; 136:89–98.

120. Evans AJ, Sostman HD, Witty LA, Paulson EK, Spritzer CE, Hertzberg BS, Carroll BA, Tapson VF, Saltzman HA, Delong DM. Detection of deep venous thrombosis: prospective comparison of MR imaging and sonography. J Magn Reson Imaging 1996; 6:44–51.

121. Laissy J-P, Cinqualbre A, Loshkajian A, Henry-Feugeas M-C, Crestani B, Riquelme C, Schouman-Claeys E. Assessment of deep venous thrombosis in the lower limbs and pelvis: MR venography versus duplex Doppler sonography. Am J Roentgenol 1996; 167:971–975.

122. Erdman WA, Jayson HT, Redman HC, Miller GL, Parkey RW, Peshock RW. Deep venous thrombosis of extremities: role of MR imaging in the diagnosis. Radiology 1990; 174:425–431.

123. Spritzer CE, Norconk JJ, Sostman HD, Coleman RE. Detection of deep venous thrombosis by magnetic resonance imaging. Chest 1993; 104:54–60.

124. Meaney JFM, Weg JG, Chenevert TL, Stafford-Johnson D, Hamilton BH, Prince MR. Diagnosis of pulmonary embolism with magnetic resonance angiography. N Engl J Med 1997; 336:1422–1427.

125. Stern J-B, Abehsera M, Grenet D, Friard S, Couderc L-J, Scherrer A, Stern M. Detection of pelvic vein thrombosis by magnetic resonance angiography in patients with acute pulmonary embolism and normal lower limb compression ultrasonography. Chest 2002; 122:115–121.

126. Hillner BE, Philbrick JT, Becker DM. Optimal management of suspected lower-extremity deep vein thrombosis: an evaluation with cost assessment of 24 management strategies. Arch Intern Med 1992; 152:165–175.

127. Lohr JM, Kerr TM, Lutter KS, Cranley RD, Spirtoff K, Cranley JJ. Lower extremity calf thrombosis: to treat or not to treat? J Vasc Surg 1991; 14:618–623.

128. Wells PS, Anderson DR, Bormanis J, Guy F, Mitchell M, Lewandowski B. SimpliRED D-dimer can reduce the diagnostic tests in suspected deep vein thrombosis. Lancet 1998; 351:1405–1406.

129. Anderson DR, Wells PS, Stiell I, MacLeod B, Simms M, Gray L, Robinson KS, Bormanis J, Mitchell M, Lewandowski B, Flowerdew G. Management of patients with suspected deep vein thrombosis in the emergency department: combining use of a clinical diagnosis model with D-dimer testing. J Emerg Med 2000; 19:225–230.

130. Farrell S, Hayes T, Shaw M. A negative SimpliRED D-dimer assay result does not exclude the diagnosis of deep vein thrombosis or pulmonary embolism in emergency department patients. Ann Emerg Med 2000; 35:121–125.

131. Anderson DR, Wells PS, Stiell I, MacLeod B, Simms M, Gray L, Robinson KS, Bormanis J, Mitchell M, Lewandowski B, Flowerdew G. Thrombosis in the emergency department: use of a clinical diagnosis model to safely avoid the need for urgent radiological investigation. Arch Intern Med 1999; 159:477–482.

132. Philbrick JT, Becker DM. Calf deep venous thrombosis. A wolf in sheep's clothing? Arch Intern Med 1988; 148:2131–2138.

133. Lohr JM, James KV, Deshmukh RM, Hasselfeld KA. Calf vein thrombi are not a benign finding. Am J Surg 1995; 170:86–90.

134. Hirko MK, Kasirajan K, Turner JJ, Rubin JR. Propagation of tibial vein thrombus in patients systematically anticoagulated or receiving antiplatelet therapy. Vasc Surg 1999; 33:251–256.

135. Gottlieb RH, Widjaja J, Mehra S, Robinette WB. Clinically important pulmonary emboli: Does calf vein US alter outcomes? Radiology 1999; 211:25–29.

136. Meissner MH, Caps MT, Bergelin RO, Manzo RA, Strandness DE. Early outcome after isolated calf vein thrombosis. J Vasc Surg 1997; 26:749–756.

137. Masuda EM, Kessler DM, Kistner RL, Eklof B, Sato DT. The natural history of calf vein thrombosis: lysis of thrombi and development of reflux. J Vasc Surg 1998; 28:67–74.

138. Lindner DJ, Edwards JM, Phinney ES, Taylor LM, Porter JM. Long-term hemodynamic and clinical sequelae of lower extremity deep vein thrombosis. J Vasc Surg 1986; 4:436–442.

139. O'Shaughnessy AM, Fitzgerald DE. Natural history of proximal deep vein thrombosis assessed by duplex ultrasound. Int Angiol 1997; 16:45–49.

140. Prandoni P, Villalta S, Bagatella P, Rossi L, Marchiori A, Piccioli A, Bernardi E, Girolami B, Simioni P, Girolami A. The clinical course of deep-vein thrombosis. Prospective, long-term follow-up of 528 symptomatic patients. Haematologica 1997; 82:423–428.

141. Koopman MM, Buller HR, ten Cate JW. Diagnosis of recurrent deep vein thrombosis. Haemostasis 1995; 25:49–57.

142. Hull RD, Carter CJ, Jay RM, Ockelford PA, Hirsch J, Turpie AG, Zielinsky A, Gent M, Powers PJ. The diagnosis of acute, recurrent, deep-vein thrombosis: a diagnostic challenge. Circulation 1983; 67:901–906.

143. Hansson P-O, Sorbo J, Eriksson H. Recurrent venous thromboembolism after deep vein thrombosis. Incidence and risk factors. Arch Intern Med 2000; 160:769–774.

144. Douketis JD, Crowther MA, Foster GA, Ginsberg JS. Does the location of thrombosis determine the risk of disease recurrence in patients with proximal deep vein thrombosis? Am J Med 2001; 110:515–519.
145. Kevorkian JP, Aparicio C, Mazoyer E, Bonnin P, Duet M, Warnet A, Elkharrat D, Beaufils P, Drouet L, Soria J, Soria C. A new clinical interest for D-dimers determination: follow-up of patients with deep vein thrombosis (abst). Thromb Haemost 2001; (suppl):abstract P725.
146. Piovella F, Crippa L, Barone M, D'Angelo SV, Serafini S, Galli L, Beltrametti C, D'Angelo A. Normalization rate of compression ultrasonography in symptomatic vs. post-surgical acute deep vein thrombosis (DVT) (abst). Thromb Haemost 2001; OC43.
147. Prandoni P, Lensing AWA, Prins MH, Simioni P, Bagatella P, Tormene D, Frulla M, Mosena L, Marchiori A, Girolami A. Residual vein thrombosis as a predictive factor of recurrent venous thromboembolism (abst). Thromb Haemost Suppl 2001; OC851.
148. Prandoni P, Lensing AWA, Bernardi E, Bagatella P, Villalta S, Frulla M, Piccioli A, Scarano L, Marchiori A, Tormene D, Benedetti L, Girolami A. A novel ultrasound protocol for the diagnosis of symptomatic recurrent deep vein thrombosis (abst). Thromb Haemost Suppl 2001; OC42.
149. Hirsh J, Lee AYY. How we diagnose and treat deep vein thrombosis. Blood 2002; 99:3102–3110.
150. Heijboer H, Jongbloets LMM, Buller HR, Lensing AWA, ten Cate JW. Clinical utility of real-time compression ultrasonography for diagnostic management of patients with recurrent venous thrombosis. Acta Radiol 1992; 33:297–300.
151. Prandoni P, Cogo A, Bernardi E, Villalta S, Polistena P, Simioni P, Noventa F, Benedetti L, Girolami A. A simple ultrasound approach for detection of recurrent proximal-vein thrombosis. Circulation 1993; 88:1730–1735.
152. Huisman MV, Buller HR, ten Cate JW. Utility of impedance plethysmography in the diagnosis of recurrent deep-vein thrombosis. Arch Intern Med 1988; 148:681–683.
153. Rathbun SW, Whitsett TL, Vesely S, Raskob GE. Utility of D-dimer in the management of suspected recurrent deep-vein thrombosis (abst). Thromb Haemost Suppl 2001; P732.
154. Murphy TP, Cronan JJ. Evolution of deep venous thrombosis: a prospective evaluation with US. Radiology 1990; 177:543–548.
155. Holmstrom M, Lindmarker P, Granqvist S, Johnsson H, Lockner D. A 6-month venographic follow-up in 164 patients with acute deep vein thrombosis. Thromb Haemost 1997; 78:803–807.
156. Peter DJ, Flanagan LD, Cranley JJ. Analysis of blood clot echogenicity. J Clin Ultrasound 1986; 14:111–116.
157. Schulman S, Rheden A-S, Lindmarker P, Carlsson A, Larfars G, Nicol P, Loogna E, Svensson E, Ljungberg B, Walter H, Viering S, Nordlander S, Leijd B, Jonsson K-A, Hjorth M, Linder O, Boberg J, and the Duration of Anticoagulation Trial Study Group. N Engl J Med 1995; 332:1661–1665.

158. Kearon C, Gent M, Hirsh J, Weitz J, Kovacs MJ, Anderson DR, Turpie AG, Green D, Ginsberg JS, Wells P, MacKinnon B, Julian JA. A comparison of three months of anticoagulation with extended anticoagulation for a first episode of idiopathic venous thromboembolism. N Engl J Med 1999; 340:901–907.

159. Hutten BA, Prins MH, Gent M, Ginsberg J, Tijssen JGP, Buller HR. Incidence of recurrent thromboembolic and bleeding complications among patients with venous thromboembolism in relation to both malignancy and achieved international normalized ratio: a retrospective analysis. J Clin Oncol 2000; 18:3078–3083.

6

Clinical Recognition of Pulmonary Embolism

JAMES E. DALEN

University of Arizona College of Medicine
Tucson, Arizona, U.S.A.

I. Introduction

The clinical diagnosis of pulmonary embolism (PE) is notoriously inaccurate; it is neither sensitive nor specific. The diagnosis of PE is not suspected in most patients who die of PE, and most patients who undergo testing for suspected PE do not have PE!

The lack of sensitivity of the clinical diagnosis is evidenced by a report by Morgenthaler and Ryu (1). In a review of autopsies at the Mayo Clinic from 1985 through 1989, 92 patients were found to have died of PE. The diagnosis had been made premortem in less than a third of the patients (1). It is estimated that only 30% of the total episodes of fatal or nonfatal PE in the United States are recognized and treated (2).

The lack of specificity of the clinical diagnosis of PE is illustrated by the fact that PE is confirmed in less than one-third of patients who undergo lung scans or pulmonary angiography because of suspected PE (3–5).

When PE is suspected, the diagnosis must be confirmed by pulmonary angiography, lung scan, or chest computed tomography (CT). The challenge for the clinician is to know when to suspect PE. What symptoms or physical findings or laboratory findings should alert the clinician to suspect PE and order an appropriate diagnostic test? A second challenge is to improve the specificity of the clinical diagnosis of PE in order to avoid unnecessary diagnostic testing.

The crux of the problem is that none of the findings that are present in patients with PE is specific for PE; they are also seen in other common conditions. The two most frequent findings in patients with documented PE are dyspnea and chest pain (6). When dyspnea or chest pain occurs in a patient with evidence of deep venous thrombosis (DVT), or with a past history of venous thromboembolism (VTE), or with risk factors for VTE, the diagnosis of PE should be strongly considered.

II. Dyspnea in Patients with Pulmonary Embolism

Dyspnea is by far the most frequent symptom reported by patients with PE. In three reports totaling 568 patients with PE documented by angiography, dyspnea was present in 80% of the patients (3,7,8). When dyspnea is due to PE, tachypnea, hypoxia, and hypocapnia are present in the vast majority of cases (6). Dyspnea is also present in the conditions most frequently confused with PE: congestive heart failure, pneumonia, and exacerbations of chronic lung disease.

Dyspnea should suggest PE when it is acute and unexplained by other conditions. Dyspnea in patients with PE occurs with effort, and with major PE, it may also occur at rest. Unlike patients with congestive heart failure, patients with PE rarely report orthopnea or paroxysmal nocturnal dyspnea. The dyspnea associated with PE is more likely to be of abrupt onset than in patients with congestive heart failure (CHF). Patients with CHF may seek help after days or weeks of dyspnea, whereas patients with PE are more likely to report dyspnea within hours or days of its onset. In patients with PE, the lungs are usually clear, unless pulmonary infarction is present, whereas in patients with CHF, rales and other signs of CHF are usually present.

In patients with chronic lung disease, new or increasing dyspnea should lead to a suspicion of PE when there is no evidence of fever, leukocytosis, change in cough or sputum production, or change in physical findings in the chest or change in chest radiographic findings. Pneumonia as the cause of dyspnea is suggested by fever, cough, leukocytosis, sputum production, the presence of rales, and chest radiographic findings.

The lack of evidence of CHF, pneumonia, or worsening of chronic lung disease in a patient with acute dyspnea should lead the clinician to suspect PE. Dyspnea is highly suggestive of PE when it is unexplained in a patient with hypoxia and hypocapnia and clear lungs by physical examination and chest radiography, especially when there is evidence of DVT, a past history of VTE, or risk factors for VTE.

III. Chest Pain in Patients with Pulmonary Embolism

Two types of chest pain may occur in patients with PE: pleuritic chest pain and central chest pain. Pleuritic chest pain is far more frequent than central chest pain. In three series reporting a total of 568 patients with PE documented by pulmonary angiography, 69% reported pleuritic chest pain (3,7,8). Pleuritic chest pain in patients with PE is due to pulmonary hemorrhage; which leads to pulmonary infarction when segmental or subsegmental pulmonary arteries are totally obstructed (8). Virchow, who in 1859 was the first to describe PE, pointed out that a given episode of PE might or may not lead to pulmonary infarction; that is, necrosis of alveolar walls (9). Patients with pulmonary infarction usually have submassive PE, and as a result, the arterial Po_2 may be normal or near normal (6). The site of pulmonary hemorrhage/infarction usually is recognized by chest radiography as a density at a pleural surface. The classic studies of Hampton and Castleman in 1940 (10) demonstrated a nearly one to one relationship between pulmonary infarction found at postmortem and an infiltrate by postmortem chest radiography. The signs and symptoms of pulmonary infarction were well described by Graham Steell in 1906 (11). Patients with pulmonary infarction may have a pleural friction rub, rales, or wheezes or an elevated hemidiaphagm (6). Hemoptysis is uncommon (12) but is highly suggestive of pulmonary infarction when it occurs in patients with pleuritic chest pain. The other causes of pleuritic chest pain, viral pleuritis and pneumonia, constitute the principal differential diagnosis. The presence of fever, leukocytosis, and/or sputum production is more consistent with pneumonia than with pulmonary infarction. Hull et al. (13) reported a series of 173 consecutive patients presenting with pleuritic chest pain. The final diagnosis was PE in 21% of the patients, viral or idiopathic pleurisy in 46%, and pneumonia in 8%. Pleuritic chest pain is most suggestive of PE when there is an infiltrate by chest radiography, and the patient is afebrile and without sputum production.

Central chest pain, similar to the chest pain of myocardial ischemia, is less common and may occur in patients with massive PE (6). The electrocardiograph (EKG) is helpful in distinguishing between these two causes of central chest pain. The absence of ischemic findings by EKG points toward PE as the cause of central chest pain. If the episode of PE is sufficiently massive (embolic obstruction of more than 60–75% of the pulmonary circulation) to cause acute cor pulmonale (14), one would expect to find EKG findings of a new S1Q3T3 pattern (14) or new incomplete right bundle branch block (15). In addition, one would expect to find evidence of cor pulmonale by physical examination: distended neck veins, a parasternal heave, tachycardia, and an S3 gallop. The chest radiography in PE patients who do not have pulmonary infarction is usually normal, and the physical examination of the lungs is normal (6).

Massive PE may present as shock or cardiac arrest with or without chest pain. In 1859, Virchow pointed out that, "in the case of very large fragments even the principal trunks of the pulmonary artery are blocked up and instantaneous asphyxia ensues" (9). In 1908, MacKenzie (16) wrote that massive PE can cause "intensive dyspnea with gradual loss of consciousness." He also noted that these patients might survive.

In addition to causing cardiac arrest or shock, massive PE may cause syncope. In a series of 132 patients with documented PE, 17 presented with syncope (17). Pulmonary angiography demonstrated obstruction of more than 50% of the pulmonary circulation in 15 of the 17 patients. Sixteen of the 17 patients had hemodynamic evidence of acute cor pulmonale, and 13 were in shock. Ten of the 17 patients had a new S1Q1T3 pattern or a new incomplete right bundle branch block. If massive PE is the cause of shock, syncope, or cardiac arrest, there usually is evidence of acute cor pulmonale by EKG and by physical examination, and arterial blood gases would demonstrate significant hypoxia and hypocapnia (6). In cases of suspected massive PE, echocardiography may be very useful and can be performed at the bedside. In addition to demonstrating right ventricular dysfunction (18), transesophageal echocardiography may confirm the presence of massive PE by visualizing emboli in the central pulmonary arteries (19).

The symptoms of dyspnea and/or chest pain should suggest the diagnosis of pulmonary embolism when there is no evidence of CHF, myocardial ischemia, pneumonia, or an exacerbation of chronic lung disease; especially if there is evidence of DVT, if the patient has a past history of VTE, or if the patient has one or more risk factors for VTE, as discussed in Chapter 2.

Once PE is suspected, the diagnosis must be confirmed or excluded. Lung scans, the most commonly used test to confirm the diagnosis, are most helpful if they are normal or if they are of high probability, demonstrating multiple segmental perfusion defects that ventilate normally, as discussed in Chapter 8. A normal lung scan essentially excludes PE, and a high probability scan is sufficiently specific to proceed to therapy without further testing. Unfortunately, in the majority of patients suspected of PE, the results of lung scanning are neither normal nor high probability; they are nondiagnostic. In the PIOPED study, the lung scan was nondiagnostic in 57% of the patients suspected to have PE, and the prevalence of PE in patients with nondiagnostic scans was 22% (3). Therefore, a nondiagnostic lung scan neither confirms nor excludes the diagnosis of PE. In the past, pulmonary angiography was frequently performed in patients with nondiagnostic scans. In order to avoid pulmonary angiography (discussed in Chapter 8) which is not available in all hospitals; some centers proceed to chest CT in these patients, and some centers proceed to chest CT without lung scan, as discussed in Chapter 8. Another diagnostic approach is to perform Doppler ultrasound of the legs in patients with nondiagnostic lung scans, as discussed in Chapter 8, or to measure D-dimers (Chapter 7). If the Doppler ultrasound of the legs is negative, or if the D-dimer test is negative in a patient with a nondiagnostic scan, most clinicians would withhold therapy.

IV. Pulmonary Embolism Prediction Models

Prediction models have been developed to estimate the probability of PE once it has been suspected. These models estimate the risk of PE as being high, intermediate, or low. If one can accurately assess the risk of PE as being low, this can be used to avoid extensive diagnostic testing. These models are especially helpful in patients suspected of PE whose lung scan results are nondiagnostic.

PE prediction models are either clinical models or score-based models. Clinical models ask clinicians to rate the probability of PE on the basis of their interpretation of the clinical signs and symptoms and relevant tests such as chest radiography, EKG, and arterial blood gases. No weighting or scoring of these variables is used; the clinician assesses the data and estimates the probability of PE as being high, intermediate, or low. Score-based prediction models evaluate a specific set of clinical or laboratory test findings and assign a numerical score for each finding. The total score is the determinant of high, intermediate, or low probability.

The PIOPED study was one of the first to estimate the probability of PE once it had been suspected (3). Prior to the performance of lung scans in patients suspected of having PE, clinicians were asked to rate the probability of PE as high (80–100%), intermediate (20–79%), or low (0–19%). These probability estimates were made after reviewing the history, physical examination, arterial blood gas analysis, chest radiographs, and EKGs. A scoring system was not used. PE was subsequently documented by angiogram in 68% of patients with a high clinical probability of PE and in only 9% in patients with a low clinical probability. However, only 10% of the patients were judged to be high probability, and only 26% were judged to be low probability. The majority (64%) of the patients were judged to be at intermediate probability; in whom the prevalence of PE was 30%. However, when the results of lung scans were combined with the clinical probability of PE, the accuracy of identifying patients with or without confirmed PE increased. Of 118 patients who had a high-probability scan, PE was confirmed in 87%. However, in patients with a high-probability scan who also had a high clinical probability, PE was documented in 96% (3). In 641 patients with a low- or intermediate-probability scan, PE was documented in 22%. However, in 158 patients with low- or intermediate-probability scans who were judged to be at low probability, PE was documented in only 4% (3).

Perrier et al. (4) also estimated the probability of PE on a clinical basis without using an algorithm. Clinicians were asked to review a checklist of clinical findings, but scores were not assigned. PE was documented in 8% of patients judged to be low probability, in 37% of those with intermediate probability, and 65% of high-probability patients. As with the PIOPED study (3), the majority of patients (56%) were judged to be of intermediate probability. The prevalence of PE in patients with the combination of a nondiagnostic scan and a low clinical probability of PE was less than 5% (4).

Two PE prediction models that use scoring systems are available to estimate the probability of PE once it has been suspected (5,20). Wells et al. (5) developed their model by reviewing the literature and coming to a consensus on a scoring system which combined risk factors for VTE, clinical signs and symptoms, and a determination by the clinician of whether an alternative diagnosis was likely. This latter determination is subjective, based on the clinician's judgment after reviewing the clinical signs and symptoms and the results of routine tests (arterial blood gas analysis, chest radiograph, and EKG). The scoring system for their prediction model is shown in Table 1.

The clinical probability is judged to be low when the score is less than 2, moderate in those with a score of 2–6, and high in patients with a score

Table 1 Scoring System for Clinical Probability of PE

Variable	Points
Signs of DVT (swelling and pain)	3
Heart rate >100	1.5
Immobilization >3 days	1.5
Previous documented VTE	1.5
Hemoptysis	1
Cancer	1
Clinical opinion that PE is most likely diagnosis	3
Total possible points =	12.5

DVT, deep venous thrombosis; PE, pulmonary embolism; VTE, venous thromboembolism.
Source: Ref. 5.

Table 2 Prevalence of PE According to Clinical Probability Score

Clinical probability	No. of patients (%)	Prevalence of PE (%)
Low	734 (59)	3.4
Moderate	403 (33)	28
High	102 (8)	78

Source: Ref. 5.

greater than 6 (5). The model was tested in a series of 1239 inpatients and outpatients with suspected PE (5). The results are shown in Table 2.

The ability of this clinical prediction model to identify 59% of the patients as having a low probability of PE (of only 3.4%) is a major achievement. This scoring model was subsequently tested in a series of 930 consecutive emergency room patients with suspected PE (21). The results were very similar to the earlier report (5). Fifty-seven percent of the patients were judged to be at low risk of PE; and the prevalence of documented PE in this group was only 1.3% (21). A potential disadvantage of the Wells model (5) is that one of the important components of the score is dependent on a subjective opinion by the clinician. Other users of the model may or may not replicate the scoring by the Wells group.

Wicki et al. (20) developed the Geneva scoring model for predicting the probability of PE by analyzing a database of 1090 emergency room patients with suspected PE; 27% of whom were found to have PE. In a multivariate analysis of their data, they found that eight factors were significantly associated with PE, as shown in Table 3.

Table 3 Factors Predictive of PE

Factor	Points
Age 60–79 years	+1
Age >80 years	+2
Previous VTE	+2
Recent surgery	+3
Pulse >.100	+1
Decreased $PaCO_2$	+1 or +2
Decreased PaO_2	+1 to +4
Chest radiograph: platelike atelectasis	+1
Chest radiograph: elevation of hemidiaphragm	+1
Maximum score =	16

Source: Ref. 20.

They classified patients with a score of 4 or less as low probability of PE, scores of 5–8 as intermediate probability, and those with a score of 9 or more as high probability (20). The percentage of patients in each of these probability categories and the prevalence of documented PE in each category is shown in Table 4.

The 10% prevalence of documented PE in patients classified at low risk by Wicki et al. (20) was higher than that reported by Wells et al. (5,21), who reported a prevalence of 3.4 and 1.3% in the patients that they predicted to be at low risk. However, the total prevalence of PE in the two patient cohorts reported by Wells et al. (5,21) was 17% (5) and 10% (21). The prevalence of PE in the patients reported by Wicki et al. (20) was much higher (27%). An advantage of the model described by Wicki et al. (20) is that all of the variables are objective, and therefore the score can be replicated by others. A disadvantage of their score-based prediction model is that it has not been verified in inpatients, and therefore they do not recommend that it be used for evaluation of inpatients (22).

The Geneva group (22) tested their prediction model on 277 patients admitted to an emergency center for suspected PE. The percentage of patients found to be at low probability (55%), intermediate (41%), and high probability (4%) was similar to the findings in their original report (20). The prevalence of PE in those judged to be at low probability by their prediction model was 13% compared to 10% in their earlier report (20). They allowed clinicians to override or disagree with the probability score based on their review of all available data. The clinicians disagreed with the Geneva score in 21% of patients; they assigned a higher probability in 36 cases and a lower probability in 21 cases. The percentage of patients assigned a low probability of PE by the clinicians (53%) was essentially the same as by the Geneva score (55%), but the prevalence of documented PE was only 5% as compared to 13% in those with low probability by the Geneva score. The 277 patients were also evaluated using the Wells score (5). Using the Wells scoring system, 58% of the patients were classified as low probability. The prevalence of PE in the patients classified as low probability by the Wells score was 12% as compared to 13% using the

Table 4 Probability of PE and Prevalence of PE

Probability of PE	No. of patients (%)	Prevalence of PE (%)
Low	486 (49)	10
Intermediate	437 (44)	38
High	63 (6)	81

Source: Ref. 20.

Geneva score in this group of patients in whom the overall prevalence of PE was 26%. Chagnon et al. (22) concluded that these two score-based prediction models were comparable.

These clinical and score-based PE prediction models do not identify a large number of patients at high risk; the number identified is 10% or less in each of the reported studies (3–5,20,21). The major achievement of these prediction models is that they identify a large number of patients suspected of PE in whom the prevalence of PE is 10% or less, as shown in Table 5.

The score-based prediction models identify more than half of PE suspects as being at low risk. The prevalence of PE in those predicted to be at low risk was 10% or less in both the clinical models and the score-based models.

The prevalence of PE in patients with a low clinical probability of PE and a nondiagnostic lung scan is even lower. In the PIOPED study, it was 4% (3), in the study by Perrier et al. (4), it was 4.4%, and in the Wells report, it was 0.5% (5). This very low prevalence of PE is sufficient to safely withhold therapy in these patients (4,5). Wells et al. (21) have reported that the combination of a low clinical probability of PE combined with a normal D-dimer also permits therapy to be withheld safely.

Further investigation of these and other prediction models should lead to even more useful techniques to identify PE suspects with a probability of PE sufficiently low to obviate extensive diagnostic testing.

If clinicians are vigilant in suspecting PE in patients with dyspnea or chest pain, especially if they occur in patients with evidence of DVT or a history of VTE or risk factors for VTE, the sensitivity of the diagnosis of PE can be improved. The use of one of the prediction models for the diagnosis of PE (3–5,20) or a future improved model will greatly increase the specificity of the clinical diagnosis of PE once it has been suspected. Improvement in the accuracy of the clinical diagnosis of PE will increase the number of patients with PE who receive appropriate therapy, and it will

Table 5 Comparison of Clinical and Score-Based Prediction Models

Report (ref. no.)	No. of patients	% PE	% Low probability	% PE
Score-based models				
5	1239	17	59	3.4
20	1090	27	49	10
21	930	10	57	1.3
Clinical models				
3	755	33	26	9
4	837	29	41	8.2

also lead to considerable cost savings by reducing the need for extensive diagnostic testing in patients suspected of having PE.

References

1. Morgenthaler TI, Ryu JH. Clinical characteristics of fatal pulmonary embolism in a referral hospital. Mayo Clin Proc 1995; 70(5):417–424.
2. Dalen JE, Alpert JS. Natural history of pulmonary embolism. Prog Cardiovasc Dis 1975; 17:259–270.
3. PIOPED Investigators. Value of the ventilation/perfusion scan in acute pulmonary embolism diagnosis. JAMA 1990; 263:2753–2759.
4. Perrier A, Miron MJ, Desmarais S. Using clinical evaluation and lung scan to rule out suspected pulmonary embolism. Arch Intern Med 2000; 160:512–516.
5. Wells PS, Ginsberg JS, Anderson DR. Use of a clinical model for safe management of patients with suspected pulmonary embolism. Ann Intern Med 1998; 129:997–1005.
6. Dalen JE. Pulmonary embolism—what have we learned since Virchow? Chest 2002; 122:1440–1456.
7. Bell WR, Simon TL, DeMets DL. The clinical features of submassive and massive pulmonary emboli. Am J Med 1977; 62:355.
8. Dalen JE, Haffajee CI, Alpert JS. Pulmonary embolism, pulmonary hemorrhage and pulmonary infraction. N Engl J Med 1977; 296:1431–1440.
9. Virchow RLK. Cellular Pathology. 1859 Special edition. London: John Churchill, 1978:204–207.
10. Hampton AO, Castleman B. Correlation of postmortem chest teleroentgenograms with autopsy findings. Am J of Roentgenol Radium Ther 1940; 43:305–326.
11. Steell G. Textbook on Diseases of the Heart. Special edition. Manchester: University Press, 1906:36–37.
12. Stein PD, Terrin ML, Hales CA. Clinical, laboratory, roentgenographic, and electrocardiographic findings in patients with acute pulmonary embolism and no preexisting cardiac or pulmonary disease. Chest 1993; 103:319–320.
13. Hull RD, Raskob GE, Carter CJ. Pulmonary embolism in outpatients with pleuritic chest pain. Arch Intern Med 1988; 148:838–844.
14. McGinn S, White S. Acute cor pulmonale resulting from pulmonary embolism. JAMA 1935; 104:1473–1480.
15. Szucs MM, Brooks HL, Grossman W. Diagnostic sensitivity of laboratory findings in acute pulmonary embolism. Ann Intern Med 1971; 74:161–166.
16. MacKenzie J. Diseases of the Heart. London: Oxford University Press, 1908: 28–29.
17. Thames MD, Alpert JS, Dalen JE. Syncope in patients with pulmonary embolism. JAMA 1977; 238:2509–2511.
18. Kasper W, Meinertz T, Henkel B. Echocardiographic findings in patients with proved pulmonary embolism. Am Heart J 1986; 112:1284–1290.

19. Wittlich N, Erbel R, Eichler A. Detection of central pulmonary artery thromboemboli by transesophageal echocardiography in patients with severe pulmonary embolism. J Am Society of Echocardiol 1992; 5:515–524.
20. Wicki J, Perneger TV, Junod AF. Assessing clinical probability of pulmonary embolism in the emergency ward. Arch Intern Med 2001; 161:92–97.
21. Wells PS, Anderson DR, Rodger M. Excluding pulmonary embolism at the bedside without diagnostic imaging: management of patients with suspected pulmonary embolism presenting to the emergency department by using a simple clinical model and d-dimer. Ann Intern Med 2001; 135:98–107.
22. Chagnon I, Bounameaux H, Aujesky D, Roy PM, Gourdier AL, Cornuz J, Perneger T, Perrier A. Comparison of two clinical prediction rules and implicit assessment among patients with suspected pulmonary embolism. Am J Med 2002; 113:269–275.

7

D-Dimer in the Diagnosis of Venous Thromboembolism

HENRI BOUNAMEAUX and ARNAUD PERRIER

University of Geneva and
University Hospitals of Geneva
Geneva, Switzerland

I. Introduction

In the past 15 years, plasma assays of several markers of activation of plasma coagulation and/or fibrinolysis have been made available for clinical use. Among these markers, D-dimer (DD), a specific degradation product of cross-linked fibrin (1), has emerged as a definite aid in the diagnostic approach of venous thromboembolism (VTE) using various immunoassays (enzyme-linked immunoassay [ELISA] or latex agglutination tests) (2,3). Its widespread use has been made possible only in recent years with the development of rapid assays that allowed result delivery within 1 hr or less after blood sampling (Table 1). However, the heterogeneity of the assays has raised uncertainty among clinicians and called for rigorous evaluation and standardization of the various tests. Uncertainty was further increased, because the usefulness of the test was also found to be dependent upon the populations to which it was applied due to variations in test specificity.

This chapter summarizes the published data on the use of rapid DD tests for diagnosing deep venous thrombosis (DVT) of the lower limbs and pulmonary embolism (PE), and puts these data in the perspective of an integrated diagnostic approach of suspected VTE.

Table 1   Some Commercially Available Rapid DD Assays

Assay	Manufacturer	Property
ELISA assays		
VIDAS DD	bioMérieux, Lyon, France	Quantitative
Nycocard	Nycomed, Oslo, Norway	Semiquantitative
Instant IA	Stago, Asnières, France	Semiquantitative
Latex assays		
SimpliRED	Agen, Acacia Ridge, QLD Australia	Semiquantitative
Minutex	Biopool, Umeå, Sweden	Semiquantitative
Liatest	Stago, Asnières, France	Quantitative
Tinaquant	Boehringer Mannheim, Mannheim, Germany	Quantitative
LPIA D–dimer	Mitsubishi Kasel, Tokyo, Japan	Quantitative
Nephelotex	Biopool, Umeå, Sweden	Quantitative
DDPlus or Advanced DD	Dade Behring, Marburg, Germany	Quantitative
Turbiquant	Dade Behring, Marburg, Germany	Quantitative
MDA assay	Organon Tecnika, Turnhout, Belgium	Quantitative

II.   Principle of DD Immunoassays

Basically, a monoclonal antibody specifically directed against the DD
epitope is attached to a solid phase. This solid phase can be the surface of
a microtiter well or a latex particle. The plasma (or whole blood in one
particular assay) sample containing the DD antigen is allowed to interact
with the antibody on the solid phase. In the case of a fixed microtiter well
(two-step sandwich-type assay or ELISA), a second DD-specific enzyme-
labeled antibody is needed for the detection, whereas use of latex particles
results in directly visible agglutination (one-step reaction).

Digestion of a fibrin clot by plasmin results in a heterogeneous population of fibrin degradation products with a highly variable number of DD
epitopes. The size distribution of these degradation products in plasma varies
from individual to individual and from disease to disease. Moreover, different monoclonal antibodies react differently with the various DD epitopes.
For these reasons, and also because different calibrators are used in com-
mercial kits, standardization of DD assays is theoretically and practically
impossible. At best, results obtained with different assays do correlate but
cannot be identical. This means that each assay has its own normal range
and needs to be validated in clinical settings for determining its appropriate
cutoff value.

III. Commercially Available Rapid DD Tests

A. Semiquantitative Tests

The *Nycocard assay* is an immunofiltration assay consisting of a laminated test card containing a thin porous membrane. A monoclonal antibody (S4H9) that is reactive against DD is bound to this membrane. A plasma sample placed on the membrane is rapidly absorbed through the membrane and DD is captured by the antibody. Subsequently, the same antibody coupled to gold particles is added that binds to other antigenic sites available on the DD molecule. Gold colloids produce an intense red staining that is proportional to the amount of DD antigen present in plasma. The color intensity is then compared with a reference chart with five different color zones corresponding to DD concentrations from 500 to 8000 ng/mL.

The *Minutex DD assay* is a semiquantitative latex agglutination test that uses latex beads covered with monoclonal antibodies directed against DD. After reagents are mixed and test plasma added, semiquantitative results are available in 3 min.

The *Instant IA test* is a rapid semiquantitative ELISA assay that utilizes two different mouse monoclonal antibodies on a membrane. The plasma sample is placed on the membrane and DD antigens are captured by the first monoclonal antibodies. The second mouse monoclonal antibody coupled to alkaline phosphatase is added and turns positive on reacting with the substrate 5-bromo-4-chloro-3-iodyl phosphate in the presence of nitroblue tetrazolium. Positive and negative controls are provided on the single-use test cartridge.

The *SimpliRED test* is a semiquantitative red cell agglutination assay that can be performed on whole blood, thus at the bedside within 2 min. It utilizes a hybrid antibody (human DD 3B6/22 and rat 1C3/86) specific for epitopes on both the DD $\gamma-\gamma$ cross-link region and red cell surface.

B. Quantitative Tests

The *Tinaquant DD* assay is a rapid quantitative test that utilizes antibodies to DD attached to latex particles. The presence of DD in plasma causes agglutination of latex particles and a subsequent increase in turbidity, which is monitored at a wavelength of 800 nm by an automated analyzer that delivers results in about 20 min.

The *LPIA DD assay* is a rapid quantitative latex photometric immunoassay that utilizes polyethylene latex particles covered with the JIF-23 monoclonal antibody, which is specific for DD. The presence of DD in plasma causes a concentration-dependent increase in turbidity that is detected at 950 nm within 10 min by an automated nephelometer.

The *Nephelotex*, the *BC DD assay* (and its developments for particular automated systems, DDPlus and Advanced DD), the *Turbiquant*, the *LIA DD test*, and the *MDA DD assay* are quantitative DD assays utilizing latex particles coated with monoclonal antibodies. The presence of DD antigen in the test plasma causes a concentration-dependent decrease in light refraction. Results are obtained in about 10–15 min with a nephelometer.

The *VIDAS DD assay* is the only rapid quantitative fluorescence-based immunoassay performed on plasma that can be performed in about half an hour. It employs two complementary murine antifibrin degradation product monoclonal antibodies and combines a sandwich immunoenzymatic method in two steps with final fluorescence detection. It requires a small automated analyzer and utilizes single-use cartridges.

IV. Performance of Rapid DD Tests for Diagnosing DVT and PE

After initial reports from the Geneva group using a classic ELISA test (4,5), the performance of these tests and that of latex tests have been reviewed in 1994 (2,3). Thereafter, the performance of various rapid DD tests for diagnosing DVT (6–30) and PE (8,20,26,28,30–42) has been further studied. The data pertaining to these more recent, rapid tests are summarized in Tables 2 and 3. Briefly, sensitivity to VTE varies from 84 to 99%, depending upon the assay used, and the lower limit of the 95% confidence interval for sensitivity exceeds 95% in very few tests: the VIDAS DD test and the Tinaquant test for DVT and the VIDAS DD test for PE.

Table 2 Performance of Rapid DD Tests for the Diagnosis of DVT

Assay (ref. no.)	n (nDVT)	Sensitivity	Specificity
		% (95% CI)	
Nycocard (6–15)	738 (311)	92.1 (89.2–94.5)	48.7 (44.8–52.6)
VIDAS DD (7,8,10,16–20)	751 (341)	97.8 (96.0–98.9)	43.1 (39.6–46.6)
Instant IA (7–11,21)	1010 (493)	92.3 (89.6–94.5)	56.8 (52.2–61.4)
SimpliRED (8,15,18,22–24)	857 (335)	84.5 (80.6–88.4)	71.3 (67.4–75.2)
Minutex (9,10,14,18,25)	565 (264)	88.6 (84.8–92.5)	58.1 (52.6–63.7)
Tinaquant (18,26)	260 (147)	98.6 (95.2–99.8)	39.8 (30.8–48.8)
DDPlus[a] (17,27,28)	315 (108)	94.4 (88.3–97.9)	50.2 (43.4–57.1)
LPIA D–Dimer (10)	87 (42)	95 (89–100)	69 (55–84)
Nephelotex (10)	87 (42)	98 (93–100)	65 (62–89)
MDA (29,30)	366 (85)	96.5 (90–99.3)	43.8 (38–49.6)

[a] DDPlus and Advanced DD are developments of the BC DD test.

Table 3 Performance of Rapid DD Tests for the Diagnosis of PE

Assay (ref. no.)	n (nPE)	Sensitivity	Specificity
		% (95% CI)	
Nycocard (8,31)	200 (26)	96.2 (80.4–99.9)	31.0 (24.2–37.9)
VIDAS DD (20,32,33)	753 (191)	100 (98.1–100)	40.0 (35.9–44.1)
Instant IA (34–36)	539 (193)	91.2 (86.3–94.8)	50.4 (45.2–55.7)
SimpliRED (31,38,39)	1446 (232)	85.8 (81.3–90.3)	67.8 (65.2–70.4)
Liatest (34,35,41,42)	1113 (370)	95.1 (92.4–97.1)	39.4 (36.0–42.9)
Tinaquant (26)	26 (15)	100 (78–100)	46 (16–77)
Turbiquant (31)	183 (19)	89 (67–99)	57 (49–65)
MDA (30)	278 (48)	96 (86–99)	45 (38–52)
DDPlus[a] (28)	166 (46)	98 (88–100)	37 (28–46)

[a] DDPlus and Advanced DD are developments of the BC DD test.

In the following sections, we discuss the conditions for evaluating a diagnostic test in the field of VTE, and we present the available data on the use of DD in large-scale management studies. Finally, we address a few practical issues pertaining to DD measurement in special patient populations or conditions.

V. Systematic Evaluation of a Test for Diagnosing VTE

Evaluation of a new diagnostic test in suspected VTE should consist of the following steps (43): (1) technical description of the method or the diagnostic strategy; (2) systematic comparison with a diagnostic standard in order to establish the values of sensitivity and specificity of the test to the presence of VTE, and if applicable, to determine the critical cutoff of a laboratory test such as DD (using receiver operating characteristics curve analysis); (3) use of the test in so-called management trials in which anticoagulation is withheld in patients in whom the test or the diagnostic strategy has ruled out the disease, with systematic, usually 3-month, follow-up to detect delayed events and establish the true diagnostic performance of the test; (4) cost-effectiveness analyses comparing the "new" strategy with other management policies.

In fact, with the development of more and more sophisticated diagnostic tools that are able to diagnose very small thrombi or emboli, the aim of a diagnostic test or strategy is less to reach diagnostic certainty than to identify a patient population that can safely be left untreated (44). This confers to the event-free follow-up the value of a new diagnostic gold standard.

VI. Management Studies Utilizing DD for Ruling Out VTE

A. D-Dimer to Rule Out DVT

In patients with clinical signs and symptoms, B-mode venous compression ultrasonography (CUS) or duplex scanning is presently used in clinical practice (45), with constrast venography still being the diagnostic gold standard. On the other hand, with increasing fear for DVT and its immediate and late consequences, PE and postthrombotic syndrome, patients are more and more referred to diagnostic centers with a low or very low clinical suspicion. This change in practice resulted in a decrease of the prevalence of DVT among clinically suspected patients, which dropped in our center from 50 to 20% or less over the past 20 years. Even though noninvasive diagnostic tests are less harmful and much cheaper than venography, they are still relatively expensive and require technical skills. A highly sensitive and simple test to be used as initial screening and allow DVT to be ruled out in a substantial proportion of individuals might save time and money.

Thus, the Geneva-Montreal study (20) enrolled 474 patients clinically suspected of DVT. One-third of them had a DD concentration below 500 μg/L (as assessed by the VIDAS DD test) and, accordingly, did not receive anticoagulant treatment. None of them developed DVT or PE during the subsequent 3-month follow-up. Admittedly, the strategy that did not include repeat CUS was associated with a 2.6% 3-month thromboembolic risk. On the other hand, Bernardi et al. (46) did not perform repeat CUS in those patients who had a negative initial CUS and a negative Instant IA DD test result, which allowed to a substantial proportion of repeat US to be saved compared to a strategy by emplying repeat CUS in all patients with a normal initial examination (47). The yield of the repeat examination at 1 week was, however, less than 1%.

The safety of the strategies including DD measurement (20,47) (Fig. 1) was similar to that of a negative venography. As displayed in Table 4, the 3-month thromboembolic risk observed with the two algorithms is widely overlapping with the 1.9% (95% confidence interval: 0.4–5.4%) reported by Hull et al. in 1981 (48) in a series of 160 patients in whom clinically suspected DVT could be ruled out by venography and who were followed up for 3 months. In addition, a formal cost-effectiveness analysis (49) showed that strategies that include DD testing are highly cost effective.

B. D-Dimer to Rule Out PE

Two diagnostic algorithms that included DD measurement have been validated in large-scale prospective outcome studies. The 3-month thromboembolic risks that were associated with these algorithms were 0.9% (95%

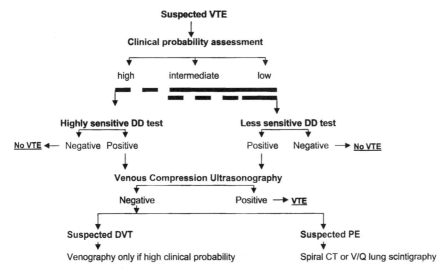

Figure 1 Examples of use of DD measurement in two diagnostic algorithms depending on the use of DD assays of high or less high sensitivity for VTE. In high clinical probability patients, there is controversy as to whether a negative DD test (even a highly sensitive one) allows VTE to be ruled out (dashed line). Thus, in that particular category of patients, DD measurement might even be skipped. Less sensitive DD tests are useful only in low and perhaps (dashed line) intermediate clinical probability patients.

Table 4 Safety of the Diagnostic Strategies Including DD Compared to Diagnostic "Gold Standards"

DD test used (ref. no.)	3-Month thromboembolic risk % (95% CI)
DVT	
Repeat US + DD (Instant IA) (47)	0.4 (0–0.9)
DD (Vidas DD) + Single CUS (20)	2.6 (0.2–4.9)
DD (Vidas DD) + Single CUS + non–high CP (20)	1.6 (0.4–5.5)
Venography (49)	1.9 (0.4–5.4)
PE	
DD (SimpliRED) (39)	0.5 (0.1%–1.3)
DD (Vidas DD) (20)	0.9 (0.2%–2.7)
Pulmonary angiography (52)	0 (0–2.2)
Perfusion lung scintigraphy (53)	0.6 (0.1–1.8)

CUS, venous compression ultrasonography; CP, clinical probability.

CI: 0.2%–2.7%) (20) or 0.5% (95% CI: 0.1%–1.3%) (39), and pulmonary angiography had to be performed in 11 or 4% of patients, respectively. These strategies allow management of the majority of patients with widely available, noninvasive diagnostic tools. Noteworthy, in the Geneva-Montreal study (20), a definitive diagnosis could be established in 46% of patients by DD and CUS alone, rendering further and more sophisticated or invasive testing unnecessary. This approach is extremely useful for the numerous smaller institutions without of nuclear medicine or pulmonary angiography facilities. Its cost effectiveness has been demonstrated in a formal analysis (50). However, formal cost-effectiveness studies comparing the two algorithms are not available yet.

The safety of these strategies (see Fig. 1) is similar to that of a negative pulmonary angiogram or normal perfusion scan. As shown in Table 4, the 3-month thromboembolic risk observed with the two new algorithms overlapps with the risks reported in two series of 167 patients (51) and 515 patients (52) in whom clinically suspected PE could be ruled out by normal pulmonary angiography or perfusion scintigraphy, respectively.

VII. Negative DD and High Clinical Probability: A Controversial Issue

In rare situations, clinicians are confronted with a negative DD test in patients with a high clinical probability. In such cases, they may be reluctant to rule out DVT or PE on the basis of this sole test. Indeed, in spite of the high sensitivity of DD to the presence of VTE, the negative predictive value of a negative test in such patients may not be sufficient to rule out the disease. In addition, preanalytical variables must be considered (e.g., blood drawn from the wrong patient or the wrong label on the test tube) as for any surprising laboratory test result. Therefore, many clinicians feel that DD measurement is useless in high clinical probability patients. For sure, an assay that is not highly sensitive to VTE has no place in the diagnostic work-up of such patients (see Fig. 1).

VIII. Usefulness of DD in Special Situations and/or Special Patient Populations

A. Prediction of Recurrent VTE

Recently, Palareti et al. (53) reported that DD has a high negative predictive value for VTE recurrence when performed after discontinuation of oral anticoagulant treatment. In a population of about 400 patients, DD was measured on the day of treatment withdrawal and 3 weeks and 3 months later. During a cumulative follow-up of more than 600 patient years, 40 recurrences were objectively confirmed (6.4% patient-year). In 39 of these 40 recurrences, DD had been measured: the level was increased in at least one measurement in 28 cases, and the negative predictive value of DD at 3 months for predicting VTE recurrence was 96%. This observation adds to the report by Sié et al. several years ago (54), demonstrating that DD returned to normal values in most patients 3 months after a thromboembolic episode, suggesting that DD measurement might be of value in the context of suspected recurrent VTE, a highly challenging and largely unresolved issue in the field.

B. Inpatients, Including Intensive Care Patients

An algorithm similar to that of the previously discussed Geneva-Montreal study (20) has been validated for inpatients (55), but DD is much less useful in that patient population owing to frequent comorbidities such as infection, malignancy, or inflammatory disease that are all associated with increased DD levels (56). Intensive care patients are also very likely to present with elevated DD levels that might even correlate with clinical outcome (57). Although the high sensitivity of the test for the presence of VTE is maintained, the reduced specificity renders the test almost useless in these populations except after exclusion of well-defined conditions (58).

C. Postoperative Patients

Several investigators have shown that there is an elevation in DD levels that persists for several days following general (59,60) or orthopedic (61) surgery. Rowbotham et al. (59) studied 135 consecutive patients undergoing major abdominal surgery. They found that DD levels (assessed with a classic ELISA test) were significantly elevated preoperatively as well as on postoperative day 1 in patients who went on to develop DVT compared with patients who did not, but the diagnostic performance of DD was poor and clinically useless. Bounameaux et al. (60) studied DD (with a classic ELISA) as a screen for DVT in 185 patients who underwent general abdominal surgery. All patients underwent venography on postoperative day 8. Using a cutoff of 3000 µg/L, the sensitivity of DD was 89% with a negative predictive value of 93%. The more favorable results in the latter study might be due to the diagnostic comparator, venography, that is certainly more sensitive than the ^{125}I-fibrinogen leg scanning that was used in the Australian study. Bongard et al. (61) looked at the diagnostic potential of DD in patients undergoing major hip surgery. They studied 173 patients who all underwent CUS on postoperative day 12. Preoperative DD levels below 500 µg/L had a sensitivity of 93% and a negative predictive value of

96%, but the specificity was low at 23%. These results must be considered with some caution because of the low sensitivity of the comparator used (CUS) in the postoperative setting in asymptomatic patients.

D. Pregnant Women

DD concentration increases during the course of pregnancy (Fig. 2), as systematically studied by Chabloz et al. (62). In a population of 144 pregnant women, the median DD plasma concentration was 341 µg/L (5th to 95th percentiles: 139–602) during the first trimester. The corresponding values during the second and third trimesters were 575 µg/L (291–1231) and 1161 µg/L (489–2217), respectively. At delivery, the median DD level was 1581 µg/L (678–5123). These figures imply that DD measurement is of no utility for ruling out VTE during the third trimester of pregnancy and at delivery, but remains a valuable tool during the first two trimesters.

E. Elderly Patients

The clinical utility of DD testing is greatly affected by age. Cadroy et al. (63) performed DD tests on 80 healthy subjects with an age range of 20–94 years. They found a linear increase in DD concentration with increasing age. Two studies evaluated DD testing in elderly patients with suspected PE. Tardy et al. (36) studied 96 consecutive outpatients who were older than 70 years. Although they excluded patients with conditions known to increase DD such

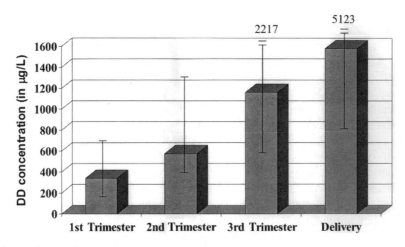

Figure 2   Median DD concentration during pregnancy (after Ref. 62). The vertical bars represent the 5th and 95th percentiles of the distribution.

Table 5 Effect of Age on Usefulness of Noninvasive Tests (DD and US) for Diagnosing PE

Age in years (n)	% With DVT on US	% With DD <500 mg/L	% With either test conclusive
<40 (196)	9	58	67
40–49 (145)	10	56	66
50–59 (142)	8	49	57
60–69 (182)	18	26	45
70–79 (205)	28	17	45
>80 (163)	25	5	30
All (1033)	18	34	52

Source: Modified from Ref. 64.

as cancer, surgery, trauma, infection, stroke, myocardial infarction, or recent VTE, the specificity was very low at 14%. Similarly, Righini et al. (64) used the Geneva database (more than 1000 patients suspected of PE) to study the effects of age on DD in patients with suspected PE. They showed that sensitivity remains unaffected by age but that specificity steadily decreases with increasing age. Nevertheless, increasing the diagnostic cutoff from 500 µg/L to higher values resulted in unacceptable loss in sensitivity (65). On the other hand, these data show that the decreasing usefulness of DD parallels an increased usefulness of systematic US search for proximal DVT (65) (Table 5), suggesting that in elderly patients, the sequence of the two tests should probably be inverted, US being performed before DD testing.

IX. Conclusions

Depending on the particular assay used, DD measurement is a sensitive to highly sensitive diagnostic tool in suspected VTE. Classic latex assays, including the rapid whole blood test SimpliRED, can be performed more rapidly but are generally less sensitive that the initial ELISA assays. Rapid assays based on the ELISA technique or automated turbidimetric methods have been developed with improved sensitivity. Such tests are increasingly being incorporated in diagnostic algorithms for VTE. Evidence is accumulating that VTE can safely been ruled out in outpatients based on a negative DD test alone, but this policy might be restricted to low or at least nonhigh clinical probability patients for safety reasons.

The usefulness of the test has mainly been demonstrated in outpatients presenting at the emergency room with clinically suspected DVT or PE. The test appears to be particularly useful in this patient population, because the prevalence of the disease among these patients has been decreasing steadily over the past 10 years with reported contemporary prevalences below 20% in diagnostic centers in Canada, Switzerland, Italy, and The Netherlands. Other patient populations such as inpatients, postoperative patients, pregnant women, and elderly subjects have higher baseline DD levels, thereby reducing the specificity for VTE, and the practical usefulness of the test in these populations in case of suspected VTE.

References

1. Kroneman R, Nieuwenhuizen W, Knot EAR. Monoclonal antibody-based plasma assays for fibrin(ogen) and derivatives, and their clinical relevance. Blood Coag Fibrinolysis 1990; 1:91–111.
2. Bounameaux H, de Moerloose P, Perrier A, Reber G. Plasma measurement of D-dimer as diagnostic aid in suspected venous thromboembolism: an overview. Thromb Haemost 1994; 71:1–6.
3. Bounameaux H, de Moerloose P, Perrier A, Miron MJ. D-dimer testing in suspected venous thromboembolism: an update. QJM 1997; 90:437–442.
4. Bounameaux H, Schneider PA, Reber G, de Moerloose P, Krahenbuhl B. Measurement of plasma D-dimer for diagnosis of deep venous thrombosis. Am J Clin Pathol 1989; 91:82–85.
5. Bounameaux H, Cirafici P, de Moerloose P, Schneider PA, Slosman D, Reber G, Unger PF. Measurement of D-dimer in plasma as diagnostic aid in suspected pulmonary embolism. Lancet 1991; 337:196–200.
6. Dale S, Gogstad GO, Brosstad F, et al. Comparison of three D-dimer assays for the diagnosis of DVT: ELISA, latex and a immunoofiltration assay (Nycocard D-dimer). Thromb Haemost 1994; 71:264–270.
7. Elias A, Aptel I, Huc B, et al. D-dimer test and diagnosis of deep-vein thrombosis: a comparative study of 7 assays. Thromb Haemost 1996; 76:518–522.
8. Freyburger G, Trillaud H, Labrouche S, et al. D-dimer strategy in thrombosis exclusion. Thromb Haemost 1998; 79:32–37.
9. Wahlander K, Tengborn L, Hellstrom M, et al. Comparison of various D-dimer tests for the diagnosis of deep vein thrombosis. Blood Coagul Fibrinolysis 1999; 10:121–126.
10. Legnani C, Pancani C, Palareti G, et al. Comparison of new rapid methods for D-dimer measurement to exclude deep vein thrombosis in symptomatic outpatients. Blood Coagul Fibrinolysis 1997; 9:296–302.
11. Scarano L, Bernardi E, Prandoni P, et al. Accuracy of two newly described D-dimer tests in patients with suspected deep venous thrombosis. Thromb Res 1997; 86:93–99.
12. Khaira HS, Mann J. Olasma D-dimer measurement in patients with suspected DVT—a means of avoiding unnecessary venography. Eur J Vasc Endovasc Surg 1998; 15:235–238.

13. Killick SB, Pnetek PG, Mercieca JE, et al. Comparison of immunofiltration assay of D-dimer with diagnostic imaging in deep vein thrombosis. Br J Haematol 1997; 96:846–849.

14. Lindhal L, Lundhal TH, Ranby M, et al. Clinical evaluation of a diagnostic strategy for deep venous thrombosis with exclusion by low plasma level of fibrin degratation product D-dimer. Scand J Clin Lab Invest 1998; 58:307–316.

15. Mayer W, Hirschwehr R, Hippman G, et al. Whole blood immunoassay (SimplRED) versus plasma immunoassay (NycoCard) for the diagnosis of clinically suspected deep vein thrombosis. Vasa 1997; 26:97–101.

16. Borg JY, Levesque H, Cailleux N, et al. Rapid quantitative D-dimer assay and the clinical evaluation for the diagnosis of clinically suspected DVT. Thromb Haemost 1997; 77:602–603.

17. Legnani C, Pancani C, Palareti G, et al. Contribution of a new, rapid, quantitative and automated method for D-dimer meaasurement to exclude deep vein thrombosis in symptomatic outpatients. Blood Coagul Fibrinolysis 1999; 10:69–74.

18. Janssen MCH, Heebels AE, de Metz M, et al. Reliability of five rapid D-dimer assays compared to ELISA in the exclusion of deep venous thrombosis. Thromb Haemost 1997; 77:262–266.

19. D'Angelo A, D'Alessandro G, Tomassini L, et al. Evaluation of a new rapid quantitative D-dimer assay in patients with clinically suspected deep vein thrombosis. Thromb Haemost 1996; 75:412–416.

20. Perrier A, Desmarais S, Miron MJ, et al. Non-invasive diagnosis of venous thromboembolism in outpatients. Lancet 1999; 353:190–195.

21. Leroyer C, Escoffre M, Moigne EL, et al. Diagnostic value of a new sensitive membrane based technique for instantaneous D-dimer evaluation in patients with clinically suspected deep venous thrombosis. Thromb Haemost 1997; 77:637–640.

22. Brenner B, Pery M, Lanir N, et al. Application of a bedside whole blood D-dimer assay in the diagnosis of deep vein thrombosis. Blood Coagul Fibrinolysis 1995; 6:219–222.

23. Turkstra F, van Beek EJR, ten Cate JW, Buller HR. Reliable rapid blood test for the exclusion of venous thromboembolism in symptomatic outpatients. Thromb Haemost 1996; 76:9–11.

24. Wells PS, Brill-Edwards P, Stevens P, et al. A novel and rapid whole-blood assay for D-dimer in patients with clinically suspected deep vein thrombosis. Circulation 1995; 91:2184–2187.

25. Tengborn L, Palmblad S, Wojciechowski J, et al. D-dimer and thrombin/ anti-thrombin III complex: diagnostic tools in deep venous thrombosis? Haemostasis 194; 24:344–350.

26. Knecht MF, Heinrich F. Clinical evaluation of an immunoturbidimetric D-dimer assay in the diagnostic procedure of deep vein thrombosis and pulmonary embolism. Thromb Res 1997; 88:413–417.

27. Scarano L, Prandoni P, Gavasso S, et al. Failure of soluble fibrin polymers in the diagnosis of clinically suspected deep vein thrombosis. Blood Coagul Fibrinolysis 1999; 10:245–250.

28. Reber G, Bounameaux H, Perrier A, de Moerloose P. Performances of a new, automated latex assay for the exclusion of venous thromboembolism. Blood Coagul Fibrinolysis 2001; 12:217–220.

29. Keeling DM, Wright M, Baker P, Sackett D. D-dimer for the exclusion of venous thromboembolism: comparison of a new automated latex particle immunoassay (MDA D-dimer) with an established enzyme-linked fluorescent assay (VIDAS D-dimer). Clin Lab Haematol 1999; 21:359–362.

30. Bates SM, Grand'Maison A, Johnston M, et al. A latex D-dimer reliably excludes venous thromboembolism. Arch Intern Med 2001; 161:447–453.

31. Veitl M, Hamwi A, Kurtaren A, et al. Comparison of four rapid D-dimer tests for diagnosis of pulmonary embolism. Thromb Res 1996; 82:399–407.

32. Miron MJ, Perrier A, Bounameaux H, et al. Contribution of noninvasve evaluation to the diagnosis of pulmonary embolism in hospitalized patients. Eur Respir J 1999; 13:1365–1370.

33. de Moerloose P, Desmarais S, Bounameaux H, et al. Contribution of a new, rapid, individual and quantitative D-dimer ELISA to exclude pulmonary embolism. Thromb Haemost 1996; 75:11–13.

34. Meyer G, Fischer AM, Collignon MA, et al. Diagnostic value of two rapid and individual D-dimer assays in patients with clinically suspected pulmonary embolism: comparison with microplate enzyme-linked immunoadsorbant assay. Blood Coagul Fibrinolysis 1998; 9:603–608.

35. Reber G, Vissac AM, de Moerloose P, et al. A new semi-quantitative and individual ELISA for rapid measurement of plasma D-dimer in patients suspected of pulmonary embolism. Blood Coagul Fibrinolysis 1995; 6:460–463.

36. Tardy B, Tardy-Poncet B, Viallon A, et al. Evaluation of D-dimer ELISA test in elderly patients with suspected pulmonary embolism. Thromb Haemost 1998; 79:38–41.

37. Ergermeyer P, Town GI, Turner JG, et al. Usefulness of D-dimer, blood gas and respiratory rate measurements for excluding pulmonary embolism. Thorax 1998; 53:830–834.

38. Ginsberg JS, Wells PS, Brill-Edwards P, et al. Application of a novel and rapid whole blood assay for D-dimer in patients with clinically suspected pulmonary embolism. Thromb Haemost 1995; 73:35–38.

39. Ginsberg JS, Wells PS, Kearon C, et al. Sensitivity and specificity of a whole-blood assay for D-dimer in the diagnosis of pulmonary embolism. Ann Intern Med 1998; 128:1006–1011.

40. Lennox AF, Nicolaides AN. Rapid D-dimer testing as an adjunct to clinical findings in excluding pulmonary embolism. Thorax 1999; 54:S33–S36.

41. Duet M, Benelhadj S, Kedra W, et al. A new quantitative D-dimer assay appropriate in emergency; reliability of the assay for pulmonary embolism exclusion diagnosis. Thromb Res 1998; 91:1–5.

42. Oger E, Leroyer C, Bressollette L, et al. Evaluation of a new, rapid, and quantitative D-dimer test in patients with suspected pulmonary embolism. Am J Respir Crit Care Med 1998; 158:65–70.

43. Büller HR, Lensing AWA, Hirsh J, ten Cate JW. Deep vein thrombosis: new non-invasive diagnostic tests. Thromb Haemost 1991; 66:133–137.

44. Perrier A, Bounameaux H. Cost-effective diagnosis of deep vein thrombosis and pulmonary embolism. Thromb Haemost 2001; 86:475–487.
45. Kearon C, Ginsberg J, Hirsh J. The role of venous ultrasonography in the diagnosis of suspected deep venous thrombosis and pulmonary embolism. Ann Intern Med 1998; 129:1044–1049.
46. Bernardi E, Prandoni P, Lensing AWA, Agnelli G, Guazzaloca G, Scannapieco G, Piovella F, Verlato F, Tomasi C, Moia M, Scarano L, Girolami A. D-dimer testing as an adjunct to ultrasonography in patients with clinically suspected deep vein thrombosis: prospective cohort study. BMJ 1998; 317:1037–1040.
47. Cogo A, Lensing AWA, Koopman MMW, Piovella F, Siragusa S, Wells PS, Villalta S, Büller HR, Turpie AGG, Prandoni P. Compression ultrasonography for diagnostic management of patients with clinically suspected deep vein thrombosis: a prospective cohort study. BMJ 1998; 316:17–20.
48. Hull R, Hirsh J, Sackett DL, Taylor DW, Carter C, Turpie AG, Powers P, Gent M. Clinical validity of a negative venogram in patients with clinically suspected venous thrombosis. Circulation 198; 64:622–625.
49. Perone N, Bounameaux H, Perrier A. Comparison of four strategies for diagnosing deep vein thrombosis: a cost-effectiveness analysis. Am J Med 2001; 110:33–40.
50. Perrier A, Buswell L, Bounameaux H, Didier D, Morabia A, de Moerloose P, et al. Cost-effectiveness of noninvasive diagnostic aids in suspected pulmonary embolism. Arch Intern Med 1997; 157:2309–2316.
51. Novelline RA, Baltarowich OH, Athanasoulis CA, Waltman AC, Greenfield AJ, McKusick KA. The clinical course of patients with suspected pulmonary embolism and a negative pulmonary angiogram. Radiology 1978; 126:561–567.
52. Hull RD, Raskob GE, Coates G, Panju AA. Clinical validity of a normal perfusion lung scan in patients with suspected pulmonary embolism. Chest 1990; 97:23–26.
53. Palareti G, Legnani C, Cosmi B, Guazzaloca G, Pancani C, Coccheri S. Risk of venous thromboembolism recurrence: high negative predictive value of D-dimer performed after oral anticoagulation is stopped. Thromb Haemost 2002; 87:7–12.
54. Sié P, Cadroy Y, Elias A, Boccalon H, Boneu B. D-dimer levels in patients with long-term antecedents of deep venous thrombosis. Thromb Haemost 1994; 72:161–162.
55. Miron MJ, Perrier A, Bounameaux H, de Moerloose P, Slosman D, Didier D, et al. Contribution of noninvasive evaluation to the diagnosis of pulmonary embolism in hospitalized patients. Eur Respir J 1999; 3:1365–1370.
56. Raimondi P, Bongard O, de Moerloose P, Reber G, Waldvogel F, Bounameaux H. D-dimer plasma concentration in various clinical conditions: Implication for the use of this test in the diagnostic approach of venous thromboembolism. Thromb Res 1993; 69:125–130.
57. 90 Kollef MH, Eisenberg PR, Shannon W. A rapid assay for the detection of circulating D-dimer is associated with clinical outcomes in critically ill patients. Crit Care Med 1998; 26:1054–1060.
58. Barro C, Bosson JL, Pernod G, Carpentier PH, Polack B. Plasma D-dimer

testing improves the management of thromboembolic disease in hospitalized patients. Thromb Res 1999; 95:263–269.

59. Rowbotham BJ, Whitaker AN, Harrison J, et al. Measurement of cross-linked fibrin derivatives in patients undergoing abdominal surgery: use in the diagnosis of postoperative venous thrombosis. Blood Coagul Fibrinolysis 1992; 3:25–30.

60. Bounameaux H, Khabiri E, Huber O, Schneider PA, Didier D, de Moerloose P, Reber G. Value of liquid crystal contact thermography and plasma level of D-dimer for screening of deep venous thrombosis following general abdominal surgery. Thromb Haemost 1992; 67:603–606.

61. Bongard O, Wicky J, Peter R, Simonovska S, Vogel JJ, de Moerloose P, Reber G, Bounameaux H. D-dimer plasma measurement in patients undergoing major hip surgery: use in the prediction and diagnosis of postoperative proximal vein thrombosis. Thromb Res 1994; 74:487–493.

62. Chabloz P, Reber G, Boehlen F, Hohlfeld P, de Moerloose P. TAFI antigen and D-dimer levels during normal pregnancy and at delivery. Br J Haematol 2001; 115:150–152.

63. Cadroy Y, Pierrejean D, Fontan B, et al. Influence of age on the hemostatic system: prothrombin fragment $F1 + 2$, thrombin antithrombin III complexes and D-dimers in 80 healthy subjects with age range from 20 to 94 years. Nouv Rev Fr Hematol 1992; 34:43–46.

64. Righini M, Goehring C, Bounameaux H, Perrier A. Influence of age on performances of common diagnostic tests in suspected pulmonary embolism. Am J Med 2000; 109:357–361.

65. Righini M, de Moerloose P, Reber G, Perrier A, Bounameaux H. Should the D-dimer cut-off value be increased in elderly patients suspected of pulmonary embolism? Thromb Haemost 2001; 85:74.

8

Chest Imaging in Pulmonary Embolism

**ROBIN L. GROSS and
MELVIN R. PRATTER**

University of Medicine and Dentistry
  of New Jersey–Robert Wood
  Johnson Medical School
and Cooper Hospital
Camden, New Jersey, U.S.A.

RICHARD S. IRWIN

University of Massachusetts Medical School
Worcester, Massachusetts, U.S.A.

I. Introduction

Pulmonary embolism (PE) is a common clinical entity. It occurs in approximately 69 people per 100,000 population in the United States (1) with an estimated 630,000 symptomatic pulmonary embolic events occurring each year (2). Untreated, the risk of recurrent PE is 30–60% (3,4) with a mortality rate of approximately 30% (2,3). When treated effectively with anticoagulation, the mortality rate of PE drops dramatically to 1.5–8% (5–7). Thus, it is imperative to make the correct diagnosis in a timely manner.

Because the signs and symptoms of PE lack both sensitivity and specificity, (5–11), physicians must maintain a high index of suspicion for PE and then rely upon a variety of imaging studies to help make the proper diagnosis. Although the postmortem prevalence of PE has not changed appreciably during the past several decades (12,13), the imaging modalities available for diagnosing the disease have undergone significant expansion and development. These technological advances hold great promise for revolutionizing our approach to diagnosing PE that hopefully will decrease both the failure of diagnosis and the mortality. In this chapter, we review the clinical utility of chest imaging in diagnosing PE and focus our discussion on chest radiography, chest ultrasonography, ventilation perfusion lung scanning, chest computed tomographic (CT) scanning, and magnetic resonance imaging (MRI). We will not discuss chest imaging in pregnancy, as this will be covered in Chapter 10.

II. Chest Radiograph

The chest radiograph (CR) is often the first chest imaging study to be performed in patients suspected of having PE. Although the CR may be within normal limits, an abnormal CR is the more common finding in patients with embolic disease. Both the spectrum and frequency of findings have varied among studies. Stein et al. (10) reviewed CRs in patients without cardiac or respiratory disease and found that the CR was abnormal 84% of the time. The most common findings were atelectasis or parenchymal abnormalities, whereas small pleural effusions were noted in almost one-half of the cases. The Urokinase in Pulmonary Embolism Trial (UPET) (5) identified hemidiaphragm elevation and parenchymal abnormality (consolidation) in 41% of patients, whereas 28% had effusions. The International Cooperative Pulmonary Embolism Registry (ICOPER) (14) identified the most common CR findings as cardiomegaly, pleural effusion, elevated hemidiaphragm, pulmonary artery enlargement, atelectasis, and parenchymal infiltrate. In this study, the investigators noted that many patients with PE also had underlying cardiopulmonary disease. Additional CR findings less commonly observed have been reported by others. Westermark (15) described PE without infarction as an area of localized oligemia (Fig. 1). Several early studies (5,16,17) identified pulmonary artery dilatation (Fleischner sign) (18), which often returns to normal size following resolution of PE (16). Signs of pulmonary infarction include Hampton's hump, which is a convex density at an area of postembolic infarction (19) and a healing infarction, which may present as a linear density ending in a nodular rounded shadow adjacent to the pleura (20).

Unfortunately, the CR findings suggestive of PE and/or infarction are not specific. This has recently been confirmed. Worsley (21) reviewed The Prospective Investigation of Pulmonary Embolism Diagnosis (PIOPED) study (22) data and identified atelectasis, lower zone parenchymal density, and pleural effusions as the most frequent findings on CR in patients with PE. However, these abnormalities occurred with equal frequency in the group with no PE. Hampton's hump and the Fleishner sign also occurred equally in both groups. Although localized oligemia occurred significantly more frequently in patients with PE, it was an uncommon finding. Similarly, Greenspan et al. (23) found that none of the expected findings on

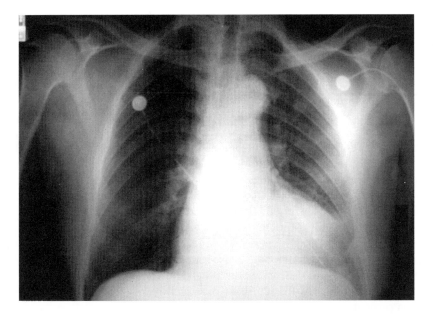

Figure 1 Westermark sign in a patient with a pulmonary embolus obstructing the right main pulmonary artery. Note the paucity of blood vessels (i.e., oligemia) in the right lung compared to the left.

CR was specific for PE. Thus, CR may be helpful to identify other pulmonary diseases, or as part of an algorithm in conjunction with other imaging techniques for the diagnostic evaluation of PE, but is never diagnostic by itself.

III. Chest Ultrasonography

Although venous ultrasonography is commonly used to diagnose deep venous thrombosis of the lower extremities, the utility of chest ultrasonography in the direct diagnosis of PE itself is limited. Findings may include hypoechoic wedge-shaped pleural-based lesions that vary with the nature of associated pleural effusion or infarction, as well as pleural changes (24,25). Ultrasonography of the chest is limited by the fact that only peripheral signs, such as parenchymal or pleural changes, are analyzable and interference from bone and air may skew findings. Echocardiography is discussed in Chapter 9.

IV. Lung Scintigraphy

Lung scintigraphy is often the second diagnostic imaging study performed following CR. In standard ventilation-perfusion ($\dot{V}/\dot{Q}$) scanning, ^{99m}Tc-macroaggregated albumin is injected intravenously with the patient in the supine position to assess perfusion. Six standard views are performed: anterior, posterior, right and left lateral, and right and left posterior oblique. The patient is scanned with a gamma camera and inhales ^{133}xenon, ^{81m}krypton, or ^{99m}Tc-DTPA (diethylentriamine pentaacetate) aerosol while breathing normally to assess ventilation. Two views are performed: anterior and posterior. The initial washin image requires a breath hold and is followed by the equilibrium and washout images (26). In 1964, Wagner (27) described perfusion findings suggested of PE as a "characteristic pattern of avascularity." When combined with ventilation scans, areas of mismatch (28) (i.e., presence of ventilation where there is decreased or absent perfusion) are thought to represent pulmonary embolism (22). However, we have learned that this is not always the case and matched areas of ventilation-perfusion defects may be due to PE (29,30). Consequently, diagnostic interpretation often presents a challenge.

There is no doubt that a normal $\dot{V}/\dot{Q}$ scan is useful, as PIOPED (22) and other studies (31,32) have demonstrated that a normal perfusion scan virtually rules out PE. This was also confirmed by Hull (33), who followed patients who received no anticoagulation for 3 months following normal perfusion scans. Venous thromboembolism (VTE) subsequently occurred in only 0.6% and symptomatic PE occurred in only 0.2% of 515 patients. A nearly normal $\dot{V}/\dot{Q}$ scan is also associated with a low risk (0–11%) of PE (34). In patients with normal/near-normal scans (i.e., those in whom disagreement existed between readers on scans read as normal, low, or very low probability) and low pretest clinical suspicion of PE (based upon investigators' interpretations of history, CR, electrocardiogram (EKG), physical examination, and arterial blood gas results with no distinct algorithm) in PIOPED (22), PE was present in only 2% of patients. A false-negative normal perfusion scan is most unusual but very rarely may occur in association with central nonobstructing PE (35), particularly when there is a relatively equal bilateral resistance to flow through both main pulmonary arteries (36).

Although a normal or near-normal $\dot{V}/\dot{Q}$ scan makes the likelihood of PE very remote, a high-probability $\dot{V}/\dot{Q}$ scan (two or more large mismatched segmental perfusion defects, two or more moderate segmental mismatched perfusion defects plus one large mismatched perfusion defect, or four or more mismatched moderate mismatched segmental perfusion defects) (22) (Fig. 2) renders the diagnosis very likely. In the PIOPED study (22), 96% of the patients with a high clinical index of suspicion and high

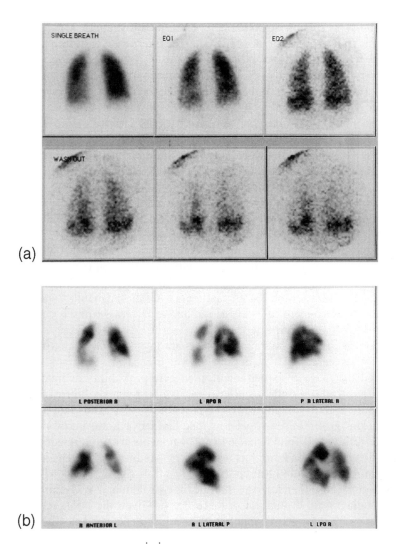

Figure 2 A high-probability V̇/Q̇ scan with a relatively normal (a) ventilation scan and a (b) perfusion scan with multiple bilateral mismatched defects.

probability perfusion scan had PE confirmed by angiogram or clinical outcome follow-up. As in normal scans, the interobserver agreement among readers was very high (95%).

Unfortunately, unless a $\dot{V}/\dot{Q}$ scan is normal/near normal or high probability (which occurs in only 27% of studies) (22), the problem with $\dot{V}/\dot{Q}$ scanning, as demonstrated by the PIOPED study, is a lack of both sensitivity and specificity. Fifty-nine percent of the patients with PE did not have high-probability $\dot{V}/\dot{Q}$ scans. Overall, 73% of the patients studied had scans interpreted as either low probability (nonsegmental perfusion defects, moderate mismatched segmental perfusion defect with normal CR, perfusion defect with larger CR abnormality, large/moderate matching segmental perfusion defects in four or less segments in one lung or three or less segments in one lung region with matching ventilation defect or normal CR, or more than three small segmental perfusion defects with a normal CR) (22) or intermediate probability (those scans not read as normal, very low-, low-, or high probability) (22) and 12% of patients with low-probability scans had PE at angiography or on outcome analysis (22). An earlier report (37) had demonstrated PE in as many as 25–40% patients with low-probability scans. Thus, further diagnostic workup such as pulmonary arteriography is clearly warranted after a nondiagnostic scan.

Unfortunately, pulmonary arteriography is often underutilized because of its perceived risk as an invasive procedure. Sostman et al. (38) reported that 42% of patients with moderate probability or indeterminate scintigrams did not undergo arteriography and remained untreated. Moreover, only 2% of patients with low-probability $\dot{V}/\dot{Q}$ scans had arteriography; in this group of seven patients, one had PE. Khorasani (39) published similar results and found that 64 of 214 patients with intermediate-probability lung scans had no further imaging studies and received no anticoagulation. Patriquin (40) reported that four of eight patients who had PE at autopsy had either low- or intermediate-probability $\dot{V}/\dot{Q}$ scans without further diagnostic evaluation prior to death. Given the hesitancy to order angiography, several investigators have advocated the use of noninvasive imaging studies of the lower extremities (41–47) following nondiagnostic scans. For example, Meyerovitz (48) demonstrated that pulmonary arteriography identified PE in only 8% of 62 patients with low-probability lung scans and negative lower extremity venous ultrasound examinations, and most of these patients (four of five) had subsegmental emboli.

Although noninvasive tests may be helpful in guiding the decision to withhold anticoagulation, the cardiopulmonary status of a patient must be considered when deciding how to proceed with the diagnostic workup following a low-probability scan. Hull et al. (49) demonstrated that if anticoagulation was withheld following a low-probability scan, mortality was significantly higher in patients with poor cardiopulmonary reserve (7.8%) than in those with normal reserve (0.14%). Thus, serial noninvasive tests would be inadequate and arteriography should be performed to rule out PE absolutely before withholding anticoagulation in this high-risk population.

Several investigators have attempted to revise the diagnostic criteria to reduce the frequency of nondiagnostic scans and increase accuracy. For example, the PIOPED investigators (29) subsequently recommended that a moderate-sized perfusion defect with or without matching ventilation should be considered intermediate rather than low probability and that two segmental $\dot{V}/\dot{Q}$ mismatched defects should be classified as intermediate-probability rather than high-probability scans. Others have also attempted to improve the diagnostic yield and interobserver agreement of $\dot{V}/\dot{Q}$ scans by use of structured protocols, (50) standardized forms (51), and anatomical reference charts (52). Also, the value of the CR prior to $\dot{V}/\dot{Q}$ scan has been reassessed, as an abnormal CR is associated with a higher prevalence of nondiagnostic $\dot{V}/\dot{Q}$ scan findings (53) (Fig. 3). Thus, perhaps another diagnostic test, such as spiral CT, should be considered following an abnormal CR if PE is still a consideration.

Other investigators have questioned the additional benefit that the ventilation scan adds to the perfusion imaging. The Prospective Investigative Study of Acute Pulmonary Embolism Diagnosis (PISA-PED) trial (54) revealed that high clinical suspicion with a perfusion scan read as "very likely" to be PE without an accompanying ventilation scan had a 99% positive predictive value. Also, there is some concern that because PE may be associated with transient bronchoconstriction, in some cases, the resultant matched defect may cause the scan to be read as having a lower probability of PE than is actually warranted (55,56). Moreover, patients with cardiopulmonary disease may have abnormalities on ventilation scans that interfere with the proper diagnosis. This is particularly true in chronic obstructive pulmonary disease (COPD), where delayed washout of ^{133}Xe due to airflow obstruction may lead to large and multiple small matched defects that are less likely to be due to PE (57,58). COPD may also be associated with perfusion defects (59,60), possibly secondary to blood vessel changes due to compression or destruction due to emphysema, or vaso-constriction (61). In these cases, the CR in conjunction with the $\dot{V}/\dot{Q}$ scan may be helpful. For example, "triple matched defects" (62) (found on CR and $\dot{V}/\dot{Q}$ scans) may be more consistent with PE if perfusion is absent rather than simply decreased. Although the frequency of indeterminate scans may be higher in patients with cardiopulmonary disease (60,63), the sensitivity and specificity of the high-probability scan appear to be similar to that in patients without cardiopulmonary disease (60,64). Therefore, although some clinicians are hesitant to order $\dot{V}/\dot{Q}$ scans in patients with

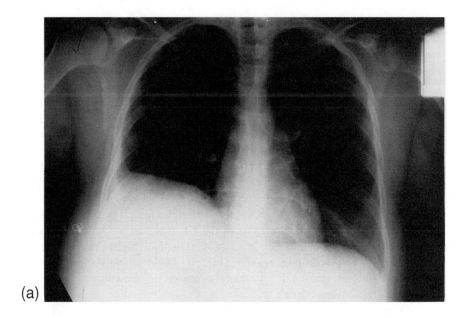

(a)

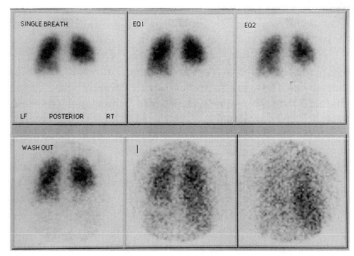

(b)

Figure 3 (a) Chest radiograph of a patient with a right pleural effusion and volume loss. The corresponding nondiagnostic $\dot{V}/\dot{Q}$ scan shows matched (b) ventilation and (c) perfusion defects in the area of abnormality.

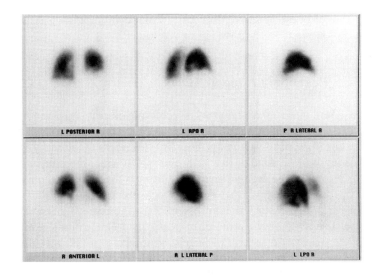

(c)

Figure 3 Continued.

cardiopulmonary disease, this technique is still probably valuable in this patient population.

Some investigators have questioned the need for ventilation scans altogether. Addressing this issue, the American College of Chest Physicians Consensus Committee on pulmonary embolism (65) has suggested that ventilation scans may not be necessary if the perfusion scan is either normal or demonstrates a characteristic defect and CR is normal. Although ^{133}Xe is generally the preferred agent, ventilation scans performed with this aerosol should be performed prior to perfusion scans. Thus, another agent must be used if the perfusion scan is the preliminary test following CR. The American Thoracic Society (66) suggests that if a perfusion defect is high probability, very low probability, or normal, a follow-up ventilation scan is not necessary.

Unfortunately, despite many attempts to improve the accuracy of $\dot{V}/\dot{Q}$ scans, the clinician is often left with nondiagnostic information in the overwhelming majority of cases. Newer techniques are therefore under investigation to improve the diagnostic yield of lung scans. One promising procedure is the $\dot{V}/\dot{Q}$ SPECT scan. Bajc (67) used a porcine model with ^{201}thallium-labeled latex emboli and reported a sensitivity and specificity of 100% each with SPECT imaging and 71 and 91% for planar scintigraphy. Scintigraphic tomography may provide better visualization than planar films and may identify other disease states (68). However, for now, as long as the frequency of nondiagnostic $\dot{V}/\dot{Q}$ scans remains high, additional studies will often be required either to rule in or rule out PE.

V. Pulmonary Arteriography

In 1963, Williams (69) described this technique of using intravenous contrast with a rapid film changer in 50 patients. This was followed by a report by Sasahara (70) using selective (pulmonary arterial) angiography, which permitted the use of a smaller dye load. Since that time, there have been many modifications of the technique. In addition to diagnosing acute PE, placement of the right heart catheter allows measurement of right heart and pulmonary arterial pressures that are essential for the assessment of patients with chronic thromboembolic disease for possible surgical embolectomy (71).

The diagnostic criteria of Sagel and Greenspan (72) are often used to document acute PE. Primary signs include an intraluminal marginal or central filling defect (Fig. 4) with the additional "trailing clot edge" in the opacified vessel if complete obstruction is present. Secondary signs include vessel cutoff (73), abrupt occlusion, oligemia, or vessel pruning. Stein (74) noted that oligemia, asymmetrical filling, prolonged arterial phase, and lower zone filling delay represented flow disturbances and were less specific, because they occurred in other diseases as well as PE. However, morphologically significant signs of filling defects, cutoffs, and vessel pruning were more specific for PE. Auger (75) described the characteristic signs of chronic thromboembolic disease as webs, bands, vascular narrowing or obstruction, intimal irregularities, and pouching (formed by a concave-shaped obstructing thrombus).

Various techniques exist for arteriography. These include selective and superselective (lobar and segmental) arteriography, which enable anatomically directed visualization. Both conventional film angiography (CFA) and digital subtraction angiography (DSA) are available and their ability to image PE has been compared. DSA produces multiple immediately available planar images and permits visualization in the cine mode; techniques that subtract overlapped anatomical structures and allow image manipulation result in better visualization (76). Also, pulsation artifact may be eliminated, and this enhances assessment of vessels in the pericardiac region (77). Less time and contrast (76,78,79) is required for this technique (78), which may also decrease cost. Generally, radiation doses of each technique are comparable. Although there is less spatial resolution with DSA (76,80), reader agreement may be higher. Van Beek et al. (78) compared DSA with CFA in patients with nondiagnostic $\dot{V}/\dot{Q}$ scans (although each patient did not receive both tests) and found > 88% reader agreement with DSA versus

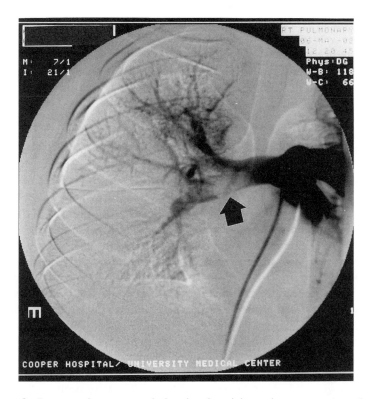

Figure 4 Large pulmonary embolus in the right pulmonary artery (arrow) presenting as a filling defect on pulmonary arteriography.

20–36% disagreement with CFA. Embolic distribution was similar in both groups, and DSA was judged to be of better quality. Johnson (77) performed both DSA and CFA on 80 patients and reported a 92 and 69% sensitivity of DSA and CFA, respectively. Although there were no statistically significant differences in sensitivity or specificity between the two techniques, reader confidence was higher with DSA. Schleuter et al. (80) compared the two techniques in a porcine model with pathological follow-up. Overall, sensitivity for film screen (conventional) angiography was 72% and for DSA 65% without a statistically significant difference. Positive predictive value (89 and 87%, respectively) and interobserver reader agreement (80 and 84%, respectively) were also similar. Since DSA is comparable to CFA, is less costly, and permits the use of less contrast as well as imaging adjustment at the workstation, we recommend DSA as the procedure of choice for the evaluation of PE. In fact, DSA has become the standard technique in most interventional radiology laboratories.

During arteriography, the patient is sedated and the catheter is guided through the femoral vein to the right heart, where right heart and pulmonary artery pressures are measured. When lung scanning has been performed prior to angiography, catheter placement is directed toward abnormal areas noted on scintigraphy. Some interventional radiology laboratories have standard protocols for discontinuation of the procedure in the setting of significant pulmonary hypertension. Approximately 50 mL of contrast is then injected into the vessels and images are obtained.

Relative contraindications to the procedure include dye allergy, recent myocardial infarction, ventricular irritability (73), and renal failure. However, these situations rarely preclude the use of angiography when truly indicated. The complication rate is low and ranges from 1 to 5% (73,81,82) with death rates of 0–0.7% (71,81–84) These rates may be higher in patients in the intensive care unit (81,84). Cardiac perforation (5,73,83), reported in earlier studies, should no longer occur, because pigtail catheters have replaced straight catheters. Although arrhythmias may occur with catheter advancement (81,83,84), they are also less likely to occur with the pigtail catheters; ventricular fibrillation secondary to ventricular irritability is usually treatable (83). Patients with known conduction delays are either paced or an external pacemaker or a pacing catheter is readily available. Bronchospasm, particularly in asthmatic patients (73), may occur, as may anaphylaxis and respiratory failure. Pulmonary arterial hypertension and right ventricular dysfunction may (82,85) or may not (71,82) be associated with increased morbidity and mortality and the risk may be less with lower osmolar and/or nonionic agents (84,86) (which are more expensive) (88). The risk of dye-induced renal failure is higher in the elderly (81), those with preexisting renal disease (85), or other risk factors, such as diabetes mellitus (87,88). Prophylactic agents such as fenoldopam (88), theophylline (89), and especially acetylcysteine (90) may be useful to prevent worsening renal failure and are currently under investigation.

The challenge in assessing the accuracy of pulmonary arteriography is that it is considered to be the reference standard in the diagnosis of PE. Baile et al. (91) used methacrylate resin emboli in pigs and found that the sensitivity and positive predictive value of angiography was only 87 and 88%, respectively, when compared with postmortem corrosion casted lungs. However, it has been generally accepted that a negative pulmonary arteriogram is associated with a very low prevalence of clinically significant PE (92). Novelline (93) followed 167 patients for 6 months following negative pulmonary angiograms for suspicious PE. Of the 20 patients who died, PE was not considered to be the cause of death (although 3 of 10 autopsies revealed small PE), and 147 patients alive at 6 months had no signs of symptoms of PE. Thus, emboli too small for detection by pulmonary arteriography were considered to be clinically insignificant. In PIOPED (22), 380 patients with negative angiograms received no anticoagulation. On 1-year follow-up (94), only 1.6% of these patients returned with PE.

Controversy still exists regarding the diagnosis of emboli in subsegmental vessels (5,80,95). In PIOPED (96), only 6% of emboli were located only in subsegmental vessels. Diffin et al. (97) found that although only 17% of 29 patients had PE isolated to the subsegmental level or smaller, interobserver agreement significantly decreased to only 45% when assessing PE at this level compared with 83% when segmental or larger vessels were analyzed. When Schleuter (80) compared DSA with film screen (conventional) angiography (FSA) in a porcine model, diagnostic sensitivity decreased in peripheral vessels with both techniques. FSA sensitivity was 91% in third-order vessels versus only 62% in fifth-order (subsegmental) vessels, and DSA sensitivity was 98 and 49% for third-order and fifth-order vessels, respectively. Interestingly, on pathological examination, 52% of emboli were fifth order or smaller. Quinn (98) reported lower reader agreement (in 13 of 15 cases) with subsegmental analysis, and suggested this may be due to the fact that injecting contrast into larger arteries results in overlapping opacified subsegmental vessels, particularly in atelectatic regions. Therefore, if PE is not detected by selective arteriography, superselective arteriography (99) may assist in the diagnosis of subsegmental PE, as vessels as small as 0.5 mm can be visualized with this technique.

Despite the difficulty in detecting smaller PE, the question as to whether they are clinically significant is a source of controversy (100,101). Novelline (93) would suggest that they are of doubtful clinical significance. However, Oser et al. (102) suggest otherwise after finding subsegmental emboli in 30% of 76 patients with positive angiograms; 17% of these patients had emboli limited to subsegmental or smaller vessels and most were multiple. Oser et al. suggest that these emboli are reflective of a larger spectrum of thromboembolic disease and should not be ignored given the mortality when the disease remains untreated. As PE is a disease with a high rate of recurrence (3,4), the clinician should be aware that subsequent embolic events following subsegmental PE may be massive and fatal.

Although pulmonary arteriography is still considered the reference standard in the diagnosis of PE, it should be appreciated that nondiagnostic pulmonary arteriograms do occasionally occur (0.9–5.0%) (54,73,79,81); they are usually related to poor image quality (73,79). For this reason and others (e.g., the study is invasive, requires skill both for performance and interpretation, and is not always available in many institutions), investigators have sought other techniques to diagnose PE. The most widely accepted alternative is spiral or helical computed tomography (CT) with contrast.

VI. Computed Tomography

Since Sinner (103) first reported the use of spiral or helical chest CT with contrast in the diagnosis of PE in 1982, this test has gained widespread acceptance as a valuable tool in the diagnostic evaluation of PE. In fact, in some instances, it is the first imaging modality used to diagnose PE. Compared to pulmonary arteriography, CT is usually available at all hours and does not require the presence of a skilled radiologist to perform the procedure. Also, CT may reveal unexpected abnormalities (104–107), such as parenchymal consolidation or pleural effusion that suggest alternate diagnoses. Similar to angiography, however, the administration of potentially nephrotoxic dye is a necessary part of the procedure. Therefore, if the CT scan is nondiagnostic, some patients may require a subsequent pulmonary arteriogram and will be subjected to another dye load, although this may not be as problematic as previously suspected. Ost recently (108) reported no difference in creatinine elevation in patients who had spiral CT alone versus spiral CT and conventional angiography. Creatinine levels returned to baseline in the few patients whose creatinine rose more than 1 mg/dL. Garg (106) reported no adverse reactions in patients who had an additional dye load when angiography and CT were both performed within 48-hr period.

During spiral CT, the patient is scanned in either the caudocranial or craniocaudal direction, and the field typically extends from the top of the aortic arch to below the inferior pulmonary veins. Contrast is injected at a constant rate following a delay that is approximately 15 sec or is extrapolated from a time-attenuation curve determined by a test dose (109). Rapid imaging occurs during a breath hold that lasts approximately 24 sec (110) while the detector rotates around the patient (111). Patients who are unable to hold their breath are instructed to breathe quietly during the procedure. In this situation, CT images are performed using a faster table feed that may result in false-positive findings at the segmental vessel level secondary to motion. This is less of a problem if the radiologist is aware of the technique used (112). Images are taken at variable collimation intervals and then reconstructed; they are best viewed and manipulated at the workstation by trained radiologists (113).

Complications are uncommon and include those associated with contrast dye, as described previously, although the dose of dye is lower than that used for arteriography (114). Protocols have been developed to prevent dye-induced anaphylaxis and contrast-induced nephropathy (Table 1). The most

Table 1 Prophylaxis for Contrast Administration

I. Chronic renal insufficiency[a]
    Acetycysteine 600 mg twice daily for 2 days
       Begin 1 day prior to contrast
    0.45 NS 1 cc/kg/hr for 12 hr before and 12 hr after contrast
II. Dye allergy or asthma
    A. Nonemergent:
        Prednisone 50 mg PO 16 hr prior to exam
                  50 mg PO 8 hr prior to exam
                  50 mg PO 1 hr prior to exam
        Cimetidine 300 mg PO 1 hr prior to exam
        Diphenhydramine 25 mg PO 1 hr prior to exam
    B. Emergent
        Solumedrol 125 mg IV prior to exam
        Cimetadine 300 mg/50 cc NS IV prior to exam
        Diphenhydramine 50 mg IV prior to exam

[a] From Ref. 115.

commonly used agent to mitigate contrast-induced nephropathy is acetyl-cysteine, which must be started the day before the procedure (115). Thus, if a spiral CT is required to rule out PE by the second day in an anticoagu-lated patient, it may be reasonable to start acetylcysteine in the patient with renal insufficiency.

Criteria for the CT diagnosis of acute PE are complete or partial filling defects (Fig. 5), secondary findings are the "railway track" sign (free-floating embolic masses that permit blood flow between the vessel wall and embolus) (111), and mural defects (110). The findings of chronic thromboembolism, like those of angiography, are eccentric defects that adhere to the vessel wall with recanalization (116,117) and a web sign (linear filling defect in a vessel of small or normal size) (106). Knowledge of the anatomy is of the utmost importance, as intersegmental (110,118) or hilar (113) lymph nodes may be mistaken for emboli. Vessels that run in an oblique, rather than vertical, direction such as those in the lingula or right middle lobe may be difficult to analyze (106,110,113,117–122). Other prob-lems include incomplete opacification, motion artifact (110,112), and poor signal-to-noise ratio (123).

In 1992, Remy-Jardin (110) first compared spiral volumetric CT with pulmonary arteriography, the gold standard for the diagnosis of PE. In this group of 42 patients, the sensitivity of spiral CT was 100% and its specificity 96%. This was followed by a subsequent report by the same investigators

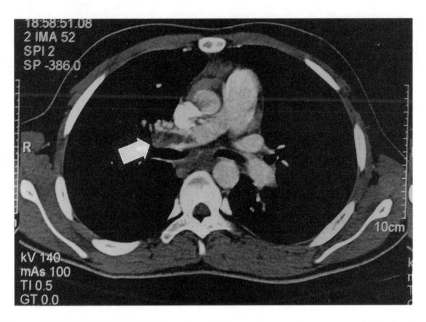

Figure 5 Spiral chest CT with contrast shows a large pulmonary embolus in the right pulmonary artery (arrow) presenting as a filling defect.

(124) on 75 patients that included inconclusive CT studies (9% of the studies) and resulted in a lower sensitivity and specificity of 91 and 78%, respectively. Van Rossum (125) found that the sensitivity of CT was 95% and specificity 97% using either high-probability $\dot{V}/\dot{Q}$ scans or pulmonary arteriography as the reference standard. In that study, patients with non-diagnostic $\dot{V}/\dot{Q}$ scans had pulmonary arteriography performed. In that subgroup, the positive predictive value of CT was 83% compared to 17% for the $\dot{V}/\dot{Q}$ scan. Therefore, this study demonstrated that the specificity of CT was considerably higher than $\dot{V}/\dot{Q}$ with comparable sensitivity. Similarly, Mayo (123) reported that the sensitivity of spiral CT was superior to scintigraphy (87 vs 65%) and the kappa statistic (κ), an indicator of inter-observer agreement, was 0.85 for spiral CT and 0.61 for $\dot{V}/\dot{Q}$ scanning.

Unfortunately, more recent studies have failed to confirm the initial high sensitivities described above. The explanation for this apparent loss of sensitivity appears to be the recognition that spiral CT often misses relatively small PE. Several investigators have addressed difficulties associated with identifying segmental and subsegmental vessels (104,105,113,120–122,126,127). Goodman (122) reported that the sensitivity of helical CT declined from 86 to 63% when subsegmental vessels were included in the analysis with central pulmonary arteries. As in arteriography, interobserver agreement declines with decreasing vessel size. Chartrand-Lefebvre (113) specifically looked at this issue in 60 patients whose CT scans were reviewed 3 months after initial presentation. Interobserver agreement was related to vessel size, as κ declined from 0.75 for lobar artery to 0.47 for segmental artery evaluation. When the same radiologists blindly reviewed these films 2 months later, intraobserver agreement revealed similar differences between larger and smaller vessels. Perrier (126) found that although interobserver agreement was excellent, false-positive rates were 38% in segmental, 15% in lobar, and 0% in main pulmonary artery readings in a series of out-patients. However, the incidence of PE in the study population was low, and many of the patients had been excluded based upon a negative d-dimer prior to CT evaluation.

Newer techniques to improve visualization in smaller vessels have resulted in higher diagnostic success rates. Using thin collimation CT (2-mm instead of 3- 5-mm collimation) increases the number of analyzable subsegments (127) as well as interobserver agreement (104). Dual section helical CT increases the z-axis (longitudinal axis) to include subsegmental vessels in the lower lobes that may be missed by routine spiral CT (114). Thinner collimation images may be reconstructed at 1.3-mm intervals and the use of overlapping lowers partial volume averaging. However, subsegmental PE may still be missed by this method. Multidetector row spiral CT scanners (128,129) have four detector arrays that simultaneously scan several images, which are then reconstructed. This technique permits shorter CT scan times. Although Raptopoulos (128) recently reported that this technique identified more subsegmental emboli than single-detector CT, these studies were not performed in the same patients; nor were they compared with arteriography results. Ghay et al. (130) recently reported that multidetector row spiral CT reconstructed scans of 1.25-mm thick sections permitted analysis of 94% subsegmental arteries versus 82% when 3-mm thick reconstructions were analyzed in the same patients. Thus, rapid scanning with thinner collimation may increase the sensitivity of multidetector spiral CT at the subsegmental level. Other CT techniques are currently in use for diagnosing PE. Electron beam CT, which is faster than spiral CT and uses less contrast (116,117), may have less motion artifact (secondary to shorter breath-holding times) and better opacification than spiral CT (121). Goldin et al. (131) recently demonstrated 86% sensitivity in detecting segmental and subsegmental emboli in a porcine model when compared with arteriography. CT with lower extremity venography (132–134) combined with CT pulmonary arteriography is currently under investigation and may be promising as diagnostic test in the evaluation of PE as well.

Because the question regarding the clinical importance of subsegmental emboli identification is still pertinent despite newer techniques, several investigators have analyzed patient outcome while withholding anticoagulation following negative CT scans (105,135). Ferretti (136), using helical CT a 5-mm collimation intervals (after intermediate-probability $\dot{V}/\dot{Q}$ scan and negative lower extremity duplex studies) reported after a 3-month follow-up that only 3 of 109 patients who did not receive treatment had recurrent PE. Overall, the false-negative rate was 5.4%, and results may have been even better had thinner sections been used. In a retrospective review, Lomis (137) followed 100 patients who had CT performed with 3-mm collimation and found that none of the 81 patients alive after 6 months had recurrent PE; none of the deaths had been attributable to thromboembolic disease. Gostäter (138) was able to identify VTE in 1.4% and death in 0.5% of 215 patients with a negative spiral CT afte a 3-month follow-up and cited a negative predictive value of 98.6% for excluding PE. Most of these patients had not had further diagnostic testing after negative spiral CT. They noted that the one death from PE occurred in a patient with severe cardiopulmonary disease. They suggested, as Hull had earlier (49), that these high-risk patients require additional workup to rule out PE, as the consequences of missing the diagnosis are potentially dire. On recent retrospective review, Swensen (139) found that the 3-month cumulative incidence of venous thromboembolism was 0.5% after a negative electron beam CT. Thus, outcomes may be comparable to those following a negative pulmonary arteriogram. As previously mentioned, because arteriography is typically used as the reference standard, it is worth noting that the sensitivity and positive predictive values for CT were comparable to arteriography in one study where pathological findings were used as the true "gold" standard (91).

Cost-analysis studies have suggested that diagnostic algorithms that include spiral CT are associated with improved survival and may be more cost effective (140,141). In clinical practice, CT scans are either obtained following nondiagnostic $\dot{V}/\dot{Q}$ scans, when $\dot{V}/\dot{Q}$ scan findings are discordant with clinical suspicion, or in lieu of $\dot{V}/\dot{Q}$ scans. Although controversy exists regarding whether CT should replace $\dot{V}/\dot{Q}$ and/or arteriography (120,140, 142,143), many physicians readily accept CT findings as fact. However, recent critical reviews (111,144) of experimental designs to evaluate CT in this setting have documented inconsistent methodology and enrollment criteria, as well as heterogeneous study populations. Thus, combined results have been uninterpretable and unless central PE is documented, accepting CT as a lone diagnostic test should be approached with caution. CT may be valuable when used as part of a diagnostic algorithm to obviate the need for pulmonary arteriography or as an initial imaging technique in the setting of an abnormal CR when there is a higher likelihood of nondiagnostic $\dot{V}/\dot{Q}$ results (53).

VII. Magnetic Resonance Imaging

The ability of magnetic resonance imaging (MRI) to detect PE has been studied for years. Even with refinements in the technique specifically to highlight the pulmonary vessels (magnetic resonance angiography [MRA]), this technique has not gained the wide acceptance of spiral CT. This is somewhat surprising, because the benefits of this technique include the lack of nephrotoxic dye and ionizing radiation (145), and like spiral CT, the lower extremities may be visualized during the same study without an additional dye load (146). Potential explanations for the lack of acceptance include patient claustrophobia in centers that do not have open MRI machines and the need to exclude patients with pacemakers, implanted metal other than titanium, or, in some centers, those requiring mechanical ventilation. In addition, one could speculate that unlike CT, MRI has never been considered to be a test that is readily available in the setting of a medical emergency.

For the detection of pulmonary emboli, early studies used T1-weighted spin-echo sequences (147). Techniques to improve visualization include respiratory and cardiac gating, dynamic cine gradient-echo scans to help distinguish clot from slow blood flow (147–149), and spatial modulation of magnetization, which uses tagging stripes to differentiate slow blood flow from embolus (150). Using a shorter single breath-hold during MRA eliminates motion artifact due to ventilation and may permit visualization of subsegmental vessels (151). Three-dimensional views with gadolinium allow better visualization of overlapping vessels (151) and images may be manipulated at a workstation. Criteria for the diagnosis of PE are an intravascular filling defect or abrupt vessel cutoff (152). Chronic thrombus presents as a low-signal–intensity mural defect (148). Factors leading to errors in diagnosis include slow flowing blood (146,153–155) and the misdiagnosis of perihilar fat or vein for clot (153,155). Gamsu (155) found that problems associated with identification of central clots injected into dogs were attributable to hilar fat and blood being mistaken for clot (in diastole). Slow flowing blood tends to be a common problem in chronic thromboembolism (145) and may present a diagnostic challenge.

In an initial study in dogs, Pope (156) reported a sensitivity of 82% and specificity of 88% (compared with pathological findings of PE) when respiratory and cardiac gating were used. False positives and negatives occurred in areas of atelectasis or infiltrate, and most of the emboli were peripheral.

Erdman et al. (153) compared MRI with arteriography and V̇/Q̇ scanning and reported a 90% sensitivity, 77% specificity, 86% positive predictive value, and 83% negative predictive value when compared with angiography. MR correctly predicted the angiographic reading in 21 of 22 indeterminate V̇/Q̇ scans. Meaney (157) reported a sensitivity of 100% and specificity of 95% when MRA was compared with pulmonary arteriography. Grist (146) compared MRA with pulmonary arteriography, high-probability V̇/Q̇ scans with positive lower extremity ultrasonography, and spiral CT and found a sensitivity of 92–100% and specificity of 62%. Gupta (152) reported an MRA sensitivity of 85% and specificity of 96% when compared with DSA, although interobserver agreement and sensitivity decreased at the subsegmental level. Schiebler (154) reported that clots smaller than 1 cm were associated with lower reader confidence and that the resolution of MRI was inferior to arteriography. Thus, MRI has the same technical difficulties in identifying subsegmental emboli as CT and arteriography.

Several studies have directly compared spiral CT with MRI. In a preliminary study, Holland (158) compared MRA with ultrafast CT in 16 patients with high-probability V̇/Q̇ scans. Results were compared with pulmonary arteriography or surgical thromboendarterectomy. For CT and MRA, the sensitivity was 92 and 79%, respectively, and specificity was 100 and 100%, respectively. Accuracy was 94% for CT and 84% for MRI. Woodard (159) compared these techniques in dogs and found that 84% of emboli documented at autopsy were detected by spiral CT, whereas only 69% were documented by MRI. As expected, the ability to detect emboli with both techniques declined with vessel size. This was confirmed in a similar study by Hurst (160), who reported CT and MRI sensitivities of 88 and 54%, respectively, with 100% specificity for both techniques. The difference in sensitivity between the techniqes persisted at the subsegmental level. Other recent studies have shown a similar detection capability of MR and CT. In a porcine model, using a pulmonary arterial tree cast as the reference, Reittner (161) reported similar sensitivity (76 and 82%) and positive predictive value (92 and 94%) for CT and MRA. In humans, Sostman (162) compared results of CT in 28 patients with MRI in 25 patients. Using positive pulmonary arteriography and high-probability V̇/Q̇ scan as reference standards, the techniques were similar when interpreted by skilled MR radiologists. Sensitivity of CT and MR were 73 and 71%, respectively, and specificity for CT and MR were both 97%. These statistics declined when radiologists with less experience interpreted the results.

In summary, although MRI/MRA may be used to diagnose PE, its sensitivity and accuracy appear to be no better than, or perhaps inferior to, spiral CT. Therefore, its utility may be restricted to the setting of an abnormal CR, when a V̇/Q̇ scan would be expected to be nondiagnostic and contraindication to contrast precludes the use of spiral CT. Furthermore, like spiral CT, skilled interpretation is necessary (159,162), and, as most centers do not routinely perform MRI for this purpose, readers may lack the experience necessary to apply this technique adequately.

Finally, promising newer techniques are emerging, such as $\dot{V}/\dot{Q}$ MRI, in which 100% oxygen is used for ventilation enhancement (163). Although this technique is in the developmental stage, it offers potential for MRI to assume a more prominent role among the diagnostic modalities used for diagnosing PE.

VIII. Diagnostic Algorithms

The fact that all of the aforementioned imaging techniques have clear limitations has led to the recommendation of an algorithmic approach to the diagnosis of PE. The primary issues are that smaller, subsegmental pulmonary emboli may not be consistently diagnosed by any of the available imaging techniques (113,122,126,154,155,159,160) and that arteriography (the gold standard) is invasive and underutilized (40,67,75) and may also miss subsegmental emboli (80,97).

To minimize the need to order chest imaging studies, many of the proposed algorithms include noninvasive imaging of the lower extremities. This is based upon the premise that up to 50% patients with PE have proximal DVT of the legs (37) and that proximal thrombi are the ones most likely to result in clinically significant PE (43). Hull (43) followed outpatients who had adequate cardiopulmonary reserve and nondiagnostic lung scans for 2 weeks with serial impedance plethysmography (IPG) of the lower extremities. Following an initial negative IPG, repeat studies were performed on days 3, 5 or 7, 10, and 14; anticoagulation was withheld if the scans remained negative. In this cohort of 711 patients, 9.5% patients had proximal vein thrombosis (DVT) on initial testing and serial testing revealed DVT in only 2.3% additional patients. During a 3-month follow-up of the remaining patients, only 1.9% of patients had VTE; a result comparable to the incidence within the population with normal lung scans. These results have been confirmed with venous ultrasonography (47,164,165). Stein (45) applied this approach using data from PIOPED and estimated that serial noninvasive leg examinations would have reduced the requirement for arteriography to 41% of 468 patients with nondiagnostic lung scans. They recommended serial noninvasive lower extremity testing or arteriography in patients with a negative initial leg test who have "adequate" cardiorespiratory reserve.

Other studies have used lower extremity imaging in conjunction with d-dimer, a cross-linked fibrin degradation product (discussed in Chapter 7).

Quinn (166) used d-dimer by the ELISA (enzyme-linked immunosorbent assay) method with lower extremity ultrasound in 36 patients with intermediate $\dot{V}/\dot{Q}$ scans and found that pulmonary arteriography remained a necessary examination, as lower extremity imaging with d-dimer diagnosed or excluded PE in only 19% of the patients. More favorable results were reported by Perrier (47), who evaluated patients in the emergency department with nondiagnostic lung scans using clinical probability, d-dimer (ELISA), and lower extremity ultrasound, followed by angiography when appropriate; patients were followed for 6 months. Of note is the fact that a nondiagnostic scan in the context of low or high clinical probability was used to rule out or diagnose PE. Using this protocol, 62% of patients with nondiagnostic scans could be diagnosed with a 1% chance of recurrent VTE during a 6-month follow-up. A follow-up study (167) revealed a 1.7% risk of VTE in untreated patients who had low clinical probability, a nondiagnostic lung scan, and normal lower extremity ultrasound. However, neither of these studies used a standardized scoring system for the clinical probability of PE.

Wells et al. (46) designed a clinical model using a scoring system for clinical signs and symptoms, EKG, CR, and risk factors for VTE to determine pretest probability in 1239 patients who then underwent scintigraphy and bilateral ultrasonography of the lower extremities. In the setting of a negative ultrasound, discordant pretest probability and $\dot{V}/\dot{Q}$ scan results required performance of contrast venography and possibly pulmonary angiography. Patients with low to moderate pretest probability and a non–high-probability $\dot{V}/\dot{Q}$ scan underwent serial lower extremity ultrasound studies for 2 weeks. Using this strategy, only 3.7% patients required venography or arteriography. The incidence of VTE on 3-month follow-up was 0.5% and none of the deaths were due to PE. A subsequent algorithm (164) required no further testing in untreated emergency department patients with a low index of suspicion for PE (by scoring system) and negative d-dimer (SimpliRed whole-blood agglutination d-dimer). Only 1 of these 437 patients had PE on 3-month follow-up. A higher clinical suspicion for PE required scintigraphy; if nondiagnostic or discordant with clinical suspicion, lower extremity ultrasonography, and possibly arteriography or serial ultrasonography were performed. Only 0.1% of patients who completed this entire protocol had VTE on follow-up. Thus, diagnostic imaging of the chest was necessary in only one-half of the population. Although the d-dimer assay used in this study had higher reported specificity, several d-dimer assays are available, and results are often variable (168). This may account for inconsistent results among studies utilizing d-dimer in an algorithmic approach to PE.

Spiral CT is a component of newer diagnostic models. Lorut (169) assessed spiral CT, $\dot{V}/\dot{Q}$ scan, d-dimer, and, if necessary, lower extremity ultrasound. Only 1% of 247 patients required arteriography for diagnosis; VTE was diagnosed in only 1.7% at 3-month follow-up and no patients died. As previously mentioned, Ferretti (136) used spiral CT as part of a diagnostic algorith and found that only 5.4% patients with a negative CT had PE.

The literature is replete with algorithms for the diagnosis of PE (44,66,143,164,170–172). Although some recommend replacing $\dot{V}/\dot{Q}$ scan with spiral CT (143,171), there are, as discussed, inherent limitations with spiral CT. Moreover, a normal or high-probability perfusion scan is diagnostic, and a nondiagnostic perfusion scan may be used to direct attention on further imaging studies, such as arteriography (173). In choosing the appropriate algorithm, several factors must be considered, such as hemodynamic stability of the patient, underlying cardiopulmonary status, clinical index of suspicion, availability of procedures, and contraindication to dye-requiring techniques. By integrating clinical skills, diagnostic acumen, and a clear understanding of the benefits and limitations of the currently available techniques to determine the presence or absence of VTE, the likelihood of accurately assessing the patient in whom PE is a diagnostic consideration should be enhanced.

References

1. Silverstein MD, Heit JA, Mohr DN, Petterson TM, O'Fallon WM, Melton LJ III. Trends in the incidence of deep vein thrombosis and pulmonary embolism: a 25-year population-based study. Arch Intern Med 1998; 158:585–593.
2. Dalen JE, Alpert JS. Natural history of pulmonary embolism. Prog Cardiovasc Dis 1975; 17:259–270.
3. Hermann RE, Davis JH, Holden WD. Pulmonary embolism: a clinical and pathologic study with emphasis on the effect of prophylactic therapy with anticoagulants. Am J Surg 1961; 102:19–28.
4. Barker NW. The diagnosis and treatment of pulmonary embolism. Med Clin North Am 1958; 42:1053–1063.
5. The urokinase pulmonary embolism trial: a national cooperative study. Circulation 1973; 47/48(suppl 2):1–108.
6. Douketis JD, Kearon C, Bates S, Duku EK, Ginsberg JS. Risk of fatal pulmonary embolism in patients with treated venous thromboembolism. JAMA 1998; 279:458–462.
7. Alpert JS, Smith R, Carlson J, Ockene IS, Dexter L, Dalen JE. Mortality in patients treated for pulmonary embolism. JAMA 1976; 236:1477–1480.
8. Sasahara AA, Cannilla JE, Morse RL, Sidd JJ, Tremblay GM. Clinical and physiologic studies in pulmonary thromboembolism. Am J Cardiol 1967; 20:10–20.
9. Anderson FA, Wheeler B, Goldberg RJ, Hosmer DW, Patwardhan NA,

Jovanovic B, Forcier A, Dalen JE. A population-based perspective of the hospital incidence and case-fatality rates of deep vein thrombosis and pulmonary embolism. Arch Intern Med 1991; 151:933–938.

10. Stein PD, Terrin ML, Hales CA, Palevsky HI, Saltzman HA, Thompson BT, Weg JG. Clinical, laboratory, roentgenographic and electrocardiographic findings in patients with acute pulmonary embolism and no pre-existing cardiac or pulmonary disease. Chest 1991; 100:598–603.

11. Moser KM. Venous thromboembolism. Am Rev Respir Dis 1990; 141:235–249.

12. Stein PD, Henry JW. Prevalence of acute pulmonary embolism among patients in a general hospital and at autopsy. Chest 1995; 108:978–981.

13. Ryu JH, Olson EJ, Pellikka PA. Clinical recognition of pulmonary embolism: problem of unrecognized and asymptomatic cases. Mayo Clin Proc 1998; 73:873–879.

14. Elliot CG, Goldhaber SZ, Visani L, DeRosa M. Chest radiographs in acute pulmonary embolism. Results from the international cooperative pulmonary embolism registry. Chest 2000; 118:33–38.

15. Westermark N. On the roentgen diagnosis of lung embolism: brief review of the incidence, pathology and clinical symptoms of lung embolism. Acta Radiol 1938; 19:357–372.

16. Chang CHJ, Davis WC. A roentgen sign of pulmonary infarction. Clin Radiol 1965; 16:141–147.

17. Davis WC. Immediate diagnosis of pulmonary embolus. Am Surg 1964; 30:291–294.

18. Fleischner FG. Pulmonary embolism. Clin Radiol 1962; 13:169–182.

19. Hampton AO, Castleman B. Correlation of postmortem chest teleroentgenograms with autopsy findings. Am J Roentgen Rad Ther 1940; 43:305–326.

20. Fleischner F, Hampton AO, Castleman B. Linear shadows in the lung. AJR Am J Roentgerol 1941; 46:610–618.

21. Worsley DF, Alavi A, Aronchick JM, Chen JTT, Greenspan RH, Ravin CE. Chest radiographic findings in patients with acute pulmonary embolism: observation from the PIOPED study. Radiology 1993; 189:133–136.

22. The PIOPED Investigators. Value of the ventilation/perfusion scan in acute pulmonary embolism. JAMA 1990; 263:2753–2759.

23. Greenspan RH, Ravin CE, Polansky SM, McLoud TC. Accuracy of the chest radiograph in diagnosis of pulmonary embolism. Invest Radiol 1982; 17:539–543.

24. Reissig A, Heyne JP, Kroegel C. Sonography of lung and pleura in pulmonary embolism. Chest 2001; 120:1977–1983.

25. Mathis G, Metzler J, Fussenegger D, Sutterlütti G, Feurstein M, Fritzsche H. Sonographic observation of pulmonary infarction and early infarctions by pulmonary embolism. Eur Heart J 1993; 14:804–808.

26. Fraser RS, Müller NL, Colman N, Paré PD. Thrombosis and thromboembolism. In: Diagnosis of Diseases of the Chest. Vol. 3. 4th ed. Philadelphia: Saunders, 1999:1800–1802.

27. Wagner HN, Sabiston DC, McAfee JG, Tow D, Stern HS. Diagnosis of massive pulmonary embolism in man by radioisotope scanning. N Engl J Med 1964; 271:377–384.

28. McNeil BJ. Ventilation-perfusion studies and the diagnosis of pulmonary embolism: concise communication. J Nucl Med 1980; 21:319–323.

29. Gottschalk A, Sostman HD, Coleman RE, Juni JE, Thrall J, McKusick KA, Froelich JW, Alavi A. Ventilation-perfusion scintigraphy in the PIOPED study: Part II. Evaluation of the scintigraphic criteria and interpretations. J Nucl Med 1993; 34:1119–1126.

30. Hull RD, Hirsh J, Carter CJ, Jay RM, Dodd PE, Ockelford PA, Coates G, Gill GJ, Turpie G, Doyle DJ, Buller HR, Raskob GE. Pulmonary angiography, ventilation lung scanning and venography for clinically suspected pulmonary embolism with abnormal perfusion lung scan. Ann Intern Med 1983; 98:891–899.

31. van Beek EJR, Kuyer PMM, Schenk BE, Brandjes PM, ten Cate JW, Büller HR. A normal perfusion lung scan in patients with clinically suspected pulmonary embolism: frequency and clinical validity. Chest 1995; 108:170–173.

32. Trujillo NP, Pratt JP, Talusani S, Quaife RA, Kumpe D, Lear JL. DTPA aerosol in ventilation/perfusion scintigraphy for diagnosing pulmonary embolism. J Nucl Med 1997; 38:1781–1783.

33. Hull RD, Raskob GE, Coates G, Panju AA. Clinical validity of a normal perfusion lung scan in patients with suspected pulmonary embolism. Chest 1990; 97:23–26.

34. Henry JW, Stein PD, Gottschalk A, Raskob GE. Pulmonary embolism among patients with a nearly normal ventilation/perfusion lung scan. Chest 1996; 110:395–398.

35. Moser KM, Harsanyi P, Rius-Garriga J, Guisan M, Landis GA, Miale A Jr. Assessment of pulmonary photoscanning and angiography in experimental pulmonary embolism. Circulation 1969; 39:663–674.

36. Wilson JE, Frenkel EP, Pierce AK, Johnson RL Jr, Winga ER, Curry GC, Mierzwiak DS. Spontaneous fibrinolysis in pulmonary embolism. J Clin Invest 1971; 50:474–480.

37. Hull RD, Hirsh J, Carter CJ, Raskob GE, Gill GJ, Jay RM, Leclerc JR, David M, Coates G. Diagnostic value of ventilation-perfusion lung scanning in patients with suspected pulmonary embolism. Chest 1985; 88:819–828.

38. Sostman HD, Ravin CE, Sullivan DC, Mills SR, Glickman MG, Dorfman GS. Use of pulmonary angiography for suspected pulmonary embolism: influence of scintigraphic diagnosis. AJR Am J Roentgenol 1982; 139:673–677.

39. Khorasani R, Gudas TF, Nikpoor N, Polak JF. Treatment of patients with suspected pulmonary embolism and intermediate-probability lung scans: is diagnostic imaging underused? AJR Am J Roentgenol 1997; 169:1355–1357.

40. Patriquin L, Khorasani R, Polak JF. Correlation of diagnostic imaging and subsequent autopsy findings in patients with pulmonary embolism. AJR Am J Roentgenol 1998; 171:347–349.

41. Dalen JE. When can treatment be withheld in patients with suspected pulmonary embolism? Arch Intern Med 1993; 153:1415–1418.

42. Stein PD, Hull RD, Saltzman HA, Pineo G. Strategy for diagnosis of patients with suspected acute pulmonary embolism. Chest 1993; 103:1553–1559.

43. Hull RD, Raskob GE, Ginsberg JS, Panju AA, Brill-Edwards P, Coates G, Pineo GF. A noninvasive strategy for the treatment of patients with suspected pulmonary embolism. Arch Intern Med 1994; 154:289–297.

44. Ginsburg JS. Management of Venous Thromboembolism. N Engl J Med 1996; 335:1816–1828.

45. Stein PD, Hull RD, Pineo G. Strategy that includes serial noninvasive leg tests for diagnosis of thromboembolic disease in patients with suspected acute pulmonary embolism based on data from PIOPED. Arch Intern Med 1995; 155:2101–2104.

46. Wells P, Ginsberg J, Anderson D, Kearon C, Gent M, Turpie A, Bormanis J, Weitz J, Chamberlain M, Bowie D, Barnes D, Hirsh J. Use of a clinical model for safe management of patients with suspected pulmonary embolism. Ann Intern Med 1998; 129:997–1005.

47. Perrier A, Bounameaux H, Morabia A, de Moerloose P, Slosman D, Didier D, Unger PF, Junod A. Diagnosis of pulmonary embolism by a decision analysis-based strategy including clinical probability, d-dimer levels, and ultrasonography: a management study. Arch Intern Med 1996; 156:531–536.

48. Meyerovitz MF, Mannting F, Polak JF, Goldhaber. Frequency of pulmonary embolism in patients with low-probability lung scan and negative lower extremity venous ultrasound. Chest 1999; 115:980–982.

49. Hull RD, Raskob GE, Pineo GF, Brant RF. The low-probability lung scan: a need for change in nomenclature. Arch Int Med 1995; 155:1845–1851.

50. Nilsson T, Måre K, Carlsson A. Value of structured clinical and scintigraphic protocols in acute pulmonary embolism. J Intern Med 2001; 250:213–218.

51. Gottschalk A, Juni JE, Sostman HD, Coleman RE, Thrall J, McKusick KA, Froelich JW, Alavi A. Ventilation-perfusion scintigraphy in the PIOPED study. Part I. Data collection and Tabulation. J Nucl Med 1993; 34:1109–1118.

52. Lensing AWA, van Beek EJR, Demers C, Tiel-van Buul MMC, Yakemchuk V, van Dongen A, Coates G, Ginsberg JS, Hirsh J, ten Cate JW, Büller HR. Ventilation-perfusion lung scanning and the diagnosis of pulmonary embolism: improvement of observer agreement by the use of a lung segment reference chart. Thromb Haemost 1992; 68:245–249.

53. Forbes KPN, Reid JH, Murchison JT. Do preliminary chest x-ray findings define the optimum role of pulmonary scintigraphy in suspected pulmonary embolism? Clin Radiol 2001; 56:397–400.

54. Miniati M, Pistolesi M, Marini C, Di Ricco G, Formichi B, Prediletto R, Allescia G, Tonelli L, Sostman HD, Giuntini C. Value of perfusion lung scan in the diagnosis of pulmonary embolism: results of the prospective investigative study of acute pulmonary embolism diagnosis (PISA-PED). Am J Respir Crit Care Med 1996; 154:1387–1393.

55. Alderson PO, Doppman JL, Diamond SS, Mendenhall KG, Barron EL, Girton M. Ventilation-perfusion lung imaging and selective pulmonary angiography in dogs with experimental pulmonary embolism. J Nucl Med 1978; 19: 164–171.

56. Kessler RM, McNeil BJ. Impaired ventilation in a patient with angiographically demonstrated pulmonary emboli. Radiology 1975; 114:111–112.

57. Biello DR, Mattar AG, McKnight RC, Siegel BA. Ventilation-perfusion studies in suspected pulmonary embolism. AJR Am J Roentgenol 1979; 133: 1033–1037.

58. Alderson PO, Biello DR, Sachariah G, Siegel BA. Scintigraphic detection of pulmonary embolism in patients with obstructive pulmonary disease. Radiology 1981; 138:661–666.

59. Robin ED. Overdiagnosis and overtreatment of pulmonary embolism: the emperor may have no clothes. Ann Intern Med 1977; 87:775–781.

60. Hartmann IJC, Hagen PJ, Melissant CF, Postmus PE, Prins MH. Diagnosing acute pulmonary embolism. Effect of chronic obstructive pulmonary disease on the performance of D-dimer testing, ventilation/perfusion scintigraphy, spiral computed tomographic angiography and conventional angiography. Am J Respir Crit Care Med 2000; 162:2232–2237.

61. Lopez-Majano V, Tow DE, Wagner HN. Regional distribution of pulmonary arterial blood flow in emphysema. JAMA 1966; 197:121–124.

62. Kim CK, Worsley DF, Alavi A. Ventilation-perfusion-chest radiograph match is less likely to represent pulmonary embolism if perfusion is decreased rather than absent. Clin Nucl Med 2000; 25:665–669.

63. Lesser BA, Leeper KV, Stein PD, Saltzman HA, Chen J, Thompson BT, Hales CA, Popovich J, Greenspan RH, Weg JG. The diagnosis of acute pulmonary embolism in patients with chronic obstructive pulmonary disease. Chest 1992; 102:17–22.

64. Stein PD, Coleman E, Gottschalk A, Saltzman HA, Terrin ML, Weg JG. Diagnostic utility of ventilation/perfusion lung scans in acute pulmonary embolism is not diminished by pre-existing cardiac or pulmonary disease. Chest 1991; 100:604–606.

65. Rodger MA, Jones G, Rasuli P, Raymond F, Djunaedi H, Bredeson CN, Wells PS. Steady-state end-tidal alveolar dead space fraction and d-dimer. Chest 2001; 120:115–119.

66. American Thoracic Society. The diagnostic approach to acute venous thromboembolism. Clinical practice guideline. Am J Respir Crit Care Med 1999; 160:1043–1066.

67. Bajc, Bitzén U, Olsson B, Perez de Sá V, Palmer J, Jonson B. Lung ventilation/ perfusion SPECT in the artificially embolized pig. J Nucl Med 2002; 43:640–647.

68. Palmer J, Bitzén U, Jonson B, Bajc M. Comprehensive ventilation/perfusion SPECT. J Nucl Med 2001; 42:1288–1294.

69. Williams JR, Wilcox C, Andrews GJ, Burns RR. Angiography in pulmonary embolism. JAMA 1963; 184:473–476.

70. Sasahara AA, Stein M, Simon M, Littmann D. Pulmonary angiography in the diagnosis of thromboembolic disease. N Engl J Med 1964; 270:1076–1081.

71. Nicod P, Peterson K, Levine M, Dittrich H, Buchbinder M, Chappuis F, Moser K. Pulmonary angiography in server chronic pulmonary hypertension. Ann Intern Med 1987; 107:565–568.

72. Sagel SS, Greenspan RH. Nonuniform pulmonary arterial perfusion. Pulmonary embolism? Radiology 1970; 99:541–548.

73. Dalen JE, Brooks HL, Johnson LW, Meister SG, Szucs MM, Dexter L. Pulmonary angiography in acute pulmonary embolism: indications, techniques and results in 367 patients. Am Heart J 1971; 81:175–185.

74. Stein PD, O'Connor JF, Dalen JE, Pur-Shahriari AA, Hoppin FG, Hammond DT, Haynes FW, Fleischner FG, Dexter L. The angiographic diagnosis of acute pulmonary embolism: evaluation of criteria. Am Heart J 1967; 73:730–741.

75. Auger WR, Fedullo PF, Moser KM, Buchbinder M, Peterson KL. Chronic major-vessel thromboembolic pulmonary artery obstruction: appearance at angiography. Radiology 1992; 182:393–398.

76. Hagspiel KD, Polak JF, Grassi CJ, Faitelson BB, Kandarpa K, Meyerovitz MF. Pulmonary embolism: comparison of cut-film and digital pulmonary angiography. Radiology 1998; 207:139–145.

77. Johnson MS, Stine SB, Shah H, Harris VJ, Ambrosius WT, Trerotola SO. Possible pulmonary embolus: evaluation with digital subtraction versus cut-film angiography-prospective study in 80 patients. Radiology 1998; 207:131–138.

78. Van Beek EJR, Bakker AJ, Reekers JA. Pulmonary embolism: interobserver agreement in the interpretation of conventional angiographic and DSA images in patients with nondiagnostic lung scan results. Radiology 1996; 198:721–724.

79. van Rooij WJJ, den Heeten GJ, Sluzewski M. Pulmonary embolism: diagnosis in 211 patients with use of selective pulmonary digital subtraction angiography with a flow-directed catheter. Radiology 1995; 195:793–797.

80. Schlueter FJ, Zuckerman DA, Horesh L, Gutierrez FR, Hicks ME, Brink JA. Digital subtraction versus film-screen angiography for detecting acute pulmonary emboli: evaluation in a porcine model. J Vasc Interv Radiol 1997; 8:1015–1024.

81. Stein PS, Athanasoulis C, Alavi A, Greenspan R, Hales CA, Saltzman HA, Vreim CE, Terrin ML, Weg JG. Complications and validity of pulmonary angiography in acute pulmonary embolism. Circulation 1992; 85:462–468.

82. Perlmutt LM, Braun SD, Newman GE, Oke EJ, Dunnick NR. Pulmonary arteriography in the high-risk patient. Radiology 1987; 162:187–189.

83. Mills SR, Jackson DC, Older RA, Heaston DK, Moore AV. The incidence etiologies and avoidance of complications of pulmonary angiography in a large series. Radiology 1980; 136:295–299.

84. Hudson ER, Smith TP, McDermott VG, Newman GE, Suhocki PV, Payne CS, Stackhouse DJ. Pulmonary angiography performed with iopamidol: complications in 1434 patients. Radiology 1996; 198:61–65.

85. Zuckerman DA, Sterling KM, Oser RF. Safety of pulmonary angiography in the 1990s. J Vasc Interv Radiol 1996; 7:199–205.

86. Smith TP, Lee VS, Hudson ER, Newman GE, Payne CS, Suhocki PV, McDermott VG, Stackhouse DJ. Prospective evaluation of pulmonary artery pressures during pulmonary angiography performed with low-osmolar nonionic contrast media. J Vasc Interv Radiol 1996; 7:207–212.

87. Schwab SJ, Hlatky MA, Pieper KS, Davidson CJ, Morris KG, Skelton TN, Bashore TM. Contrast nephrotoxicity: a randomized controlled trial of a nonionic and an ionic radiographic contrast agent. N Engl J Med 1989; 320: 149–153.

88. Tumlin JA, Wang A, Murray PT, Mathur VS. Fenoldopam mesylate blocks reductions in renal plasma flow after radiocontrast dye infusion: a pilot trial in the prevention of contrast nephropathy. Am Heart J 2002; 143:894–903.

89. Huber W, Ilgmann K, Page M, Hennig M, Schweigart U, Jeschke B, Lutilsky L, Weiss W, Salmhofer H, Classen M. Effect of theophylline on contrast material-induced nephropathy in patients with chronic renal insufficiency: controlled, randomized, double-blinded study. Radiology 2002; 223:772–779.

90. Diaz-Sandoval LJ, Kosowsky BD, Losordo DW. Acetylcysteine to prevent angiography-related renal tissue injury (the APART trial). Am J Cardiol 2002; 89:356–358.

91. Baile EM, King GG, Müller NL, D'Yachkova Y, Coche EE, Paré PD, Mayo JR. Spiral computed tomography is comparable to angiography for the diagnosis of pulmonary embolism. Am J Respir Crit Care Med 2000; 161:1010–1015.

92. van Beek EJR, Brouwers EMJ, Song B, Stein PD, Oudkerk M. Clinical validity of a normal pulmonary angiogram in patients with suspected pulmonary embolism—a critical review. Clin Radiol 2001; 56:838–842.

93. Novelline RA, Baltarowich OH, Anthanasoulis CA, Waltman AC, Greenfield AJ, McKusick KA. The clinical course of patients with suspected pulmonary embolism and a negative pulmonary arteriogram. Radiology 1978; 126:561–567.

94. Henry JW, Relyea B, Stein PD. Continuing risk of thromboemboli among patients with normal pulmonary angiograms. Chest 1995; 107:1375–1378.

95. Stein PD, Henry JW, Gottschalk A. Reassessment of pulmonary angiography for the diagnosis of pulmonary embolism: relation of interpreter agreement to the order of the involved pulmonary arterial branch. Radiology 1999; 210:689–691.

96. Stein PD, Henry JW. Prevalence of acute pulmonary embolism in central and subsegmental pulmonary arteries and relation to probability intepretation of ventilation/perfusion lung scans. Chest 1997; 111:1246–1248.

97. Diffin DC, Leyendecker JR, Johnson SP, Zucker RJ, Grebe PJ. Effect of anatomic distribution of pulmonary emboli on interobserver agreement in the interpretation of pulmonary antiography. AJR Am J Roentgenol 1988; 171: 1085–1089.

98. Quinn MF, Lundell CJ, Klotz TA, Finck EJ, Pentecost M, McGehee WG, Garnic JD. Reliability of selective pulmonary arteriography in the diagnosis of pulmonary embolism. AJR Am J Roentgenol 1987; 149:469–471.

99. Bookstein JJ. Segmental arteriography in pulmonary embolism. Radiology 1969; 93:1007–1012.

100. Gurney JW. No fooling around: direct visualization of pulmonary embolism. Radiology 1993; 188:618–619.

101. Oudkerk M, van Beek EJR. Diagnosis of pulmonary embolism: no fooling around (letter). Radiology 1993; 191:288–289.

102. Oser RF, Zuckerman DA, Gutierrez FR, Brink JA. Anatomic distribution of pulmonary emboli at pulmonary angiography: implications for cross-sectional imaging. Radiology 1996; 199:31–35.

103. Sinner WN. Computed tomography of pulmonary thromboembolism. Eur J Radiol 1982; 2:8–13.

104. Remy-Jardin M, Remy J, Baghaie F, Gribourg M, Artaud D, Duhamel A. Clinical value of thin collimation in the diagnostic workup of pulmonary embolism. AJR Am J Roentgenol 2000; 175:407–411.

105. Garg K, Sieler H, Welsh CH, Johnson RJ, Russ PD. Clinical validity of helical CT being interpreted as negative for pulmonary embolism: implications for patient treatment. AJR Am J Roentgen 1999; 172:1627–1631.

106. Garg K, Welsh CH, Feyerabend AJ, Subber SW, Russ PD, Johnston RJ, Durham JD, Lynch DA. Pulmonary embolism: diagnosis with spiral CT and ventilation-perfusion scanning-correlation with pulmonary angiographic results or clinical outcome. Radiology 1998; 208:201–208.

107. Cross JJL, Kemp PM, Walsh CG, Flower CDR, Dixon AK. A randomized trial of spiral CT and ventilation perfusion scintigraphy for the diagnosis of pulmonary embolism. Clin Radiol 1998; 54:177–182.

108. Ost D, Rozenshtein A, Saffran L, Snider A. The negative predictive value of spiral computed tomography for the diagnosis of pulmonary embolism in patients with nondiagnostic ventilation-perfusion scans. Am J Med 2001; 110:16–21.

109. Goodman LR. CT of acute pulmonary emboli: where does it fit? RadioGraphics 1997; 17:1037–1042.

110. Remy-Jardin M, Remy J, Wattinne L, Giraud F. Central pulmonary thromboembolism: diagnosis with spiral volumetric CT with the single-breath-hold tecnique-comparison with pulmonary angiography. Radiology 1992; 185:381–387.

111. Rathbun S, Raskob GE, Whitsett TL. Sensitivity and specificity of helical computed tomography in the diagnosis of pulmonary embolism: a systematic review. Ann Intern Med 2000; 132:227–232.

112. Remy-Jardin M, Remy J, Artaud D, Fribourg M, Beregi JP. Spiral CT of pulmonary embolism: diagnostic approach, interpretive pitfalls and current indications. Eur Radiol 1998; 8:1376–1390.

113. Chartrand-Lefebvre C, Howarth N, Lucidarme O, Beigelman C, Cluzel P, Mourey-Gérosa I, Cadi M, Grenier P. Contrast-enhanced helical CT for

pulmonary embolism detection: inter- and intraobserver agreement among radiologists with variable experience. Am J Radiol 1999; 172:107–112.

114. Qanadli SD, Hajjam ME, Mesurolle B, Barré, Bruckert F, Joseph T, Mignon F, Vieillard-Baron A, Dubourg O, Lacombe P. Pulmonary embolism detection: prospective evaluation of dual-section helical CT versus selective pulmonary arteriography in 157 patients. Radiology 2000; 217:447–455.

115. Tepel M, Van der Giet M, Schwarzfeld C, Laufer U, Liermann D, Zidek W. Prevention of radiographic-contrast-agent-induced reductions in renal function by acetylcysteine. N Engl J Med 2000; 343:180–184.

116. Teigen CL, Maus TP, Sheedy PF II, Johnson CM, Stanson AW, Welch TJ. Pulmonary embolism: diagnosis with electron-beam CT. Radiology 1993; 188: 839–845.

117. Teigen CL, Maus TP, Sheedy PF II, Stanson AW, Johnson CM, Breen JF, McKusick MA. Pulmonary embolism: Diagnosis with contrast-enhanced electron beam CT and comparison with pulmonary angiography. Radiology 1995; 194:313–319.

118. Van Rossum AB, Pattynama PMT, Ton ERT, Treurniet FEE, Arndt JW, van Eck B, Kieft GJ. Pulmonary embolism: validation of spiral CT angiography in 149 patients. Radiology 1996; 201:467–470.

119. Blachere H, Latrabe V, Montaudon M, Valli N, Couffinhal T, Raherisson C, Leccia F, Laurent F. Pulmonary embolism revealed on helical CT angiography: comparison with ventilation-perfusion radionuclide lung scanning. AJR Am J Roentgenol 2000; 174:1041–1047.

120. Velmahos GC, Pantelis V, Wilcox A, Hanks SE, Salim A, Harrel D, Palmer S, Demetriades D. Spiral computed tomography for the diagnosis of pulmonary embolism in critically ill surgical patients: a comparison with pulmonary angiography. Arch Surg 2001; 136:505–510.

121. Schoepf UJ, Helmberger T, Holzknecht N, Kang DS, Bruening RD, Aydemir S, Becker CR, Muehling O, Knez A, Haberl R, Reiser MF. Segmental and subsegmental pulmonary arteries: evaluation with electron-beam versus spiral CT. Radiology 2000; 14:433–439.

122. Goodman LR, Curtin JJ, Mewissen MW, Foley WD, Lipchik RJ, Crain MR, Sagar KB, Collier BD. Detection of pulmonary embolism in patients with unresolved clinical and scintigraphic diagnosis: helical CT versus angiography. AJR Am J Roentgenol 1995; 164:1369–1374.

123. Mayo JR, Remy-Jardin M, Müller NL, Remy J, Worsley DF, Hossein-Foucher C, Kwong JS, Brown MJ. Pulmonary embolism: prospective comparison of spiral CT with ventilation-perfusion scintigraphy. Radiology 1997; 205:447–452.

124. Remy-Jardin M, Remy J, Deschildre F, Artaud D, Beregi JP, Hossein-Foucher C, Marchandise X, Duhamel A. Diagnosis of pulmonary embolism with spiral CT: comparison with pulmonary angiography and scintigraphy. Radiology 1996; 200:699–706.

125. Van Rossum AB, Treurniet FEE, Kieft GJ, Smith SJ, Schepers-Bok R. Role of spiral volumetric computed tomographic scanning in the assessment of patients

with clinical suspicion of pulmonary embolism and an abnormal ventilation/ perfusion lung scan. Thorax 1996; 51:23–28.

126. Perrier A, Howarth N, Didier D, Loubeyre P, Unger PF, de Moerloose P, Slosman D, Junod A, Bounameaux H. Performance of helical computed tomography in unselected outpatients with suspected pulmonary embolism. Ann Intern Med 2001; 135:88–97.

127. Remy-Jardin M, Remy J, Artaud D, Deschildre F, Duhamel A. Peripheral pulmonary arteries: optimization of the spiral CT acquisition protocol. Radiology 1997; 204:157–163.

128. Raptopoulos V, Boiselle PM. Multi-detector row spiral CT pulmonary angiography: comparison with single-detector row spiral CT. Radiology 2001; 221:606–613.

129. Schoepf UJ, Holzknect N, Helmberger TK, Crispin A, Hong C, Becker CR, Reiser MF. Subsegmental pulmonary emboli: improved detection with thin-collimation multi-detector row spiral CT. Radiology 2002; 222:483–490.

130. Ghaye B, Szapiro D, Mastora I, Delannoy V, Duhamel A, Remy J, Remy-Jardin M. Peripheral pulmonary arteries: how far in the lung does multi-detector row spiral CT allow analysis? Radiology 2001; 219:629–636.

131. Goldin JG, Yoon HC, Greaser LE III, Nishimura EK. Detection of pulmonary emboli at the segmental and subsegmental level with electron-beam CT: validation in a porcine model. Acad Radiol 1998; 5:503–508.

132. Coche EE, Hamoir XL, Hammer FD, Hainaut P, Goffette PP. Using dual-detector helical CT angiography to detect deep venous thrombosis in patients with suspicion of pulmonary embolism: diagnostic value and additional findings. AJR Am J Roentgenol 2001; 176:1035–1039.

133. Loud PA, Katz DS, Klippenstein DL, Shah RD, Grossman ZD. Combined CT venography and pulmonary angiography in suspected thromboembolic disease: diagnostic accuracy for deep venous evaluation. Am J Roentgen 2000; 174:61–65.

134. Ciccotosto C, Goodman L, Washington L, Quiroz F. Indirect CT venography following CT pulmonary angiography: spectrum of CT findings. J Thorac Imag 2002; 17:18–27.

135. Goodman LR, Lipchik RJ, Kuzo RS, Liu Y, McAuliffe TL, O'Brien DJ. Subsequent pulmonary embolism: risk after a negative helical CT pulmonary angiogram-prospective comparison with scintigraphy. Radiology 2000; 215: 535–542.

136. Feretti GR, Bosson JL, Buffaz PD, Ayanian D, Pison C, Blanc F, Carpentier F, Carpentier P, Coulomb M. Acute pulmonary embolism: role of helical CT in 164 patients with intermediate probability at ventilation-perfusion scintigraphy and normal results at duplex US of the legs. Radiology 1997; 205: 453–458.

137. Lomis NNT, Yoon HC, Moran AG, Miller FJ. Clinical outcomes of patients after a negative spiral CT pulmonary arteriogram in the evaluation of acute pulmonary embolism. J Vasc Interv Radiol 1999; 10:707–712.

138. Gottsäter A, Berg A, Centergård J, Frennby B, Nirhov H, Nyman U. Clini-

cally suspected pulmonary embolism: is it safe to withhold anticoagulation after a negative spiral CT? Eur Radiol 2001; 11:65–72.

139. Swensen SJ, Sheedy PF, Ryu JH, Pickette DD, Schleck CD, Ilstrup DM, Heit JA. Outcomes after withholding anticoagulation from patients with suspected acute pulmonary embolism and negative computed tomographic findings: a cohort study. Mayo Clin Proc 2002; 77:130–138.

140. Paterson DI, Schwartzman. Strategies incorporating spiral CT for the diagnosis of acute pulmonary embolism. A cost-effective analysis. Chest 2001; 119:1791–1800.

141. van Erkel AR, van Rossum AB, Bloem JL, Kievit J, Pattynama PMT. Spiral CT angiography for suspected pulmonary embolism: a cost-effective analysis. Radiology 1996; 201:29–36.

142. van Rossum AB, Pattynama PMT, Mallens WMC, Hermans J, Heijerman HGM. Can helical CT replace scintigraphy in the diagnostic process in suspected pulmonary embolism? A retrolective-prolective cohort study focusing on total diagnostic yield. Eur Radiol 1998; 8:90–96.

143. Goodman LR, Lipchik RJ. Diagnosis of acute pulmonary embolism: time for a new approach. Radiology 1996; 199:25–27.

144. Mullins MD, Becker DM, Hagspiel KD, Philbrick JT. The role of spiral volumetric computed tomography in the diagnosis of pulmonary embolism. Arch Intern Med 2000; 160:293–298.

145. Krüger S, Haage P, Hoffmann R, Breuer C, Bücker A, Hanrath P, Günther RW. Diagnosis of pulmonary arterial hypertension and pulmonary embolism with magnetic resonance angiography. Chest 2001; 120:1556–1561.

146. Grist TM, Sostman HD, MacFall JR, Foo TK, Spritzer CE, Witty L, Newman GE, Debatin JF, Tapson V, Saltzman HA. Pulmonary angiography with MR imaging: preliminary clinical experience. Radiology 1993; 189:523–530.

147. Gefter WB, Hatabu H. Evaluation of pulmonary vascular anatomy and blood flow by magnetic resonance. J Thorac Imaging 1993; 8:122–136.

148. Gefter WB, Hatabu H, Dinsmore BJ, Axel L, Palevsky H, Reichek N, Schiebler ML, Kressel HY. Pulmonary vascular cine MR imaging: a non-invasive approach to dynamic imaging of the pulmonary circulation. Radiology 1990; 176:761–770.

149. Gefter WB, Hatabu H, Holland GA, Gupta KB, Henschke CI, Palevsky HI. Pulmonary thromboembolism: recent developments in diagnosis with CT and MR imaging. Radiology 1995; 197:561–574.

150. Hatabu H, Gefter WB, Axel L, Palevsky HI, Cope C, Reichek N, Dougherty L, Listerud J, Kressel HY. MR imaging with spatial modulation of magnetization in the evaluation of chronic central pulmonary thromboemboli. Radiology 1994; 190:791–796.

151. Rubin GD, Herfkens RJ, Pelc NJ, Foo TKF, Napel S, Shimakawa A, Steiner RM, Bergin CJ. Single breath-hold pulmonary magnetic resonance angiography. Optimization and comparison of three imaging strategies. Invest Radiol 1994; 29:766–772.

152. Gupta A, Frazer CK, Ferguson JM, Kumar AB, Davis SJ, Fallon MJ, Morris

JT, Drury PJ, Cala LA. Acute pulmonary embolism: diagnosis with MR angiography. Radiology 1999; 210:353–359.

153. Erdman WA, Peshock RM, Redman HC, Bonte F, Meyerson M, Jayson HT, Miller GL, Clarke GD, Parkey RW. Pulmonary embolism: comparison of MR images with radionuclide and angiographic studies. Radiology 1994; 190:499–508.

154. Schiebler ML, Holland GA, Hatabu H, Listerud J, Foo T, Palevsky H, Edmunds H, Gefter WB. Suspected pulmonary embolism: prospective evaluation with pulmonary MR angiography. Radiology 1993; 189:125–131.

155. Gamsu G, Hirji M, Moore EH, Webb WR, Brito A. Experimental pulmonary emboli detected using magnetic resonance. Radiology 1984; 153:467–470.

156. Pope CF, Sostman D, Carbo P, Gore JC, Holcomb W. The detection of pulmonary emboli by magnetic resonance imaging: evaluation of imaging parameters. Invest Radiol 1987; 22:937–946.

157. Meaney JFM, Weg JG, Chenevert TL, Starrford-Johnson D, Hamilton BH, Prince MR. Diagnosis of pulmonary embolism with magnetic resonance angiography. N Engl J Med 1997; 336:1422–1427.

158. Holland GA, Gefter WB, Baum RA, Gupta KB, Cope C, Kressel HY. Prospective comparison of pulmonary MR angiography and ultrafast CT for diagnosis of pulmonary thromboembolic disease [abstract]. Radiology 1993; 189(P):234.

159. Woodard PK, Sostman HD, MacFall JR, DeLong DM, McDonald JW, Foo TKF, Patz EF, Goodman PC, Spritzer CE. Detection of pulmonary embolism: comparison of contrast-enhanced spiral CT and time-of-flight MR techniques. J Thorac Imaging 1995; 10:59–72.

160. Hurst DR, Kazerooni EA, Stafford-Johnson D, Williams DM, Platt JF, Cascade PN, Prince MR. Diagnosis of pulmonary embolism: comparison of CT angiography and MR angiography in canines. J Vasc Interv Radiol 1999; 10:309–318.

161. Reittner P, Coxson HO, Nakano Y, Heyneman L, Ward S, King GG, Baile EM, Mayo JR. Pulmonary embolism: comparison of gadolinium-enhanced MR angiography with contrast-enhanced spiral CT in a porcine model. Acad Radiol 2001; 8:343–350.

162. Sostman HD, Layish DT, Tapson VF, Spritzer CE, DeLong DM, Trotter P, MacFall JR, Patz EF, Goodman PC, Woodard PK, Foo TK, Farber JL. Prospective comparison of helical CT and MR imaging in clinically suspected acuted pulmonary embolism. J Magn Reson Imaging 1996; 6:275–281.

163. Nakagawa T, Sakuma H, Murashima S, Ishida N, Matsumura K, Takeda K. Pulmonary ventilation-perfusion MR imaging in clinical patients. J Magn Reson Imaging 2001; 14:419–424.

164. Wells PS, Anderson DR, Rodger M, Stiell I, Dreyer JF, Barnes D, Forgie M, Kovacs G, Ward J, Kovacs MJ. Excluding pulmonary embolism at the bedside without diagnostic imaging: management of patients with suspected

pulmonary embolism presenting to the emergency department by using a simple clinical model and d-dimer. Ann Intern Med 2001; 135:98–107.

165. Kearon C, Ginsberg J, Hirsh J. The role of venous ultrasonography in the diagnosis of suspected deep venous thrombosis and pulmonary embolism. Ann Intern Med 1998; 129:1044–1049.

166. Quinn RJ, Nour R, Butler SP, Glenn DW, Travers PL, Wellings G, Kwan YL. Pulmonary embolism in patients with intermediate probability lung scans: diagnosis with Doppler venous US and D-dimer measurement. Radiology 1994; 190:509–511.

167. Perrir A, Miron MJ, Desmarais S, de Moerloose P, Slosman D, Didier D, Unger PF, Junod A, Patenaude JV, Bounameaux H. Using clinical evaluation and lung scan to rule out suspected pulmonary embolism. Arch Intern Med 2000; 160:512–516.

168. Pérez-Rodriguez E, Jimenez D, Diaz G, Flores J. D-dimer and pulmonary embolism: is there a good interpretation? Arch Intern Med 2000; 160:2217–2218.

169. Lorut C, Ghossains M, Horellou MH, Achkar A, Fretault J, Laaban JP. A noninvasive diagnostic strategy including spiral computed tomography in patients with suspected pulmonary embolism. Am J Respir Crit Care Med 2000; 162:1413–1418.

170. Wood KE. Major pulmonary embolism. Review of a pathophysiologic approach to the golden hour of hemodynamically significant pulmonary embolism. Chest 2002; 121:877–905.

171. Wolfe TR, Hartsell SC. Pulmonary embolism: making sense of the diagnostic evaluation. Ann Emerg Med 2001; 37:504–514.

172. Hirsh J, Hoak J. Management of deep vein thrombosis and pulmonary embolism. Circulation 1996; 93:2212–2245.

173. Miniati M, Prediletto R, Formichi B, Marini C, DiRicco G, Tonelli L, Alescia G, Pistolesi M. Accuracy of clinical assessment in the diagnosis of pulmonary embolism. Am J Respir Crit Care Med 1999; 159:864–871.

9

Echocardiography in the Diagnosis of Pulmonary Thromboembolism

JOHN A. PARASKOS and DENNIS A. TIGHE

University of Massachusetts Medical School
Worcester, Massachusetts, U.S.A.

I. Introduction

Short of direct inspection, pulmonary angiographic delineation of a tubular intra-arterial filling defect is generally accepted as the most reliable antemortem indicator of pulmonary thromboembolism. The search for a less invasive yet reliable diagnostic tool has been intense for over four decades. The use of chest radiography in conjunction with radionuclide pulmonary perfusion and ventilation scintigraphy has been widely accepted as a useful alternative to angiography in most cases of suspected pulmonary embolism. Yet, scintigraphic evidence highly consistent with pulmonary embolism is found in a minority of suspected cases (1). This leaves the clinician to undertake treatment based on less reliable data or to go on to more definitive imaging techniques (2). The clinical acumen of the physician in ascertaining the pretest likelihood of pulmonary embolism (see Chapter 6) is central in giving proper weight to less reliable laboratory and imaging data (3). In Chapter 8, advances in nonultrasonic imaging techniques are discussed that are often very useful in persuading the clinician for or against the diagnosis of pulmonary embolism.

Ultrasonic techniques have been proven to be an important tool in the clinician's evaluation of the patient suspected of pulmonary embolism. The value of two-dimensional imaging of leg veins in conjunction with Doppler imaging of venous flow is of great value in determining the presence of deep venous thrombosis and is discussed in Chapter 5. Although the absence of in situ thrombi in the deep veins of the thigh does not exclude pulmonary embolism, its presence constitutes important evidence supporting the diagnosis. Echocardiography has been proven to be a useful tool in managing patients suspected of pulmonary embolism. Although a normal echocardiographic study does not exclude the diagnosis, visualization of the morphology and function of the right and left side of the central circulation is often invaluable in leading toward or away from the diagnosis. The finding or the exclusion of other cardiovascular diseases that may explain the patient's presentation will be central to the clinician's treatment decisions. Finally, echocardiography in some cases will provide direct imaging of emboli in the central pulmonary arteries or in transit through the right side of the circulation, or even traversing a patent foramen ovale. Intravascular ultrasound through catheter transducers allows more direct evidence of central thrombi but has only limited application during specialized catheterization studies. Finally, the use of ultrasonic scanning of the intercostal spaces allows some inferences to be made about the state of the underlying pulmonary and pleural structures and its potential value in imaging suspected embolized lung is being studied.

II. Direct Imaging of a Thromboembolus

As the great majority of pulmonary thromboemboli arise from the deep capacitance veins of the thigh, the demonstration of a residual thrombus in the legs is indirect evidence in support of a suspected diagnosis of embolic disease. A thrombus may also develop in the pelvic veins, venae cavae, right atrium, or ventricle, and under circumstances of severe pulmonary hypertension or hypercoagulable state (such as sickle cell anemia) in the pulmonary arteries themselves. Echocardiography has been useful in documenting thrombi in all areas of the venous circulation. In 1977, Covarrubias et al. (4) first reported an M-mode recording of a mass apparently attached to or trapped in the tricuspid valve. The patient died 48 hr later and autopsy confirmed a large pulmonary embolus. Kasper et al. (5) studied 105 patients with documented pulmonary embolism, using two-dimensional transthoracic echocardiography, and found right pulmonary artery masses in 11 and right ventricular masses in 3 patients.

Thrombi of intracardiac origin are occasionally seen in the right atrium or in the right ventricle with right ventricular infarction or adherent to indwelling catheters or pacemaker and defibrillator electrodes. These masses tend to be globular and usually appear attached or are mural in location. They are either immobile or restricted with limited motion of fronds at their free surfaces. In a multicenter retrospective study, 40% of 57 patients with such masses had evidence of pulmonary embolism, but none was fatal irrespective of treatment (6). These thrombi need to be distinguished from myxomata (Fig. 1), other tumors, and vegetations. When mobile, yet adherent to valve structures, the possibility of vegetation is much increased. The distinction will be guided by the clinical presentation and occasionally by surgical intervention.

Thrombi that are mobile and snakelike in structure are much more likely to represent emboli arising in large veins (7). In the same multicenter study reported above (5), 98% of 48 patients with such snakelike mobile masses developed symptoms of pulmonary embolism and 13 proved fatal; one-third of the fatalities occurred within 24 hr of the echocardiographic finding. Such thrombi often appear trapped in a Chiari network, eustachian valve, or patent foramen ovale. Unattached, free-floating thrombi can

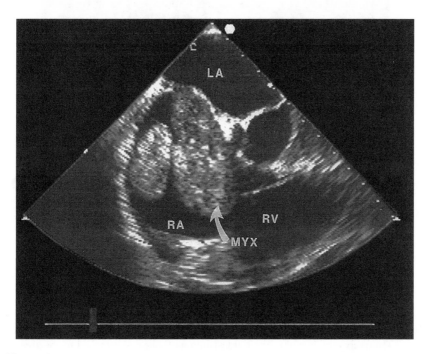

Figure 1 Transesophageal echocardiogram demonstrating a large bilobed globular right atrial mass (MYX) apparently attached to the interatrial septum. This mass is characteristic of an intracardiac tumor; a myxoma was diagnosed at pathology. LA, left atrium; RA, right atrium; RV, right ventricle.

sometimes be seen tumbling in the right atrium or prolapsing into the right ventricle with each diastole, and have been observed to traverse the right ventricle to reach the pulmonary arteries. Whether a thrombus appeared trapped or was freely moving did not seem to make a difference in outcome in a meta-analysis of cases reported up to 1989 (8). Although asymptomatic transit of such thrombi to the pulmonary artery has occasionally been noted (9), patients with mobile thrombi are clearly at high risk for early embolism and death. Immediate aggressive treatment is advised without delay for additional imaging modalities.

Although most cases of right heart thrombi have been detected by transthoracic echocardiography, the improved image resolution of transesophageal echocardiography allows better visualization of proximal pulmonary arteries and right-sided structures, particularly in patients with poor transthoracic ultrasonic "windows" (Figs. 2 and 3). Hunter et al. (10) re-

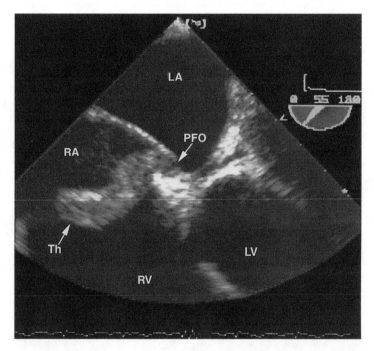

Figure 2 Transesophageal echocardiogram demonstrating a large serpiginous mass (Th) freely mobile within the right atrium with one end attached to the area of the foramen ovale (PFO). This mass is characteristic of a thromboembolus arising in the large veins of the lower extremity and threatening to traverse the PFO to the systemic circulation.

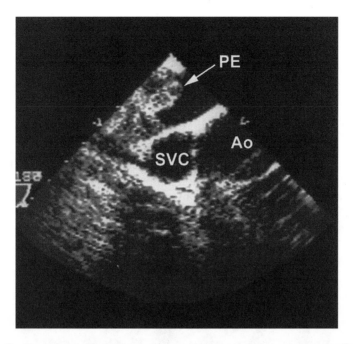

Figure 3 Transesophageal echocardiogram intermediate between longitudinal and transverse planes. The arrow points to a somewhat globular mass (PE) within the right pulmonary artery. The mass was somewhat mobile and more likely to be thromboembolic in origin. Ao, aorta; SVC, superior vena cava.

ported a case in which transesophageal echocardiography revealed a mobile right atrial thrombus that had failed to be seen on transthoracic imaging. Bashir et al. (11) reported that whereas 14% of patients undergoing transesophageal echocardiography for planned cardioversion of atrial fibrillation had spontaneous echo contrast, less than 1% had evidence of right atrial thrombus; presumably from clot forming within the right atrium. During orthopedic surgery, transesophageal monitoring has been reported to demonstrate the transit of pulmonary thromboemboli (12). Parmet et al. (13) monitored 35 total knee arthroplasties with intra-operative transesophageal echocardiography and pulmonary hemodynamics. No abnormalities were noted during anesthesia induction, tourniquet inflation on the operated leg, or during cementing. All procedures were associated with showers of echogenic material traversing the right heart upon deflation of the tourniquet on the operated leg. In 9 patients the echogenic masses were described as "miliary" and in 26 "large" echogenic masses were also seen. Only in the latter group was there a rise in pulmonary vascular resistance index.

Transesophageal echocardiographic monitoring has been used to modify orthopedic procedures to minimize thromboemboli as well as fat and marrow emboli (14,15). Systemic emboli of pulmonary origin have also been demonstrated by this technique. In cases of blunt thoracic trauma, transesophageal echocardiography has revealed showers of echogenic material consistent with systemic air embolism during lung insufflation (16). The investigators suggest that such air embolism can be minimized by decreasing airway pressure and lowering tidal volume. Transesophageal echocardiographic monitoring has demonstrated such showers in all cases of valve surgery and half of the cases of coronary artery bypass grafting (17). The source seems to be air trapped in the pulmonary veins.

Transthoracic echocardiography usually allows reasonable imaging of the main pulmonary artery and the proximal segments of the right and left pulmonary arteries (Figs. 3 and 4). Nevertheless, central pulmonary thromboemboli are often missed by this technique (18,19). Transesophageal echocardiography has had a slightly better record. Pruszczyk et al. (20) have

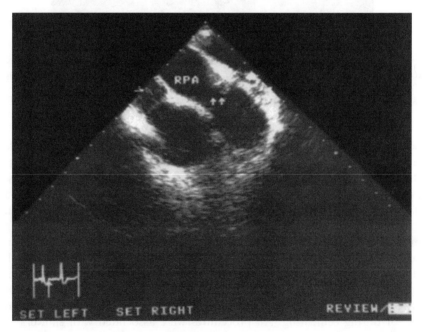

Figure 4 Transesophageal echocardiogram in the transverse plane. The arrows point to a rounded lesion within the right pulmonary artery (RPA) apparently totally adherent to the arterial wall. This could represent arterial plaque, in situ thrombus, or old organized thromboembolus. (From Ref. 24.)

reported central thrombi demonstrated in 63 of 113 patients with suspicion of pulmonary embolism and right ventricular volume overload. Wittlich et al. (21) noted central thrombi in 35 of 60 patients with massive pulmonary embolism. Krivec et al. (22) demonstrated central pulmonary clots in 12 of 24 patients with unexplained shock and distended neck veins by transesophageal echocardiography. Sixteen of 19 patients with right ventricular volume overload and central clots by helical computed tomography (CT) showed clots on transesophageal echocardiography, but only one of six clots in the left pulmonary artery could be detected (23). In several studies, transesophageal echocardiography was much less successful, revealing thrombi in only 3 of 22 patients with central pulmonary emboli detected by helical CT (18) in 1 and 3 of 37 patients with severe pulmonary embolism in another (19). In a study of 25 patients with chronic obstructive lung disease, Russo et al. (24) described central mobile masses suggestive of emboli in three patients, whereas nine patients had adherent masses that may have represented pulmonary arterial plaque or in situ thrombi (see Fig. 4).

Transesophageal echocardiography has been used during cardiac arrest in an attempt to ascertain the cause. In one study, 6 of 48 patients evidenced massive pulmonary emboli (25). Using transesophageal echocardiography, Comess et al. (26) found pulmonary emboli in 8 of 25 patients with pulseless electrical activity. None of the 11 patients with asystole or ventricular arrhythmias had evidence for pulmonary emboli.

The likelihood that echocardiography, transthoracic or transesophageal, will visualize thrombi in a patient with pulmonary embolism is unknown. It is apt to be very low. However, its positive predictive accuracy is high, and if a thrombus is seen, it contributes greatly to the diagnosis of pulmonary embolism. When no thrombus is seen, the likelihood of the diagnosis is not significantly affected.

III. Evidence for Acute Cor Pulmonale

Acute cor pulmonale can be defined as right ventricular dysfunction caused by sudden afterloading of the right ventricle from acute obstruction of the pulmonary vasculature and a marked increase in impedance to right ventricular outflow. Although this is often caused by massive or submassive thromboembolic obstruction, it can also occur with overwhelming pneumonia or acute respiratory distress syndrome. In patients with a clinical syndrome suspicious for pulmonary embolism, echocardiographic evidence for such right ventricular dysfunction serves as strong indirect evidence in support of the diagnosis. This evidence may be structural, with right ventricular dilatation or right ventricular wall motion abnormalities. Alternatively,

Doppler studies may demonstrate evidence for abnormal filling patterns and ejection patterns that are consistent with elevated impedance to right ventricular outflow.

As originally reported by McGinn and White (27), massive or submassive obstruction is required to bring about acute cor pulmonale. The sudden increase in impedance to right ventricular outflow (afterload) results in an abrupt decrease in right ventricular fractional shortening. Concomitantly, the acute pulmonary vascular obstruction decreases the left ventricle's preload, and left ventricular fractional shortening may be increased. Although right-sided pressures rise only minimally, the right side dilates and becomes dysfunctional. Dalen et al. (28) demonstrated that with angiographically demonstrated acute massive obstruction of the pulmonary vasculature, the expected hemodynamic changes are a rise in right atrial pressure and fall in cardiac output. The previously normal right ventricle is unable to generate significantly increased systolic pressures before dilating. As the right ventricle dilates, there is a dramatic increase in wall stress and in right ventricular oxygen demand (29). Chronic cor pulmonale caused by unresolved thromboemboli is unusual in patients who have been adequately anticoagulated (30), and the hemodynamic abnormalities usually resolve in a matter of weeks (28). Evidence of right ventricular ischemia and infarction has been reported in acute pulmonary embolism, and in some cases occult coronary artery disease contributes to these findings (31).

Structural evidence of acute cor pulmonale has been reported in patients with suspected or documented pulmonary embolism (32–37). An increased right ventricular end-diastolic dimension with leftward bulging of the intraventricular septum in diastole were the signs most often reported (Fig. 5). The right ventricular end-diastolic diameter is best observed in the apical four-chamber view (Fig. 6), and in the adult is between 0.9 and 2.6 cm with a mean of 1.9 cm (38). In acute pulmonary embolism, the right ventricular end-diastolic diameter has been reported to be greater than 2.7 cm (33,39). It must be noted that similar findings have been described in acute respiratory distress syndrome (40).

The extent to which structural abnormalities are seen in patients with acute pulmonary embolism is unknown. Obviously, such changes will depend on the extent of pulmonary vascular obstruction. Small emboli that are asymptomatic, or that become clinically manifest only by causing pulmonary infarcts, are likely to be associated with no echocardiographic abnormalities. Right ventricular dilatation has been reported by Kasper et al. in 75% of patients with symptomatic pulmonary embolism (41), and in 92% of patients with massive pulmonary embolism (42). In contrast, Ribeiro et al. (43) reported on 126 patients with acute pulmonary embolism. Nineteen percent had a normal study. Forty-four percent had no or only

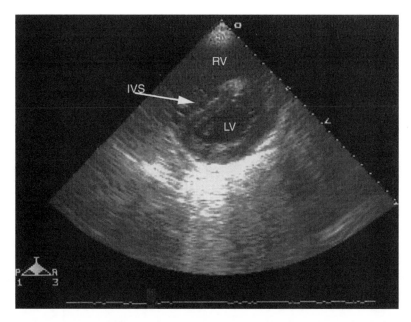

Figure 5 Acute cor pulmonale caused by massive pulmonary embolism. Enlargement of the right ventricle (RV) and reduction of the left ventricle (LV) can be seen in the short-axis end-diastolic views. This view also demonstrates "flattening" of the interventricular septum (IVS) brought about by leftward displacement.

slight right ventricular dysfunction, whereas 56% had moderate to severe right ventricular dysfunction. The presence of right ventricular dysfunction was associated with an increased mortality rate.

In acute cor pulmonale, the ratio of RV to LV end-diastolic diameter (RVED/LVED) has been found to be increased. Jardin et al. found the ratio of right to left ventricular end-diastolic area (RVEDA/LVEDA) in the long axis was also increased in acute cor pulmonale (44). Vieillard-Baron et al. defined acute cor pulmonale as an RVEDA/LVEDA of greater than 0.6 associated with paradoxical septal motion in the short axis. Only 61% of 161 patients with massive pulmonary embolism had such findings (45). Moreover, the presence or absence of these echocardiographic findings did not correlate with prognosis. A low inspiratory collapse for the inferior vena cava of less than 40% is also common and signifies an elevated RA pressure (35). In 1993, Kasper et al. (36) noted asynergy of the right ventricular free wall in 81% of 36 patients with massive or submassive pulmonary embolism. In 1996, McConnell reported on 14 patients with acute pulmonary

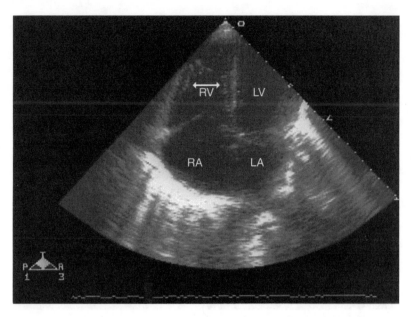

Figure 6 Apical four-chamber view in a transthoracic echocardiogram. The RV diastolic diameter at the mid free wall is mildly dilated (2.9 cm) in a patient with acute cor pulmonale. LA, left atrium; LV, left ventricle; RA, right atrium; RV, right ventricle.

embolism, compared to 18 normal subjects and 9 patients with primary pulmonary hypertension (46). Patients with acute pulmonary embolism had a characteristic pattern of right ventricular dysfunction in which the apex and base were spared and the mid free wall was hypokinetic or akinetic. This was in contrast to primary pulmonary hypertension in which the apex was affected along with the mid free wall. The positive predictive value of this finding among 85 patients with right ventricular dysfunction of any cause was 71% and the negative predictive value 96%. Significant improvement in regional right ventricular function was observed after thrombolysis (47,48). (Figs. 7–9).

Doppler recordings of a tricuspid regurgitant jet can be recorded in the majority of subjects with acute cor pulmonale and allows an assessment of systolic tricuspid pressure gradient, using the modified Bernoulli equation, $P = 4 \times V^2$ (49). The addition of (measured or estimated) right atrial pressure to this gradient gives an approximation of the right ventricular systolic pressure—and in the absence of pulmonic stenosis—of the pulmonary artery systolic pressure. It should be noted, however, that Doppler-derived estimates may be lower than simultaneous high-fidelity catheter-tipped

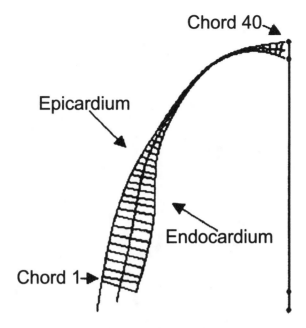

Figure 7 Qualitative wall motion scores were assigned by McConnell et al. at 40 locations in the right ventricular free wall. (From Ref. 46.)

pressure recordings (50). If the quality of the tricuspid regurgitant envelope is inadequate, it can often be enhanced by the injection of an echo-contrast agent, such as agitated saline (51). In acute cor pulmonale, however, the level of the pulmonary systolic pressure is a poor predictor of the severity of the pulmonary obstruction. The tricuspid velocity was greater than 2.6 m/sec in all 60 patients suspected of pulmonary embolism studied by Cheriex et al. (35). This corresponds to a mild to moderate elevation of PA systolic pressure (27 mmHg plus RA pressure). Indeed, with massive pulmonary embolism, pulmonary pressures may even be reduced, as right ventricular dysfunction leads to a drop in cardiac output. If the patient has been previously volume depleted, the likelihood of a normal or low PA systolic pressure will be increased. An early study of tricuspid regurgitant velocity in 18 patients with acute pulmonary embolism failed to show a correlation between tricuspid velocity and percentage of pulmonary obstruction (52). However, patients with velocities greater than 3.5 m/sec (49 mmHg plus the RA pressure) had evidence for preexisting chronic cor pulmonale. Miniati et al. used echocardiography to evaluate 110 consecutive patients with suspected pulmonary embolism (53). They accepted either a dilated hypokinetic right ventricle or

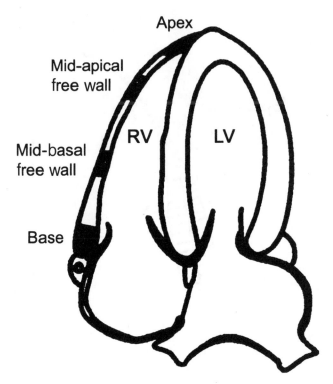

Figure 8 A diagram of the four-chamber transthoracic view with the four areas of particular interest. (From Ref. 46.)

evidence for pulmonary hypertension (tricuspid velocity of > 2.7 m/sec; 30 mmHg plus RA pressure) as evidence for cor pulmonale. Using these rather loose criteria, 50% of the 43 patients with confirmed pulmonary embolism had neither. Using similar criteria, Perrier et al. (54) examined 50 consecutive patients with suspected pulmonary embolism; in 18, the diagnosis was confirmed. As in the study by Maniati et al. (53), the absence of both criteria did not allow the exclusion of pulmonary embolism; the presence of both had high predictive value only in patients with an already high pretest likelihood of pulmonary embolism.

The presence of pulmonary valve regurgitation allows an estimate of the pulmonary artery diastolic pressure in a method analogous to that described above (55). The difference between the gradients of tricuspid regurgitation and pulmonary regurgitation should approximate the pulmo-

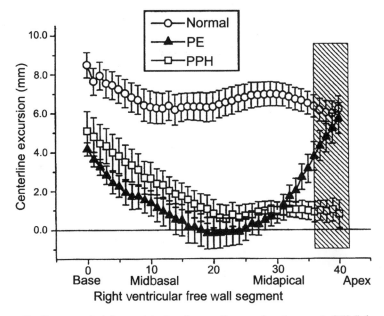

Figure 9 Segmental right ventricular free wall excursion (mean ± SEM) by centerline analysis. Wall excursion in patients with acute pulmonary embolism was near normal at the apex, but abnormal at the mid free wall and base. Wall excursion in patients with primary pulmonary hypertension was reduced compared to normals in all segments. (From Ref. 46.)

nary artery pulse pressure (Fig. 10). Nakayama et al. (56) reported that among 35 patients with pulmonary hypertension and pulmonary regurgitation on echocardiogram, 19 had chronic pulmonary thromboembolism and 16 were considered to have primary pulmonary hypertension. Patients with chronic pulmonary thromboembolism had higher normalized pulse pressures than those with primary pulmonary hypertension; possibly due to the more central nature of the obstruction with more rapid pulmonary capillary runoff. Whether such a distinction can help distinguish chronic embolic pulmonary hypertension from other etiologies remains to be seen. It is worth reiterating that pulmonary artery pressures (both systolic and diastolic) are often not significantly increased in acute pulmonary embolism. The normal right ventricle when suddenly faced with an increase in outflow impedance and pulmonary vascular resistance is unable to generate significantly high pressures. In cases of chronic pulmonary vascular disease

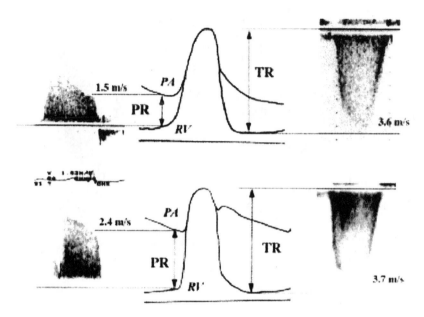

Figure 10 Continuous wave Doppler measurements of pulmonary regurgitation envelopes taken in the right ventricular outflow tract on the left. On the right are tricuspid regurgitation envelopes taken in the right atrium. In the central panel are schematic diagrams of PA and RV pressure waveforms. The top panels from representative patient with chronic pulmonary thromboembolism and the bottom panels from a representative patient with primary pulmonary hypertension. (From Ref. 55.)

of any etiology, elevations of pulmonary artery pressures are demonstrated along with right ventricular hypertrophy. Although such findings aid in the diagnosis of long-standing pulmonary vascular disease, they do not help in identifying the cause.

The Doppler recording of systolic blood velocity in the right ventricular outflow tract and main pulmonary artery have been analyzed in patients with various etiologies of right-sided failure. The normal Doppler velocity curve in the right ventricular outflow tract and pulmonary artery peaks in mid ejection. In the presence of significant pulmonary hypertension, the curve begins to resemble the left-sided velocity curves with a shorter acceleration time. In severe pulmonary hypertension, there is often a biphasic curve with a mid systolic reduction in velocity (Fig. 11). Torbicki et al. (57) found that patients with acute pulmonary embolism had the shortest systolic acceleration time and time to midsystolic deceleration despite having the lowest tricuspid regurgitant velocities. An acceleration time of less than 60 msec in

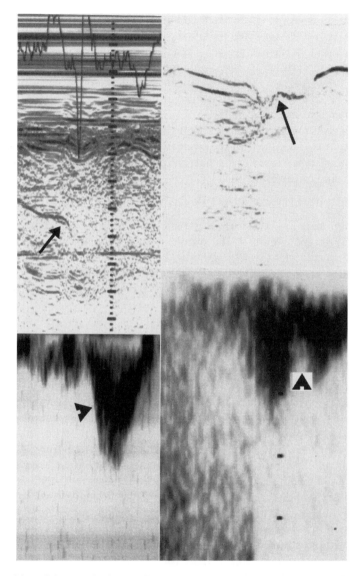

Figure 11 Right ventricular outflow tract Doppler signals (bottom) and M-mode of pulmonary valve (top). On the left panel are normals and on the right are tracings from a patient with pulmonary hypertension caused by recurrent and unresolved pulmonary thromboemboli. Note the midsystolic notching in the right-hand tracings (on both Doppler and M-mode) typically seen in severe pulmonary hypertension.

patients with tricuspid gradients of less than 60 mmHg had a 98% specificity and 48% sensitivity for acute pulmonary embolism in a group of 86 patients with tricuspid gradients greater than 27 mmHg. Yoshinaga et al. (58) examined the systolic acceleration time divided by the right ventricular ejection time (AcT/RVET) in 16 patients with acute pulmonary embolism. They observed a poor correlation with mean pulmonary artery pressure (r = −0.68; $P < .05$) and total pulmonary resistance (r = −0.66; $P < .05$). This correlation disappeared after treatment, although in the chronic phase, there was a slight correlation with the severity of residual obstruction. The AcT/RVET has also been used to estimate the mean pulmonary artery pressure by the following formula (59–61):

$$Log_{10}(mPAP) = -2.8(AcT/RVET) + 2.4$$

Pulmonary artery flow characteristics have been studied in lung disease. The velocity-time integral of the systolic flow in the main pulmonary artery may reflect the right ventricular stroke output and the mean systolic acceleration may reflect right ventricular outflow impedance (62). The value of these measurements in the diagnosis of patients with suspected pulmonary embolism is as yet unknown.

IV. Echocardiography in the Diagnosis of Paradoxical Embolism

It is an axiom of cardiovascular diagnostics that paradoxical embolism must be strongly suspected whenever any of the symptoms or findings of acute pulmonary embolism coexist with those of acute arterial occlusion. Approximately a quarter of the population have a probe-patent foramen ovale. When one of these individuals develops acute cor pulmonale from pulmonary thromboembolism, the elevated right atrial pressures facilitate opening of the foramen and place the subject at risk for additional thromboemboli to cross to the systemic arterial circuit. Large thromboemboli arising in the venous periphery have been demonstrated traversing the foramen ovale by both transthoracic and transesophageal echocardiography (Figs. 12–14) (63–67). Some may become trapped there for a time and spawn smaller clots to embolize both the pulmonary and systemic circulation. Some may remain trapped to seal the patent foramen so that contrast studies and indicator dilution techniques no longer provide evidence of a right-to-left shunt.

The echocardiogram may prove to be very useful in the evaluation of the patient suspected of both pulmonary and paradoxical embolism. A potential right to left shunt at the atrial level may be documented either by Doppler color mapping or by adequate opacification of the right atrium

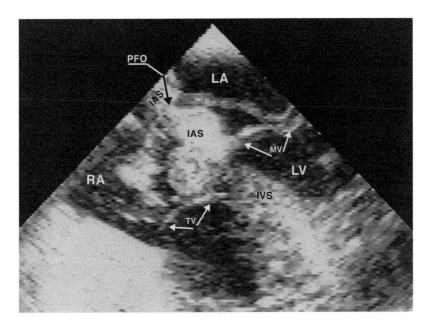

Figure 12 Transesophageal echocardiogram demonstrating cylindrical echo densities in the right atrium (RA) attached to the area of the fossa ovalis with a thinner serpiginous echodensity in the left atrium (LA) arising from the area of the fossa ovalis. The right atrial mass could be seen to prolapse through the tricuspid valve (TV) into the right ventricle (RV) during diastole. This is most consistent with a thromboembolism arising from the deep veins of the leg and caught traversing a patent foramen ovale. IAS, interatrial septum; IVS, interventricular septum; PFO, patent foramen ovale; LV, left ventricle; MV, mitral valve.

with contrast (e.g., agitated saline). During opacification, the right atrial pressures must be momentarily increased above those of the left atrium on release of the Valsalva maneuver or with forceful cough or abdominal compression. If contrast is not seen crossing the atrial septum or not seen opacifying the left side within several beats, a patent foramen ovale is very unlikely. As mentioned earlier, an embolus can occasionally be documented caught within the foramen ovale; in which case the diagnosis is essentially corroborated and streaming of contrast right to left is not to be expected. Evidence for thromboemboli in the proximal pulmonary arteries or evidence for acute cor pulmonale is, of course, evidence for concomitant pulmonary embolism, although ultrasonic evidence for deep venous thrombi also support the diagnosis.

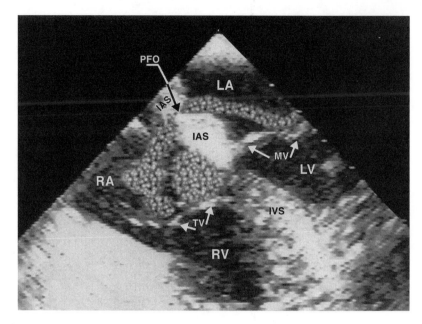

Figure 13   The same echo frame as in Figure 12. The hypermobile echoes consistent with thrombus are stippled. See Figure 12 for abbreviations.

In recent years, it has become evident that many people experience paradoxical embolism without having signs or symptoms of pulmonary embolism. Of course, it should have been suspected that this would be the case. Unless pulmonary embolism is massive or submassive, it is unlikely to cause acute cor pulmonale (27); and because of the bronchial arterial supply to the lung, pulmonary injury or infarction does not occur unless distal pulmonary arterial branches are totally occluded (68). Therefore, most small pulmonary emboli remain silent. Furthermore, even in the absence of pathological elevations of right atrial pressure, there is momentary streaming of blood right to left across a patent foramen ovale, during release of a Valsalva maneuver, cough, and even during the normal respiratory cycle (69). Therefore, clots too small to affect the pulmonary circuit may pass to the systemic arteries where they may present as transient or permanent arterial occlusions. Transient ischemic neurological events, cryptogenic strokes (70), acute myocardial infarctions (71,72), and other arterial ischemic events have been described in patients with patent foramen ovale. As a quarter of the population have such potential openings, it is difficult to establish paradoxical embolism as the etiology, especially if another poten-

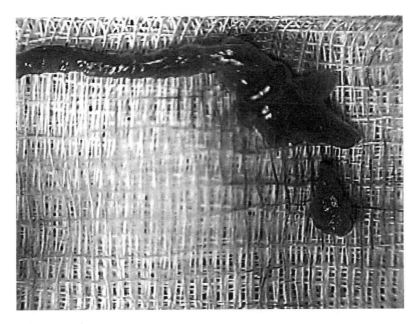

Figure 14 A large thrombus removed from the right brachial artery in a patient who sustained a paradoxical embolism via a patent foramen ovale.

tial etiology such as vasculitis or atherosclerosis coexists. It has been found that patients below the age of 50 years with cryptogenic strokes have a higher than usual incidence of patent foramen ovale by contrast study with echocardiography (73) or a large right-to-left shunt demonstrated by transcranial Doppler (74,75). It has become common to intervene in patients with arterial emboli and evidence of a shunt with lifelong anticoagulation (76) or closure of the patent foramen ovale with surgery (77,78) or catheter device (79,80).

V. Intravascular Ultrasound

Pandian et al. (81) described in vivo intravascular ultrasound recordings of normal pulmonary arteries in dogs and in humans. Subsequently, intravascular ultrasound has been used to observe experimental pulmonary emboli in dogs (82), as well as to document pulmonary emboli in patients with both acute (83,84) and chronic (85–87) pulmonary embolism. Gorge et al. (85) examined 11 patients with documented pulmonary embolism and found ultrasonic evidence for embolism in all. One hundred sixty-eight pulmonary segments were studied and ultrasound images compared to the angiographic appearance. Ultrasound indicated thrombi in 38 (34%) of 112 angiographically normal segments; missed thrombi in 3 (6%) of 49 angiographically partially occluded segments; and confirmed all of the 7 angiographically completely occluded segments. Intravascular ultrasound was therefore more sensitive than angiography in detecting thrombis. Continued refinement of equipment (88–91) and comparison of ultrasonic images with histologic findings (92,93), promise to improve the clinical usefulness of this invasive tool as a complement to pulmonary angiography and, possibly, angioscopy (94,95).

Intravascular ultrasound has a possible role in the treatment of pulmonary embolism, as inferior vena cava filters have been inserted and deployed successfully in the intensive care unit under the guidance of intravascular ultrasound (96–98).

VI. Thoracic Sonography of the Lung

With the use of special transducers, the same equipment used for echocardiography can be used to scan along intercostal spaces and obtain ultrasonic recordings of subjacent structures, pleura, lung, and associated pathology. In 1966, Joyner et al. (99–101) produced pulmonary embolism in 21 dogs with autologous clot. Using a primitive ultrasonic device they reported that they observed a deeper penetration of echoes in the interspace overlying ischemic lung parenchyma. They stated that they located 99% of embolized areas. They also reported finding the same ultrasonic pattern in 64 patients with suspected pulmonary embolism out of a total of 183 patients at the Hospital of the University of Pennsylvania. Of the 64 patients, however, only 13 had the diagnosis confirmed by angiography, surgery, or autopsy. They also noted that similar patterns were observed in patients with other pathologies (102). While a fellow at the Peter Bent Brigham Hospital, in the laboratory of Dr. Lewis Dexter, the author (J.A.P.) was unable to duplicate these results in either the laboratory or the clinic.

In 1993, Mathis and Derschmid reported on a characteristic wedge-shaped or lobular hypoechoic pattern when scanning infarcted lung at autopsy (103). Subsequently, similar patterns have been reported in patients with suspected or confirmed pulmonary embolism (104–106) (Fig. 15). Lechleitner et al. (104) found 33% of subjects with normal lung scans had similar findings. Although this is a promising technique, much additional work needs to be done to improve the technology, refine the technique, and establish any potential usefulness in the diagnosis of pulmonary pathology (107).

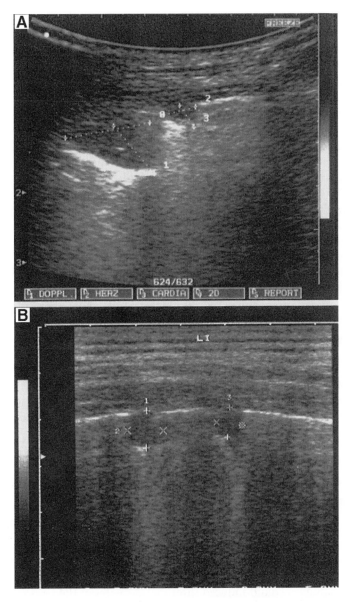

Figure 15   Representative intercostal sonograms associated with pulmonary embolism. (A) Two triangular hypoechoic pleura-based parenchymal lesions. (B) Two rounded hypoechoic pleura-based parenchymal lesions. (From Ref. 106.)

VII. Future Applications of Echocardiography in Pulmonary Thromboembolism

Owing to its low sensitivity for the diagnosis of pulmonary thromboembolism, echocardiography will remain, for the foreseeable future, a test used primarily in patients with compromised hemodynamic status (108). Some investigators have used echocardiography selectively in hemodynamically stable patients to document right heart dysfunction, estimate the extent of pulmonary vascular obstruction, and monitor therapy (109,110). Algorithms recommending fibrinolysis as primary therapy in normotensive patients with evidence of right ventricular dysfunction have been proposed (109,110). However, large-scale randomized trials comparing this approach to heparin anticoagulation are not yet available (111,112). If such studies are initiated, echocardiography will play a central role in identifying patients and monitoring their response to therapy.

As described in the previous section, recent reports have demonstrated the ability of transthoracic sonography to identify parenchymal changes caused by peripheral pulmonary emboli with high concordance with established diagnostic procedures (104–106). The potential advantages of this technique include wide availability, bedside performance, earlier diagnosis, and avoidance of radiation exposure. However, large-scale prospective studies are not available and, therefore, its clinical utility remains to be determined.

Continuing technological advances in three-dimensional echocardiography offer the potential of improved delineation of cardiac structures with enhanced identification of abnormalities (113). The additional information promises to allow more accurate characterization of intracardiac masses and prediction of their histology and origin than can be obtained by currently available two-dimensional techniques (113,114).

An account of the future of ultrasound in pulmonary thomboembolism would be incomplete without a passing remark about its potential value in therapy. In addition to its diagnostic capabilities, ultrasound—at higher energy—may prove to enhance the treatment of pulmonary thromboembolism (115,116). With concomitant administration of fibrinolytic agents, in vitro and in vivo studies have demonstrated that ultrasonic energy, delivered transcutaneously or by means of an intravascular catheter, can facilitate thrombolysis and vessel recanalization (117–119). The use of microbubbles to potentiate ultrasound-induced thrombolysis without the need for fibrinolytic agents has also been explored (120). Delivery of therapeutic ultrasound without adjunctive pharmacological agents has also been reported to facilitate thrombolysis (121). Study of the clinical applications of therapeutic ultrasound is in its infancy; ongoing work is required to determine optimal insonation frequencies and duration of exposure to maximize thrombolysis and minimize tissue injury.

References

1. PIOPED Investigators. Value of the ventilation/perfusion scan in acute pulmonary embolism. JAMA 1990; 263:2753–2759.
2. Khorasani R, Gudas TF, Nikpoor N, Polak JF. Treatment of patients with suspected pulmonary embolism and intermediate-probability lung scans: is diagnostic imaging underused? AJR Am J Roentgenol 1997; 169:1355–1357.
3. Wolfe TR, Hartsell SC. Pulmonary embolism: making sense of the diagnostic evaluation. Ann Emerg Med 2001; 37:504–514.
4. Covarrubias EA, Sheikh MU, Fox LM. Echocardiography and pulmonary embolism. Ann Intern Med 1977; 87:720–721.
5. Kasper W, Meinertz T, Henkel B, Eisnner D, Hahn K, Hofman T, Zeiher A, Just H. Echocardiographiic findings in patients with proved pulmonary embolism. Am Heart J 1986; 112:1284–1290.
6. The European Working Group on Echocardiography. The European cooperative study on the clinical significance of right heart thrombi. Eur Heart J 1989; 10:1046–1059.
7. Malloy PC, Gore JM, Rippe JM, Paraskos JA, Benotti JR, Ockene IS, Alpert JS, Dalen JE. Transient right atrial thrombus resulting in pulmonary embolism detected by two-dimensional echocardiography. Am Heart J 1984; 108:1047–1049.
8. Kinney EL, Wright RJ. Efficacy of treatment of patients with echocardiographically detected right-sided thrombi: a meta-analysis. Am Heart J 1989; 110:569–573.
9. Tsoukas A, Athanasopoulos G, Koliandris I, Koutelou M, Ritsou M, Christakos S, Cokkinos DV. Silent pulmonary embolism of a large right atrial thrombus. Echocardiography 1998; 15:503–506.
10. Hunter JJ, Johnson KR, Karagianes TG, Dittrich HC. Detection of massive pul-monary embolus-in-transit by transesophageal echocardiography. Chest 1991; 100:1210–1214.
11. Bashir M, Asher CR, Garcia MJ, Abdella I, Jasper SE, Murray RD, Grimm RA, Thomas JD, Klein AL. Right atrial spontaneous echo contrast and thrombi in atrial fibrillation: a transesophageal echocardiographic study. J Am Soc Echocardiogr 2001; 14:122–127.
12. Mohanty N, Campbell D, McGrath B, Hsla J. Transesophageal echocardiographic visualization of pulmonary emboli during orthopedic surgery. Circulation 1992; 86(suppl 1):193.
13. Parmet JL, Horrow JC, Singer R, Berman AT, Rosenberg H. Echogenic emboli upon tourniquet release during total knee arthroplasty. Anesth Analg 1994; 79:940–945.

14. Coles RE, Clements FM, Lardenoye JW, Wermeskerken GV, Hey LA, Nunley JA, Levin LS, Pearsall AW IV. Transesophageal echocardiography in quantitation of emboli during femoral nailing: reamed versus unreamed techniques. J South Orthop Assoc 2000; 9:98–104.

15. Koessler MJ, Fabiani R, Hamer H, Pitto RP. The clinical relevance of embolic events detected by transesophageal echocardiography during cemented total hip arthroplasty: a randomized clinical trial. Anesth Analg 2001; 92:49–55.

16. Saada M, Goarin JP, Riou JJ, Jacquens Y, Guesda R, Viars P. Systemic gas embolism complicating pulmonary contusion. Diagnosis and management using transesophageal echocardiography. Am J Respir Crit Care Med 1995; 152:812–815.

17. Tingleff J, Joyce FS, Pettersson G. Intraoperative echocardiographic study of air embolism during cardiac operations. Ann Thorac Surg1995; 673–677.

18. Steiner P, Lund GK, Debatin JF, Steiner D, Nienaber C, Nicolas V, Bucheler E. Acute pulmonary embolism: value of transthoracic and transesophageal echocardiography in comparison with helical CT. AJR Am J Roentgenol 1996; 167:931–936.

19. Otmani A, Tribouilloy C, Leborgne L, Vermes E, Trojette F, Beckers C, Remond A, Fonroget J, Rey JL, Lesbre JP. Valeur diagnostique de l'échographie cardiaque et de l'angioscanner thoracique hélicoïdal pour le diagnostic de l'embolie pulmonaire aiguë. Ann Cardiol Angéiol 1998; 47:707–715.

20. Pruszczyk P, Torbicki A, Kuch-Wocial A, Szulc M, Pacho R. Diagnostic value of transoesophageal echocardiography in suspected haemodynamically significant pulmonary embolism. Heart 2001; 85:628–634.

21. Wittlich N, Erbel R, Eichler A, Schuster S, Jakob H, Iversen S, Oelert H, Meyer J. Detection of central pulmonary artery thromboemboli by trans-esophageal echocardiography in patients with severe pulmonary embolism. J Am Soc of Echocardiogr 1992; 5:515–524.

22. Krivec B, Voga G, Zuran I, Skale R, Pereznik R, Podbregar M, Noc M. Diagnosis and treatment of shock due to massive pulmonary embolism: approach with transesophageal echocardiography and intrapulmonary throm-bolysis. Chest 1997; 112:1310–1316.

23. Vieillard-Baron A, Qanadli SD, Antakly Y, Fourme T, Loubieres Y, Jardin F, Dubourg O. Transesophageal echocardiography for the diagnosis of pulmo-nary embolism with acute cor pulmonale: a comparison with radiological procedures. Intensive Care Med 1998; 24:429–433.

24. Russo A, DeLuca M, Vigna C, DeRito V, Pacilli M, Lombardo A, Armillotta M, Fanelli R, Loperfido F. Central pulmonary artery lesions in chronic ob-structive pulmonary disease. Circulation 1999; 100:1808–1815.

25. van der Wouw PA, Koster RW, Delemarre BJ, de Vos R, Lampe-Schoenmaeckers AJ, Lie KI. Diagnostic accuracy of transesophageal echo-cardiography during cardiopulmonary resuscitation. J Am Coll Cardiol 1997; 30:780–783.

26. Comess KA, DeRook PA, Russell ML, Tognazzi-Evans TA, Beach KW. The incidence of pulmonary embolism in unexplained sudden cardiac arrest with pulseless electrical activity. Am J Med 2000; 109:351–356.

27. McGinn S, White PD. Acute cor pulmonale resulting from pulmonary embolism. JAMA 1935; 104:1473–1480.
28. Dalen JE, Banas JS Jr, Brooks HL, Evans GL, Paraskos JA, Dexter L. Resolution rate of acute pulmonary embolism in man. N Engl J Med 1969; 280:1194–1199.
29. Brooks H, Kirk ES, Vokonas PS, Urschel CW, Sonnenblick EH. Performance of the right ventricle under stress: relation to right coronary flow. J Clin Invest 1971; 50:2176–2183.
30. Paraskos JA, Adelstein SJ, Smith RE, Rickman FD, Grossman W, Dexter L, Dalen JE. Late prognosis of acute pulmonary embolism. N Engl J Med 1973; 289:55–58.
31. Adams JE III, Siegel BA, Goldstein JA, Jaffe AS. Elevations of CK-MB following pulmonary embolism: a manifestation of occult right ventricular infarction. Chest 1992; 101:1203–1206.
32. Steckley R, Smith CW, Robertson RM. Acute right ventricular overload: an echocardiographic clue to pulmonary thromboembolism. Johns Hopkins Med J 1978; 143:122–125.
33. Come PC. Echocardiographic recognition of pulmonary arterial disease and determination of its cause. Am J Med 1988; 84:384–394.
34. Casazza F, Centonze F, Chirico M, Marzegalli M, Bongarzoni A, Piane C, Morpurgo M. Diagnosi ecocardiografica precoce di embolia polmonare massiva. G Ital Cardiol 1994; 24:483–490.
35. Cheriex EC, Sreeram N, Eussen YF, Pieters FA, Wellens HJ. Cross-sectional Doppler echocardiography as the initial technique for the diagnosis of acute pulmonary embolism. Br Heart J 1994; 72:52–57.
36. Kasper W, Konstantinides S, Geibel A, Tiede N, Krause T, Just H. Prognostic significance of right ventricular afterload stress detected by echocardiography in patients with clinically suspected pulmonary embolism. Heart 1997; 77:346–349.
37. Jardin F, Dubourg O, Bourdarias JP. Echocardiographic pattern of acute cor pulmonale. Chest 1997; 111:209–217.
38. Feigenbaum H. Echocardiography. 4th ed. Philadelphia: Lea & Febiger, 1986: 622.
39. Metz D, Chapoutot L, Ouzan J. Doppler echocardiographic assessment of the severity of acute pulmonary embolism: a correlative angiographic study in forty-eight adult patients. Am J Noninvas Cardiol 1991; 5:223–228.
40. Vieillard-Baron A, Schmitt JM, Augarde R, Fellahi JL, Prin S, Page B, Beauchet A, Jardin F. Acute cor pulmonale in acute respiratory distress syndrome submitted to protective ventilation: incidence, clinical implications, and prognosis. Crit Care Med 2001; 29:1641–1642.
41. Kasper W, Meinertz T, Henkel B, Eissner D, Hahn K, Hofmann T, Zeither A, Just H. Echocardiographic findings in patients with proved pulmonary embolism. Am Heart J 1986; 112:1284.
42. Kasper W, Geibel A, Tiede N, Bassenge D, Kauder E, Konstantinides S, Meinertz T, Just H. Distinguishing between acute and subacute massive pulmonary embolism by conventional and Doppler echocardiography. Br Heart J 1993; 70:352–356.

43. Ribeiro A, Lindmarker P, Juhlin-Dannfelt A, Johnsson H, Jorfeldt L. Echocardiography Doppler in pulmonary embolism: right ventricular dysfunction as a predictor of mortality rate. Am Heart J 1997; 134:479–487.

44. Jardin F, Dubourg O, Gueret P, Delorme G, Bourdarias JP. Quantitative two-dimensional echocardiography in massive pulmonary embolism: emphasis on ventricular interdependence and leftward septal displacement. J Am Coll Cardiol 1987; 10:1201–1206.

45. Vieillard-Baron A, Page B, Augarde R, Prin S, Qandli S, Beauchet A, Dubourg O, Jardon F. Acute cor pulmonale in massive pulmonary embolism: incidence, echocardiographic pattern, clinical implications and recovery rate. Intensive Care Med 2001; 27:1481–1486.

46. McConnell MV, Solomon SD, Rayan ME, Come PC, Goldhaber SZ, Lee RT. Regional right ventricular dysfunction detected by echocardiography in acute pulmonary embolism. Am J Cardiol 1996; 78:469–473.

47. Come PC, Kim D, Parker JA, Goldhaber SZ, Braunwald E, Markis JE. Early reversal of right ventricular dysfunction in patients with acute pulmonary embolism after treatment with intravenous tissue plasminogen activator. J Am Coll Cardiol 1987; 10:971–988.

48. Nass N, McConnell MV, Goldhaber SZ, Chyu S, Solomon SD. Recovery of regional right ventricular function after thrombolysis for pulmonary embolism. Am J Cardiol 1999; 83:804–806.

49. Yock PG, Popp RL. Noninvasive estimation of right ventricular systolic pressure by Doppler ultrasound in patients with tricuspid regurgitation. Circulation 1984; 70:657–662.

50. Becker SJ, Gibbs JS, Fox KM, Yacoub MH, Gibson DG. Comparison of Doppler derived haemodynamic variables and simultaneous high fidelity pressure measurements in severe pulmonary hypertension. Br Heart J 1994; 72:384–389.

51. Himelman R, Stulbarg M, Kircher B, Lee E, Kee L, Dean NC, Golden J, Wolfe CL, Schiller NB. Noninvasive evaluation of pulmonary artery pressure during exercise by saline-enhanced Doppler echocardiography in chronic pulmonary disease. Circulation 1989; 79:863–871.

52. Metz D, Chapoutot L, Pollet E, Jolly D, Chabert JP, Elaerts J, Bajolet A. Intérêt diagnostique et pronostique du doppler continu dans l'embolie pulmonaire. Arch Mal Coeur Vaiss 1988; 81:1087–1091.

53. Miniati M, Monti S, Prateli L, Di Ricco G, Marini C, Formichi B, Prediletto R, Michelassi C, Di Lorenzo M, Tonelli L, Pistolesi M. Value of transthoracic echocardiography in the diagnosis of pulmonary embolism: results of a prospective study in unselected patients. Am J Med 2001; 110:528–535.

54. Perrier A, Tamm C, Unger PF, Lerch R, Sztajzel J. Diagnostic accuracy of Doppler-echocardiography in unselected patients with suspected pulmonary embolism. Int J Cardiol 1998; 65:101–109.

55. Masuyama T, Kodama K, Kitabatake A, sato H, Nanto S, Inoue M. Continuous-wave Doppler echocardiographic detection of pulmonic regurgitation and its application to noninvasive estimation of pulmonary artery pressure. Circulation 1986; 74:484–492.

56. Nakayama Y, Sugimachi M, Nakanishi N, Takaki H, Okano Y, Satoh T, Miyatake K, Sunagawa K. Noninvasive differential diagnosis between chronic pulmonary thromboembolism and primary pulmonary hypertension by means of Doppler ultrasound measurement. J Am Coll Cardiol 1998; 31:1367–1371.

57. Torbicki A, Kurzyna M, Ciurzynski M, Pruszczyk P, Pacho R, Kuch-Wocial A, Szulc M. Proximal pulmonary emboli modify right ventricular ejection pattern. Eur Respir J 1999; 13:616–621.

58. Yoshinaga T, Ikeda S, Nishimura E, Shioguchi K, Shikuwa M, Miyahara Y, Kohno S. Diagnostic value of pulsed Doppler echocardiography in acute pulmonary thromboembolism—comparison with pulmonary angiography and pulmonary artery pressure. Jpn Circ J 2001; 65:171–176.

59. West JB. Ventilation-perfusion relationship. In: West JB, ed. Respiratory Physiology–the Essentials. 2d ed. Baltimore: William & Wilkins, 1979:51–68.

60. Schumacker PT. Ventilation-perfusion relationship. In: Leff AR, Schumacker PT, eds. Respiratory Physiology. Philadelphia: Saunders, 1993:93–110.

61. Shioya T, Kagaya M, Sasaki M, Hasegawa H, Kibira S, Miura M. Clinical importance of AaDO2 and pulmonary artery pressure as predicted by pulsed Doppler echocardiography at bedside in diagnosing pulmonary embolism. Angiology 1998; 49:33–40.

62. Schmitt JM, Vieillard-Baron A, Augarde R, Prin B, Jardin F. Positive end-expiratory pressure titration in acute respiratory distress syndrome patients: impact on right ventricular outflow impedance evaluated by pulmonary artery Doppler flow velocity measurements. Crit Care Med 2001; 29:1154–1158.

63. Nellessen U, Daniel WG, Matheis G, Oelert H, Depping K, Lichtlen PR. Impending paradoxical embolism from atrial thrombus: correct diagnosis by transesophageal echocardiography and prevention by surgery. J Am Coll Cardiol 1985; 5:1002–1004.

64. Nelson CW, Snow FR, Barnett M, McRoy L, Wechsler AS, Nixon JV. Impending paradoxical embolism: echocardiographic diagnosis of an intra-cardiac thrombus crossing a patent foramen ovale. Am Heart J 1991; 122:859–862.

65. DeCastro S, Cartoni D, Conti G, Beni S. Continuous monitoring by biplane transesophageal echocardiography of pulmonary and paradoxical embolism. J Am Soc Echocardiogr 1995; 8:217–220.

66. Mathew TC, Ramsaran EK, Aragam JR. Impending paradoxic embolism in acute pulmonary embolism: diagnosis by transesophageal echocardiography and treatment by emergent surgery. Am heart J 1995; 129:826–827.

67. Quere JP, Tribouilloy C, Adam MC, Juracan E, Rey JL, Lesbre JP. Paradoxical embolism following acute pulmonary embolism: diagnosis and outcome. Int J cardiol 1998; 64:131–135.

68. Dalen JE, Haffajee CI, Alpert JS, Howe JP, Ockene IS, Paraskos JA. Pulmonary embolism, pulmonary hemorrhage and pulmonary infarction. N Engl J Med 1977; 296:1431–1435.

69. Langholz D, Louis EK, Konstadt SN, Rao TL, Scanlon PJ. Transesophageal echocardiographic demonstration of distinct mechanisms for right to left

shunting across a patent foramen ovale in the absence of pulmonary hypertension. J Am Coll Cardiol 1991; 18:1112–1117.

70. Isayev Y, Chan RK, Pullicino PM. "Economy class" stroke syndrome? Neurology 2002; 58:960–961.

71. Crump R, Shandling AH, Van Natta B, Ellestad M. Prevalence of patent foramen ovale in patients with acute myocardial infarction and angiographically normal coronary arteries. Am J cardiol 2000; 85:1368–1370.

72. Gersmony DR, Kim SH, Di Tullio M, Fard A, Rabbani L, Homma S. Acute myocardial infarction caused by paradoxical coronary embolization in a patient with a patent foramen ovale. J Am Soc Echocardiogr 2001; 14:1227–1229.

73. Lehcat P, Mas JL, Lascault G, Loron P, Theard M, Klimczac M, Drobinski G, Thomas D, Grosgogeat Y. Prevalence of patent foramen ovale in patients with stroke. N Engl J Med 1988; 318:1148–1152.

74. Klotzsch C, Janssen G, Berlit P. Transesophageal echocardiography and contrast-TCD in the detection of a patent foramen ovale: experience with 111 patients. Neurology 1994; 44:1603–1606.

75. Serena J, Segura T, Perez-Ayuso MJ, Bassaganyas J, Molins A, Davalos A. The need to quantify right-to-left shunt in acute ischemic stroke: a case-control study. Stroke 1998; 29:1322–1328.

76. Homma S, Sacco RL, Di Tullio MR, Sciacca RR, Mohr JP. Effect of medical treatment in stroke patients with patent foramen ovale. Circulation 2002; 105:2625–2631.

77. Devuyst G, Bogousslavsky J, Ruchat P, Jeanrenaud X, Despland PA, Regli F, Aebischer N, Karpuz HM, Castillo V, Guffi M, Sadeghi H. Prognosis after stroke followed by surgical closure of patent foramen ovale: a prospective follow-up study with brain MRI and simultaneous transesophageal and transcranial Doppler ultrasound. Neurology 1996; 47:1162–1166.

78. Dearani JA, Ugurlu BS, Danielson GK, Daly RC, McGregor CG, Mullany CJ, Puga FJ, Orszulak TA, Anderson BJ, Brown RD Jr, Schaff HV. Surgical patent foramen ovale closure for prevention of paradoxical embolism-related cerebrovascular ischemic events. Circulation 1999; 100:II171–II175.

79. Dhillon R, Thanopoulos B, Tsaousis G, Triposkiadis F, Kyriakidis M, Redington A. Transcatheter closure of atrial septal defects in adults with Amplatzer septal occluder. Heart 1999; 82:559–562.

80. Hung J, Landzberg MJ, Jenkins KJ, King ME, Lock JE, Palacios IF, Lang P. Closure or patent foramen ovale for paradoxical emboli: intermediate-term risk of recurrent neurological events following transcatheter device placement. J Am Coll Cardiol 2000; 35:1311–1316.

81. Pandian N, Weintraub A, Kreis A, Schwartz S, Konstam M, Salem D. Intracardiac, intravascular, two-dimensional, high frequency ultrasound imaging of pulmonary artery and its branches in humans and animals. Circulation 1990; 81:2007–2012.

82. Tapson VF, Davidson CJ, Gurbel PA, Sheikh KH, Kisslo KB, Stack RS. Rapid and accurate diagnosis of pulmonary emboli in a canine model using intravascular ultrasound imaging. Chest 1991; 100:1410–1413.

83. Gorge G, Erbel R, Schuster S, Ge J, Meyer J. Intravascular ultrasound in patients with acute pulmonary embolism: comparison to angiography. J Am Coll Cardiol 1992; 19:314A.

84. Tapson VF, Davidson CJ, Kisslo KB, Stack RS. Rapid visualization of massive pulmonary emboli utilizing intravascular ultrasound. Chest 1994; 105:888–890.

85. Gorge G, Schuster S, Ge J, Meyer J, Erbel R. Intravascular ultrasound in patients with acute pulmonary embolism after treatment with intravenous urokinase and high dose heparin. Heart 1997; 77:73–77.

86. Ricou F, Nicod PH, Moser KM, Peterson KL. Catheter-based intravascular ultrasound imaging of chronic thromboembolic pulmonary disease. Am J Cardiol 1991; 67:749–752.

87. Scott PJ, Essop AR, al-Ashab W, Deaner A, Parsons J, Williams G. Imaging of vascular disease by intravascular ultrasound. Int J Card Imaging 1993; 9:179–184.

88. Gorge G, Ge J, Haude M, Baumgart D, Buck T, Erbel R. Initial experience with a steerable intravascular ultrasound catheter in the aorta and pulmonary artery. Am J Card Imaging 1995; 9:180–184.

89. Kimura BJ, Bhargava V, Palinski W, Russo RJ, DeMaria AN. Distortion of intravascular ultrasound images because of nonuniform angular velocity of mechanical-type transducers. Am Heart J 1996; 132:328–336.

90. Hiro T, Hall P, Maiello L, Itoh A, Colombo A, Jang YT, Salmon SM, Tobis JM. Clinical feasibility of 0.018-inch intravascular ultrasound imaging device. Am Heart J 1998; 136:1017–1020.

91. Oshima A, Itchhaporia D, Fitzgerald P. New developments in intravascular ultrasound. Vasc Med 1998; 3:281–290.

92. Stahr P, Rupprecht HJ, Voigtlander T, Otto M, Rudigier K, Erbel R, Kearney P, Meyer J. Comparison of normal and diseased pulmonary artery morphology by intravascular ultrasound and histological examination. Int J Card Imaging 1999; 15:221–231.

93. Nakamoto A, Yoshitake J, Hase T, Harasawa H, Okamoto S, Fuse D, Kawasaki R, Kuga H, Kishiro I, Machida S, Oshiro H, Totsuka M, Kaneko N. Intravascular ultrasound imaging of the pulmonary arteries in primary pulmonary hypertension. Respirology 2000; 5:71–78.

94. Uchida Y, Oshima T, Hirose J, Sasaki T, Morizuki S, Morita T. Angioscopic detection of residual pulmonary thrombi in the differential diagnosis of pulmonary embolism. Am Heart J 1995; 130:854–859.

95. Dartevelle P, Fadel E, Chapelier A, Macchiarini P, Cerrina J, Parquin F, Simonneau F, Simonneau G. Angioscopic video-assisted pulmonary endarterectomy for post-embolic pulmonary hypertension. Eur J Cardiothorac Surg 1999; 16:38–43.

96. Oppat WF, Chiou AC, Matsumura JS. Intravascular ultrasound-guided vena cava filter placement. J Endovasc Surg 1999; 6:285–287.

97. Matsumura JS, Morasch MD. Filter placement by ultrasound technique at the bedside. Semin Vasc Surg 2000; 13:199–203.

98. Ebaugh JL, Chiou AC, Morasch MD, Matsumura SJ, Pearce WH. Bedside vena cava filter placement guided with intravascular ultrasound. J Vasc Surg 2001; 34:21–26.

99. Dudrick SJ, Joyner CR, Miller LD, Eskin DJ, Knight DH. Ultrasound in the early diagnosis of pulmonary embolism. Surg Forum 1966; 17:117–118.

100. Joyner CR Jr, Miller LD, Dudrick SJ, Eskin DJ, Knight DH. Reflected ultrasound in the detection of pulmonary embolism. Trans Assoc Am Physicians 1966; 79:262–277.

101. Joyner CR Jr, Miller LD, Dudrick SJ, Eskin DJ, Bloom P. Reflected ultrasound in the study of diseases of the chest. Trans Am Clin Climat Assoc 1967; 78:28–37.

102. Miller LD, Joyner CR Jr, Dudrick SJ, Eskin DJ. Clinical use of ultrasound in the early diagnosis of pulmonary embolism. Ann Surg 1967; 166:381–393.

103. Mathis G, Dirschmid K. Pulmonary infarction: sonographic appearance with pathologic correlation. Eur J Radiol 1993; 17:170–174.

104. Lechleitner P, Raneburger W, Gamper G, Riedl B, Benedikt E, Theurl A. Lung sonographic findings in patients with suspected pulmonary embolism. Ultraschall Med 1998; 19:78–82.

105. Mathis G, Bitschnau R, Gehmacher O, Sheier M, Kopf A, Schwarzler B, Amann T, Doringer W, Hergan K. Chest ultrasound in diagnosis of pulmonary embolism in comparison to helical CT. Ultraschall Med 1999; 20:54–59.

106. Reissig A, Heyne JP, Kroegel C. Sonography of lung and pleura in pulmonary embolism. Chest 2001; 120:1977–1983.

107. Koh DM, Burke S, Davies N, Padley SPG. Transthoracic ultrasound of the chest: clinical uses and applications. Radiographics 2002; 22:e1.

108. Goldhaber SZ. Echocardiography in the management of pulmonary embolism. Ann Intern Med 2002; 136:691–700.

109. Goldhaber SZ, Haire WD, Feldstein ML, Miller M, Toltzis R, Smith JL, Taveira da Silva AM, Come PC, Lee RT, Parker JA, Mogtader A, McDonough TJ, Braunwald E. Alteplase versus heparin in acute pulmonary embolism: randomized trial assessing right-ventricular function and pulmonary perfusion. Lancet 1993; 341:507–511.

110. Konstantinides S, Geibel A, Olschewski M, Heinrich F, Grosser K, Rauber K, Iversen S, Redecker M, Kienast J, Just H, Kasper W. Association between thrombolytic treatment and the prognosis of hemodynamically stable patients with major pulmonary embolism. Results of a multicenter registry. Circulation 1997; 96:882–888.

111. Davidson BL, Lensing AWA. Should echocardiography of the right ventricle help determine who receives thrombolysis for pulmonary embolism? Chest 2001; 120:6–8.

112. Goldhaber SZ. Thrombolysis in pulmonary embolism. A large-scale clinical trial is overdue. Circulation 2001; 104:2876–2878.

113. Roelandt JR. Three-dimensional echocardiography: the future today. Acta Cardiol 1998; 53:323–336.

114. Borges AC, Witt C, Bartel T, Muller S, Konertz W, Baumann G. Preoperative

two-dimensional and three-dimensional echocardiographic assessment of heart tumors. Ann Thorac Surg 1996; 61:1163–1167.

115. Porter TR, Xie F. Ultrasound, microbubbles, and thrombolysis. Prog Cardiovasc Dis 2001; 44:101–110.

116. Francis CW. Ultrasound-enhanced thrombolysis. Echocardiography 2001; 18:239–246.

117. Kudo S. Thrombolysis with ultrasound effect. Tokyo Med J 1989; 104:1005–1012.

118. Siegel RJ, Atar S, Fishbein MC, Brasch AV, Peterson TM, Nagai T, Pal D, Nishioka T, Chae JS, Birnbaum Y, Zanelli C, Luo H. Noninvasive, transthoracic, low-frequency ultrasound augments thrombolysis in a canine model of acute myocardial infarction. Circulation 2000; 101:2026–2029.

119. Suchkova VN, Baggs RB, Francis CW. Effect of 40-kHz ultrasound on acute thrombotic ischemia in a rabbit femoral artery thrombosis model. Enhancement of thrombolysis and improvement in capillary muscle perfusion. Circulation 2000; 101:2296–2301.

120. Birnbaum Y, Luo H, Nagai T, Fishbein MC, Peterson TM, Li S, Kricsfeld D, Porter TR, Seigel RJ. Non-invasive in vitro clot dissolution without a thrombolytic drug. Recanalization of thrombosed iliofemoral arteries by transcutaneous ultrasound combined with intravenous infusion of microbubbles. Circulation 1998; 97:130–134.

121. Rosenschein U, Furman V, Kerner E, Fabian I, Bernheim J, Eschel Y. Ultrasound imaging-guided noninvasive ultrasound thrombolysis. Preclinical results. Circulation 2000; 102:238–245.

10

Venous Thromboembolism and Pregnancy

JOHN BONNAR

Trinity College
and St. James's Hospital
Dublin, Ireland

I. Introduction

In Europe and North America, venous thromboembolism (VTE) is the most serious complication of pregnancy and childbirth. In the British Isles, VTE has been the leading cause of maternal death since 1985. The Confidential Enquiries into maternal death (2001), entitled Why Mothers Die, reported 35 deaths from VTE in the years 1997–1999 and accounted for 33% of direct maternal deaths (1). This was a substantial reduction from 48 maternal deaths from VTE, which were reported for the years 1994–1996 (2). The reduction in deaths from VTE was mainly due to a dramatic fall in deaths after cesarean section, which followed the publication in 1995 of the Royal College of Obstetricians and Gynaecologists (RCOG) Guidelines on Thromboprophylaxis and Cesarean Section (Fig. 1) (3). In recent years, therefore, VTE has accounted for as many maternal deaths as the combined deaths from hypertension (eclampsia), hemorrhage, and sepsis (Table 1).

VTE can occur without warning in low-risk women, but in the main, the complication arises in the presence of multiple risk factors. The Confidential Enquiries have shown that in many cases care was suboptimal—mainly a failure to appreciate the significance of risk factors, failure to provide

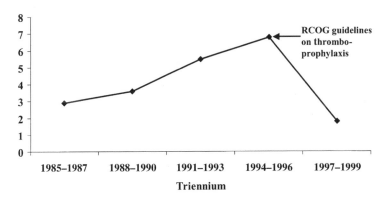

Figure 1 Deaths from pulmonary embolism following cesarean section, rate per million maternities, United Kingdom, 1985–1999. (From Ref 1.)

prophylaxis, and a failure of diagnosis and treatment when VTE occurred. The most recent report recommends that all women undergoing cesarean section should receive prophylaxis against VTE and the most effective method of prophylaxis, heparin at appropriate doses, should be used (1).

The risk factors of VTE in pregnancy include both genetic and acquired conditions. Inherited thrombophilia is now recognized as an important risk factor for VTE arising in pregnancy, during the puerperium, and with oral contraception. Current evidence suggests that genetic factors account for up to 50% of VTE in pregnancy. Major advances have occurred in identifying the gene mutations in coagulation and fibrinolytic proteins which predispose to VTE (4–6). This information in conjunction with the knowledge of acquired risk factors provide a rational basis for

Table 1 Causes of Direct Maternal Deaths in the United Kingdom (1982–1999)

Years	Thromboembolism (%)	Hypertension (%)	Hemorrhage (%)	Sepsis (%)
1982–1984	25 (18.1)	25 (18.1)	9 (6.5)	2 (1.4)
1985–1987	32 (23.0)	27 (19.4)	10 (7.2)	6 (4.3)
1988–1990	33 (22.8)	27 (18.6)	22 (15.2)	7 (4.8)
1991–1993	35 (27.1)	20 (15.5)	15 (11.6)	9 (7.0)
1994–1996	48 (35.8)	20 (14.9)	12 (8.9)	14 (10.4)
1997–1999	35 (30.0)	15 (14.2)	7 (6.6)	14 (13.2)

recognizing high-risk patients and using effective prophylactic treatment. Currently, this would seem to be the only feasible approach to reducing death from VTE, as most patients with fatal pulmonary embolism die within 2 hrs before diagnosis and treatment is possible. The weeks following childbirth are the time of greatest risk, particularly in patients delivered by cesarean section.

II. Epidemiology

A study of 72,000 pregnancies in Scotland based on objective diagnosis reported an incidence of deep vein thrombosis of 0.71 per 1000 deliveries and an incidence of pulmonary embolism of 0.15 per 1000 deliveries (7). If the Scottish data are calculated in women-years, the incidence of thrombotic events during pregnancy was 0.97 per 1000 pregnant woman years and postpartum 7.19 per 1000 women-years. This represents a 2.5-fold increase in the risk of thrombotic events during pregnancy and a 20-fold increase in the puerperium relevant to nonpregnant women of the same age. Table 2 from the Confidential Enquiries analyzed 190 deaths from pulmonary embolism between 1982 and 1999; 87 deaths occurred after abortion or during pregnancy and 99 deaths in the puerperium with 1 death recorded during labor. Again, using pregnant women–years, the incidence of fatal pulmonary embolism is seven to eight times higher in the puerperium than during pregnancy. Cesarean section is associated with over 60% of deaths from fatal pulmonary embolism following delivery. The frequency of fatal pulmonary embolism was 9 to 10 times greater after cesarean section than vaginal delivery. Clearly, the puerperium is the time of greatest risk of VTE;

Table 2 Time of Maternal Deaths from VTE in the United Kingdom (1982–1999)

Years	Total	After abortion or during pregnancy	Death in labor	After vaginal delivery	After cesarean section
1982–1984	29	13	0	4	12
1985–1987	30	17	0	6	7
1988–1990	24	13	0	3	8
1991–1993	30	12	1	4	13
1994–1996	46[a]	18	0	10	15
1997–1999	31	14	0	10	7
	190	87	1	37	62

[a] Includes three deaths for which details were not available.

postpartum thromboprophylaxis for women identified as being at increased risk could have a major impact in reducing maternal death from VTE.

III. Pathogenesis

The physiology of pregnancy results in increased venous distensibility, which is apparent from the first trimester. In addition, the pressure of the gravid uterus impedes venous return from the lower limbs with a greater effect on the left side due to the anatomical arrangement of the common iliac vessels. Using duplex Doppler ultrasound, a marked decrease in blood flow velocity was shown during pregnancy and for 6 weeks following delivery (8,9). The reduced flow velocity is much greater in the left common femoral vein than in the right, which probably explains why around 85% of deep vein thromboses during pregnancy occur in the left leg compared with 55% in nonpregnant women (7,10).

In contrast with the nonpregnant woman, the majority of deep vein thrombosis in pregnancy involves the ileofemoral segment, which is more likely to embolize. The rates of venous insufficiency are also much higher following deep vein thrombosis in pregnancy than observed in nonpregnant women. A Swedish study showed that 65% of women with deep vein thrombosis in pregnancy developed venous insufficiency in the affected leg within 3–10 years of the event despite appropriate anticoagulant therapy (10).

Normal pregnancy involves an increased concentration of coagulation factors, I, VII, VIII, IX, X, XII, von Willebrand's factor antigen, and ristocetin cofactor activity, the functional assessment of von Willebrand's factor (11). During pregnancy, acquired resistance to activated protein C appears to develop, and in the second half of pregnancy, a marked reduction in protein S occurs (12). Fibrinolytic activity shows progressive impairment during pregnancy with a rapid return to normal following delivery. The impairment of fibrinolysis appears to be the result of the production of plasminogen activator inhibitor type 2 by the placenta.

The changes in coagulation and fibrinolysis may be physiological developments to protect the integrity of the maternal and fetal circulations. They also provide a physiological preparation for the hemostatic challenge of placental separation from the uterus when a blood flow of around 800 mL/min has to be stanched. Damage to the endothelium in the uteroplacental vasculature occurs during normal delivery, and additional damage to pelvic vasculature during operative delivery will occur, especially at cesarean section. Pregnancy and delivery, therefore, provide all the predisposing factors of Virchow's triad of venous stasis, hypercoagulability, and vascular damage.

IV. Inherited Thrombophilia in Pregnancy

The hypercoagulable state of pregnancy presents special problems for the women with inherited or acquired thrombophilia. A study in Scotland compared the prevalence of thrombophilia in 75 women with VTE during pregnancy or the puerperium to determine the prevalence of thrombophilia (13) (Table 3). The general population incidence of thrombophilia was antithrombin deficiency type 1, 1 in 5000, type 2, 3 in 2000, factor V Leiden 2.2%, prothrombin mutation 20210A, 2.2%, and the MTHFR mutation (homozygous C677T) 12%. In pregnant women who had had VTE, the odds ratio of an increased incidence for antithrombin deficiency type 1 was 282 and for type 2 was 28, for factor V Leiden 4.5, and for the prothrombin mutation 4.4; the MTHFR mutation, did not have an increased frequency (odds ratio 0.45). This study concluded that both the factor V Leiden and the prothrombin mutation were associated with maternal VTE, but not the MTHFR mutation, and as the odds ratio for the prothrombin mutation was similar to factor V Leiden, routine population screening for this

Table 3 Prevalence of Antithrombin Deficiency, Factor V Leiden, Prothrombin 20210A, and the C677T Mutation in the MTHFR Gene in 75 Women with VTE Related to Pregnancy Compared to General Population in Scotland

Thrombophilia	Cases	General population	Odds ratio	95% CI
Antithrombin				
Type 1 deficiency				
Present	4	1	282	31–2552
Absent	71	4999		
Type 11 deficiency				
Present	3	3	28	5.5–142
Absent	72	1997		
Factor V Leiden				
Present	7	5	4.4	2.1–14.5
Absent	68	219		
Prothrombin 20210A				
Present	5	5	4.5	1.2–16.0
Absent	50	219		
MTHFR				
Homozygous	3	19	0.45	0.13–1.58
Heterozygous or normal allele	49	139		

Source: Ref. 13.

mutation was not indicated. However, based on these findings, it was recommended that women with a personal or strong family history of VTE should be screened for the prothrombin mutation in addition to screening for other thrombophilias (14). Ideally, this should be carried out before pregnancy to allow time to plan pregnancy management with joint consultation between the hematologist and the obstetrician. Women with a history of recurrent fetal loss, fetal growth restriction, and severe preeclampsia and placental abruption should also be screened for inherited and acquired thrombophilia (4,6).

The risk of VTE in pregnancy with underlying thrombophilia will depend on the thrombophilic defect, the history of thrombotic events, and acquired risk factors. Pregnancy and the puerperium often trigger the first thrombotic event in women with deficiencies of antithrombin, protein C, and protein S. Occurrence rates of VTE of 32–40% have been reported in Europe for pregnant women with antithrombin deficiency (5,6). For pregnant women with abnormalities of the protein C and protein S systems, the risk is substantially lower and postpartum VTE is more common than antepartum VTE. The risk of VTE in pregnancy is 3–10% for protein C deficiency and 0–6% for protein S deficiency. In postpartum women, the risk for protein C deficiency is 7–19% and for protein S deficiency is 7–22%. These studies are based on investigations in women with venous thromboembolism and do not reflect the risk of thrombosis in previously symptom-free women with the mutations. In the Scottish study of 72,000 pregnancies, the risk of VTE in pregnancy was 1 in 437 for factor V Leiden, 1 in 113 for protein C deficiency, 1 in 2.8 for type 1 antithrombin deficiency, and 1 in 42 for type 2 antithrombin deficiency (7).

V. Acquired Risk Factors

The Confidential Enquiries have shown that when a maternal death occurs from VTE, one or more of the following risk factors were present in approximately 80% of women:

- Inherited or acquired thrombophilia
- Previous VTE related to pregnancy, surgery, or contraceptive pill use
- Cesarean section: risk of VTE increased 9- to 10-fold (see Table 2)
- Obesity: exceeding 80 kg (176 lb or body mass index over 30 kg/m^2
- Over 35 years old
- Immobility
- Surgical procedures during pregnancy
- Sickle cell anemia
- Air travel

VI. Clinical Features and Diagnosis

The clinical diagnosis of VTE during pregnancy is unreliable, and fewer than half of all cases of leg vein thrombosis involving major proximal veins are identified clinically. Venous thrombosis will almost invariably cause more symptoms in one leg than the other, and in pregnancy will usually be in the left leg. A diagnosis of deep vein thrombosis is almost certain when physical signs are present such as definite tenderness or induration of the calf muscle, leg edema, and increased skin temperature. Clinical evaluation should identify the patient at risk and objective methods should be used to confirm the diagnosis. If a pregnant woman has chest or leg symptoms, duplex ultrasound and ventilation-perfusion (V/Q) lung scanning should be used to exclude the presence of VTE. These investigations are of no significant risk to the mother or fetus. Individual hospitals should have an agreed protocol for the objective diagnosis of suspected VTE during pregnancy. Most pregnant women with ileofemoral thrombosis show evidence on lung scanning of small symptomless pulmonary emboli.

Magnetic resonance imaging (MRI) has the advantage of direct imaging of thrombi in the pulmonary arteries and the large veins. The lack of ionizing radiation makes MRI attractive for use in pregnancy.

In the investigation of suspected VTE in pregnancy, duplex ultrasound and V/Q scanning will usually provide a diagnosis. If these are negative in the presence of a high degree of clinical suspicion, treatment with anticoagulant therapy should be considered and the tests repeated after an interval of 1 week. If the repeat investigations are negative, treatment can be discontinued.

A. d-Dimer

The levels of d-dimer are usually raised in normal pregnancy and increased levels are found in the puerperium and with complications such as pre-eclampsia. This being so, a raised d-dimer is of doubtful diagnostic value during pregnancy or the puerperium, but a low or normal d-dimer would help to rule out VTE.

VII. Anticoagulant Therapy During Pregnancy

Both unfractionated heparin and low molecular weight heparin (LMWH) do not cross the placenta and thus do not carry a risk of teratogenesis or fetal hemorrhage. The disadvantages of heparin treatment are the need for parenteral administration and complications such as heparin-induced thrombocytopaenia, allergy, and osteoporosis can occur with prolonged use. LMWH has been shown to be safe and effective in nonpregnant women and is associated with fewer side effects than unfractionated heparin in the treatment of VTE (14,15).

Coumarin derivatives such as warfarin should be avoided during pregnancy; the drug crosses the placenta and warfarin embryopathy may occur in 4–5% of fetuses exposed to the drug between 6 and 9 weeks of gestation (16). Warfarin embryopathy can be avoided by substitution of heparin for warfarin during the first trimester. Central nervous system abnormalities have also been reported with warfarin exposure in the fetus; most likely caused by spontaneous intracerebral bleeding during pregnancy. The fetal liver is immature and the levels of vitamin K–dependent coagulation factors are low in the fetus. Warfarin therapy in the optimal range for the mother will result in excessive anticoagulation in the fetus. If warfarin is used in pregnancy, it should also be avoided after 36 weeks' gestation because of the risk of hemorrhage in both mother and baby. Women who are taking long-term oral anticoagulant prophylaxis because they have a mechanical prosthatic heart valve should be informed of the risks of fetal complications if they become pregnant. They should be advised to avoid pregnancy and to contact their physician immediately if pregnancy is likely. Self-administered heparin should be substituted for warfarin as soon as possible after conception and before 6 weeks' gestation.

VIII. Management of VTE in Pregnancy

Although the objective diagnosis of VTE during pregnancy is important, treatment should be commenced on clinical grounds if objective tests cannot be performed quickly. Extensive clinical experience has established heparin to be the safest anticoagulant to use during pregnancy. Immediate treatment of VTE with heparin is important to reduce the morbidity and mortality from pulmonary embolism and arrest the extension of deep vein thrombosis, therefore reducing long-term morbidity from postthrombotic venous insufficiency.

Recommended treatment in antenatal VTE has three options: intravenous unfractionated heparin, subcutaneous unfractionated heparin, or LMWH. If intravenous heparin is used, 5000 IU or 75 IU/kg body weight should be given slowly over 3–5 min followed by 15–25 IU/kg/hr by continuous intravenous infusion to prolong the activated partial thromboplastin time to 1.5–2.5 times the control. Intravenous therapy is usually continued for 5–7 days. Treatment with subcutaneous unfractionated heparin is given by injection into the flank of the anterior abdominal wall; dosage of subcutaneous heparin of 10,000–15,000 IU at 8- to12-hr intervals will usually provide adequate anticoagulation.

In late pregnancy, heparin resistance occurs that is most likely due to increased physiological activation of the coagulation system and raised levels of factor VIII and fibrinogen. If available, measurement of the anti Xa activity to monitor the dose of heparin is recommended and will allow better control of heparin dosage. Therapeutic treatment with heparin should be continued for at least 6 weeks followed by a prophylactic dosage of subcutaneous heparin and reduction or cessation of heparin during labor and delivery. Patients usually have no difficulty in learning to self-administer subcutaneous heparin into the lateral aspect of the anterior abdominal wall. Subcutaneous heparin is best avoided in the arms and legs, as painful bruising is more likely in these areas.

LMWH is used increasingly in pregnant women (17). Experience has been gained with enoxaparin and tinzaparin for treatment of antenatal VTE. Enoxaparin is given as a dose of 1 mg/kg (40–80 mg) subcutaneously 12-hr intervals. With tinzaparin, the recommended dosage is 175 IU/kg (10,000 IU) once daily by subcutaneous injection. Until further experience is published, treatment is best monitored by measuring anti-Xa activity and the recommended therapeutic range is between 0.35 and 1.0 IU/mL at 3–4 hr postinjection. As with standard heparin, LMWH is reduced or discontinued for labor and delivery.

If a woman is anticoagulated during labor, epidural or spinal anesthesia should be avoided because of the risk of hematoma formation during insertion and removal of the indwelling cannula. If heparin has been discontinued for 12 hr and the platelet count and activated partial thromboplastin time (aPPT) are normal, epidural or spinal anaesthesia should not be associated with any increased risk of bleeding. Similar precautions are recommended in the use of LMWH, and the insertion and removal of a cannula for epidural or spinal anaesthesia should be delayed until 12 hr after LMWH has been administered (18).

Anticoagulant prophylaxis should resume within 4–8 hr following delivery using either subcutaneous standard heparin or LMWH. The puerperium is the time of greatest risk; if standard heparin is used, 5000–10,000 units every 12 hr is advisable. Warfarin therapy can begin postpartum with 7 mg on the first and second days and 5 mg on the third day. Both heparin and warfarin are safe for nursing mothers to use. Heparin can be discontinued when the international normalized ratio (INR) has increased to a therapeutic range of 2–3 for 2 consecutive days. Warfarin therapy should be continued for at least 3 months. If there is a severe underlying thrombophilic problem such as antiphospholipid antibody syndrome, the INR should be maintained at between 3.0 and 3.5. Following 3 months of anticoagulant treatment, the patient should be referred for thrombophilia screening tests if these have not previously been carried out.

If the mother has inherited thrombophilia, the child has a 50% chance of being affected. In symptomatic families with inherited thrombophilia, screening tests before puberty are recommended (4). This allows time to discuss with young women the possible risks of oral contraceptives and pregnancy before sexual activity begins. The mother should also be advised that screening for thrombophilia should be done at an earlier age if the child experiences any major illness or injury.

A. Vena Cava Filters

Inferior vena cava filters have been used successfully during pregnancy (19). Indications for use are similar to those in the nonpregnant patient and include contraindication to anticoagulant therapy, complications of anticoagulation and recurrent pulmonary embolism in patients with adequate anticoagulation.

B. Fibrinolytic Agents

Recent surgery or childbirth is a contraindication to thrombolytic therapy. Pulmonary emboli are lysed more rapidly with streptokinase or recombinant tissue plasminogen activator than with conventional anticoagulation, and these agents should be considered in massive pulmonary embolism during pregnancy. The treatment can result in placental bleeding and abruption. Thrombolysis should be avoided if delivery is imminent or within 1 week of childbirth, as severe hemorrhage from the placental site is to be expected. Likewise, extensive bleeding will occur from any genital tract lacerations, episiotomies, and cesarean section wounds.

C. Pulmonary Embolectomy

Pulmonary embolectomy should be considered in pregnant women with massive pulmonary embolism who fail to respond to medical treatment within 1–2 hrs. The use of cardiopulmonary bypass has improved the results of the surgical approach to massive thromboembolism. The decision must be based upon the clinical and hemodynamic state of the patient as well as the ready availability of the surgical team and required facilities. If the patient survives long enough to be put on cardiopulmonary bypass, embolectomy is likely to be successful.

IX. Thromboprophylaxis in Pregnancy and the Puerperium

No randomized control trials to determine optimal management have been reported. Advice is therefore based on observational studies and expert opinion. Given the lack of randomized controlled trials of antithrombotic prophylaxis in pregnancy, the need for prophylactic therapy in women with a previous history of a single episode of deep vein thrombosis with no additional risk factors has been questioned (20). This approach would reserve prophylaxis for women with additional risk factors such as inherited or acquired thrombophilia, postthrombotic venous insufficiency, and recurrent thrombosis. However, previous deep vein thrombosis is a proven risk factor for further thrombosis in pregnancy. At present, maternal deaths from VTE are the major cause of maternal mortality and 50% of these deaths occur antenatally. This being so, probably a safer approach is to advise thromboprophylaxis in women with previous thrombosis, particularly where this has occurred during pregnancy even when current screening tests for both inherited and acquired thrombophilia are negative.

In assessing the thrombotic risk in the individual patient, acquired risk factors as well as genetic predisposition should be considered. A personal and family history of venous thrombosis would be a major factor in the decision. The issues of prophylaxis and its risks should be discussed with the patient before or during early pregnancy and a management policy based on the individual assessment agreed and recorded. Each hospital should have agreed guidelines for the management of women at an increased risk of VTE in pregnancy. In 1995, the Royal College of Obstetricians and Gynaecologists (RCOG) in London published recommendations for prophylaxis against thromboembolism in obstetrics and gynecology (3). These recommendations would appear to have had a dramatic effect in reducing maternal mortality for thromboembolism, particularly in patients undergoing cesarean section (Table 4).

Based on a combination of inherited and acquired risk factors, pregnant women can be classified as being at very high risk, high risk, moderate risk, or low risk of VTE (4–7) (Table 5).

A. Women at Very High Risk

Women at very high risk are those currently on anticoagulants for a previous episode of VTE irrespective of the presence or absence of underlying thrombophilia, VTE in the current pregnancy, and those with antithrombin deficiency with type 1 or certain type 2 defects. In this group, anticoagulants should be used throughout pregnancy with treatment changed to heparin before the sixth week of pregnancy. In women who are not already on anticoagulants, heparin should be commenced as soon as pregnancy is confirmed and continued throughout pregnancy and for at least 3 months after delivery.

In this group, adjusted-dose heparin is used in conjunction with antiembolic stockings throughout pregnancy and the postpartum period. Ad-

Table 4 RCOG Risk Assessment Profile for Thromboembolism in Cesarean Section

Low Risk: early mobilization and hydration
  Elective cesarean section—uncomplicated pregnancy and no other risk factors
Moderate risk: consider one of a variety of prophylactic measures:
  Age over 35 years
  Obesity (80 kg or greater)
  Parity four or more
  Labor 12 hrs or more
  Gross varicose veins
  Current infection
  Preeclampsia
  Immobility prior to surgery (4 days or more)
  Major current illness; e.g., heart or lung disease, cancer, inflammatory bowel
    disease, nephrotic syndrome
  Emergency cesarian section in labor
High risk: heparin prophylaxis with or without leg stockings
  A patient with three or more moderate risk factors from above
  Extended major pelvic or abdominal surgery; e.g., cesarean hysterectomy
  Patients with personal or family history of DVT, pulmonary embolism or
    thrombophilia, paralysis of lower limbs
  Patients with antiphospholipid antibody (cardiolipin antibody or lupus
    anticoagulant)

Table 5 Risk Assessment and Prophylaxis for VTE in Pregnancy

Group	Patients	Management
Very high risk	Antithrombin deficiency. Previous VTE on anticoagulants. VTE in current pregnancy.	Adjusted-dose heparin anti-embolism stockings.
High risk	Protein C deficiency and family history of VTE. Homozygous factor V Leiden. Prothrombin mutation. Combined thrombophilia. Previous VTE not on treatment.	Fixed-dose heparin from 20–24 weeks or 4–6 weeks before gestation of previous event. Postpartum oral anticoagulation for 12 weeks.
Moderate risk	Family history of VTE and heterozygous factor V Leiden, prothrombin mutation, or protein S deficiency.	Antenatal antiembolism stockings. Monitor for other VTE risks. Postpartum oral anticoagulation for 6 weeks.
Low risk	No personal or family history of VTE and heterozygous factor V Leiden or prothrombin mutation.	Monitor for additional risk for VTE.

Source: Ref. 6.

justed-dose heparin can be given as standard heparin or LMWH to achieve a peak anti-Xa activity of 0.3–1.0 IU/ml 3–4 hr after injection. This will usually require a dosage of 7500–12,500 IU of standard heparin twice daily in the first half of pregnancy and 10,000–15,000 IU twice daily in the second half of pregnancy. LMWH can be given according to body weight. Suggested dosage regimens for LMWH are enoxaparin 40 mg every 12 hr, or tinzaparin 175 IU/kg (10,000 IU) daily. In women with a body weight of less than 50 kg, satisfactory heparin levels can be achieved with lower doses of standard heparin or LMWH. Likewise, if renal function is impaired, a lower dose of heparin will be required.

B. Women at High Risk

Women at high risk are those who have had a previous VTE but are not on anticoagulant therapy or have a protein C deficiency plus a family history of thromboembolism, homozygous factor V Leiden, prothrombin mutation, and combined thrombophilia. In this group, thromboprophylaxis is introduced 4–6 weeks before the gestational age of the event in a previous pregnancy or from 20 to 24 weeks of gestation in the others. Anticoagulation may be given earlier if additional risk factors for VTE are present. Heparin prophylaxis may be given as standard heparin 7500 IU every 12 hr until 30 weeks and 10,000 IU every 12 hr for the remainder of the pregnancy. Once-daily LMWH may be given as enoxaparin 40 mg daily or tinzaparin (4500–7500 IU) per day to achieve anti-Xa levels of 0.1–0.5 IU/mL 3–4 hr postinjection. Postpartum oral anticoagulation should be continued for 12 weeks together with the use of antiembolism stockings.

C. Women at Moderate Risk

Women at moderate risk include patients with heterozygous factor V Leiden, prothrombin mutation, or protein S deficiency and a family history of VTE. Antiembolism stockings are recommended in the antenatal period. Anticoagulation is given for 6 weeks during the puerperium starting with heparin 4–8 hr after delivery and continuing with warfarin. Anticoagulation is used in late pregnancy if additional risk factors such as age, obesity, or restricted activity are present.

D. Women at Relatively Low Risk

Women at relatively low risk are those with factor V Leiden or prothrombin mutation who have no personal or family history of VTE. These patients may be detected as the result of routine screening for thrombophilia. If no other risk factors for VTE during pregnancy are present, such as preeclampsia or cesarean section, these patients are not offered antenatal thrombo-prophylaxis but are reviewed regularly to determine if additional thrombotic risk factors have developed during pregnancy.

E. Management of Labor and Delivery

In women at increased risk of VTE, the additional risk of cesarean section makes spontaneous labor and delivery preferable. In general, women can continue on heparin prophylaxis and discontinue the treatment at the onset of labor, with heparin prophylaxis being resumed 4–8 hr after delivery.

In a patient receiving therapeutic intravenous heparin, the infusion should be stopped for labor and delivery. Heparin activity should fall to safe levels within 1 hour. A protamine sulfate infusion can be used if needed to neutralize the heparin activity. If a woman fully anticoagulated on warfarin starts labor, she should be given a concentrate of factors II, IX, X (prothrombin complex concentrate). The dose depends on the INR, and for patients with an INR of 2.0–3.9, 25 U/kg is recommended. If concentrates are not available, solvent detergent (SD) plasma should be used in an initial dose of 12–15 mL/kg. Following delivery, the baby should be given fresh plasma and vitamin K and screened by ultrasound for any signs of hemorrhage in the head and abdomen.

Women who have been on antenatal standard heparin may have an epidural or spinal anesthesia providing their coagulation and platelet count are normal. LMWH does not prolong the APPT to the same extent as standard heparin. Monitoring the effect of LMWH requires an anti-Xa assay, which is not widely available. Peak levels of anti-Xa occur 2–4 hr after subcutaneous LMWH or standard heparin is administered. The optimal time for insertion and removal of a spinal or epidural catheter would be at least 12 hr after the last dose (18).

Women with antithrombin deficiency are at very high risk for VTE, and in this group, the use of antithrombin concentrate should be considered in order to increase the antithrombin levels to normal for labor and delivery. Increasing the plasma antithrombin activity to 80–120% is recommended on the day of delivery by infusion of 0.6–0.7 U antithrombin concentrate per kilogram of maternal weight. This allows the heparin level to be reduced or discontinued (21).

X. Thromboprophylaxis and Cesarean Section

Almost two-thirds of the postpartum deaths from thromboembolism in the years 1982–1999 in the United Kingdom followed delivery by cesarean section. Because of the increased risk associated with cesarean section, the

Report of the Confidential Enquiry published in 2001 (1) recommended that all women undergoing elective or emergency cesarean section should have a risk assessment for VTE and prophylaxis instituted as appropriate (Table 3). Table 3 provides a useful risk assessment profile, which can be used as a basis for guidelines. Some obstetrical units have incorporated the risk assessment profile into the obstetrical record for use when the patient is admitted for cesarean section. Patients in the moderate- and high-risk categories should receive prophylaxis with standard heparin in a dose of 5000 units every 12 hr by subcutaneous injection or low molecular weight heparin, tinzaparin (3500–4500 IU), or enoxaparin 20–49 mg) as a single daily dose starting during the operation if the patient has regional anesthesia. Treatment should be given for a minimum of 5 days and can be self-administered. In the woman with inherited or acquired thrombophilia, anticoagulation should be continued in the postpartum period for at least 6–12 weeks. In this group, oral anticoagulants can be commenced 1–2 days following delivery, and the heparin can be discontinued once the INR has been in the therapeutic range for 4 consecutive days. Anticoagulant therapy in the patient undergoing cesarean section is likely to increase the risk of wound hematomas; care should be taken to ensure that subcutaneous heparin is injected subcutaneously in the flank as far away as possible from the wound.

XI. Conclusions

Our first priority must be to bring proven prophylactic methods to obstetrical patients who are at increased risk of VTE complications. No method is likely to be 100% effective, but present evidence indicates that both LMWH and standard heparin confer a high degree of protection against VTE and can be used by the woman herself throughout pregnancy.

The time of greatest danger is the immediate puerperium, particularly in the patient who has been delivered by cesarean section. Prophylaxis with low-dose heparin or LMWH should be given to all mothers in the moderate- or high-risk category for VTE complications. This includes all women undergoing emergency cesarean section. In addition to reducing the number of maternal deaths from pulmonary embolism, the judicious use of prophylactic methods should also decrease the incidence of deep vein thrombosis and the postphlebitic syndrome.

Major advances have occurred in identifying women at increased risk of VTE in pregnancy as a result of both inherited and acquired risk factors. Every woman with a personal or family history of VTE should be screened for both inherited and acquired thrombophilia. In addition to increasing the risk of VTE in pregnancy, inherited and acquired thrombophilia may be partly responsible for recurrent fetal death and intrauterine growth restriction. Wider use of thromboprophylaxis and thorough investigation of symptoms of VTE are urgently required (22). All women undergoing cesarean section should be assessed for prophylaxis against VTE.

References

1. Why Mothers Die. Confidential Enquiries into Maternal Deaths in the United Kingdom. London: RCOG Press, 2000:49–75.
2. Department of Health, Welsh Office, Scottish Home and Health Department and Department of Health and Social Services, Northern Ireland. Confidential Enquiries into Maternal Deaths in the United Kingdom 1994–1996. London: Stationery Office, 1998.
3. Royal College of Obstetricians and Gynaecologists. Report of the RCOG Working Party on Prophylaxis against Thromboembolism in Gynaecology and Obstetrics. London: RCOG, 1995.
4. Bonnar J, Green R, Norris L. Inherited thrombophilia and pregnancy: the obstetric perspective. Semin Thromb Hemost 1998; 24(suppl 1):49–53.
5. Greer IA. Thrombosis in pregnancy: maternal and fetal issues. Lancet 1999; 353:1258–1265.
6. McColl MD, Walker ID, Greer IA. The role of inherited thrombophilia in venous thromboembolism associated with pregnancy. Br J Obstet Gynaecol 1999; 106:756–766.
7. McColl MD, Ramsay JE, Tait RC, Walker ID, McCall F, Conkie JA, Carty MJ, Greer IA. Risk factors for pregnancy associated venous thromboembolism. Thromb Hemost 1997; 78:1183–1188.
8. Macklon NS, Greer IA. The deep venous system in the puerperium: an ultrasound study. Br J Obstet Gynaecol 1997; 104:198–200.
9. Macklon NS, Greer IA, Bowman AW. An ultrasound of gestational and postural changes in the deep venous system of the leg in pregnancy. Br J Obstet Gynaecol 1997; 104:191–197.
10. Linghagen A, Bergqvist A, Bergqvist D, Hallbrook T. Late venous function in the leg after deep venous thrombosis occurring in relation to pregnancy. Br J Obstet Gynaecol 1986; 93:348–352.
11. Greer IA. Epidemiology, risk factors and prophylaxis of venous thromboembolism in obstetrics and gynecology. Bailliere's Clin Obstet Gynecol 1997; 11: 403–430.
12. Clark P, Brennand J, Conkie JA, McCall F, Greer IA, Walker ID. Activated protein C sensitivity, protein C, protein S and coagulation in normal pregnancy. Thromb Haemost 1998; 79:1166–1170.
13. McColl MD, Ellison J, Reid F, Tait RC, Walker ID, Greer IA. Prothrombin 20210G-A MTHFR C677T mutations in women with venous thromboembolism associated with pregnancy. Br J Obstet Gynaecol 2000; 107:565–569.

14. Hull RD, Raskob GE, Pineo GF, Green D, Trowbridge A, Elliott CG, Lerner RG, Hall J, Sparling T, Brettell HR, Norton J, Carter CJ, George R, Merli G, Ward J, Mayo W, Rosenbloom D, Brant R. Subcutaneous low-molecular weight heparin compared with continuous intravenous heparin in the treatment of proximal vein thrombosis. N Engl J Med 1992; 326(15):975–982.

15. Simmoneau G, Sors H, Charbonnier B, Page Y, Laaban J, Azarian R, Laurent M, Hirsch J, Ferrari E, Bosson J, Mottier D, Beau B. A comparison of low molecular weight heparin with unfractionated heparin for acute pulmonary embolism. N Engl J Med 1997; 337:663–669.

16. Bates SM, Ginsberg JS, Greer IA, eds. Anticoagulants in pregnancy: fetal defects. In: Bailliere's Clinical Obstetrics and Gynecology. Thromboembolic Disease in Obstetrics and Gynecology. London: Bailliere Tindall, 1997:479–488.

17. Thomson AJ, Walker ID, Greer IA. Low molecular weight heparin for the immediate management of thromboembolic disease in pregnancy. Lancet 1998; 352:1904.

18. Bonnar J, Norris LA, Greene R. Low molecular weight heparin for thrombo-prophylaxis during cesarean section. Thromb Res 1999; 96:317–322.

19. Narayan H, Cullimore J, Krarup K, Thurston H, MacVicar J, Bolia A. Experience with the cardial inferior vena cava filter as prophylaxis against pulmonary embolism in pregnant women with extensive deep venous thrombosis. Br J Obstet Gynecol 1992; 99:637–640.

20. Brill-Edwards P, Ginsberg JS, Gent M, Hirsh J, Burrows R, Kearon C, Geerts W, Kovacs M, Weitz JI, Robinson KS, Whittom R, Couture G. Safety of withholding heparin in pregnant women with a history of venous thromboembolism. N Engl J Med 2000; 343:1439–1444.

21. Walker ID. Inherited coagulation disorders and thrombophilia and pregnancy. In: Bonnar J, ed. Recent Advances in Obstetrics and Gynaecology. Edinburgh: Churchill Livingstone, 1998:35–64.

22. Bonnar J. Can more be done in obstetric and gynecologic practice to reduce morbidity and mortality associated with venous thromboembolism? Am J Obstet Gynecol 1999; 180(4):784–791.

11

Anticoagulant Therapy of Venous Thromboembolism

THOMAS M. HYERS

St. Louis University School of Medicine
St. Louis, Missouri, U.S.A.

I. Introduction

Heparin has been commercially available for some 70 years, but widespread use of the drug for treatment of venous thromboembolism (VTE) has only been employed for about 50 years. For the first 15–20 years after heparin (now called unfractionated heparin [UH]) became clinically available, there was considerable controversy about the benefit of anticoagulation in the treatment and prevention of acute VTE. During that time, some clinicians argued that the risk of hemorrhage associated with anticoagulants outweighed any therapeutic benefit.

The timeline shown in Figure 1 begins with the seminal clinical trial testing heparin and oral anticoagulation against no anticoagulation in medical and surgical patients with acute pulmonary embolism (PE) (1). In retrospect, this small trial has obvious flaws, but the high rate of autopsy-confirmed fatal PE (25%) in the untreated patients remains persuasive. The benefit of anticoagulation in preventing fatal pulmonary embolism far outweighed the risk of bleeding.

The timeline is neither exhaustive nor precise. Major clinical trials and drug introductions that changed practice patterns are emphasized. For anticoagulation treatment of VTE, UH and several oral anticoagulants were

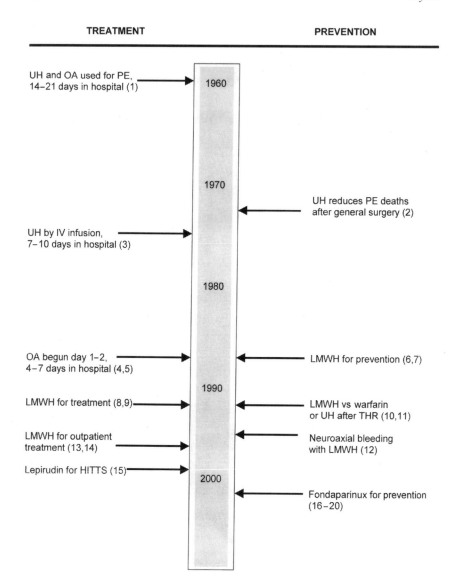

Figure 1   Time line for major developments in prevention and treatment of venous thromboembolism. See text for details.

the only effective therapeutic agents available for the first two decades of the timeline. Low molecular weight heparin (LMWH) was introduced in Europe in the early 1980s, but did not achieve widespread use for VTE prevention and treatment until about 10 years later. In the last decade, the pace of development has accelerated with introduction of several new anticoagulants and regimens. In the vanguard of these new anticoagulants are the direct thrombin inhibitors (DTIs) and the indirect factor Xa inhibitor fondaparinux. The first DTI was recombinant hirudin (lepirudin), which was introduced in the United States in 1999 for treatment of the heparin-induced thrombocytopenia thrombosis syndrome (HITTS). After that, argatroban was introduced for treatment of HITTS and bivalirudin was approved for anticoagulation in acute coronary syndromes.

The evolution of UH has seemingly culminated in fondaparinux, a synthetic pentasaccharide (MW 1726 Ds) whose structure is similar to the heparin sequence that binds to antithrombin (AT) and enhances its inhibitory activity. Fondaparinux was recently introduced in both the United States and Europe for the prevention of VTE in major hip and knee surgeries.

Since 1960, the clinical evaluation and validation of antithrombotic drugs has been accomplished by randomized controlled trials. More effective drugs and shorter hospitalizations with attendant cost savings have been the hallmarks of management advances. This chapter highlights the history of current anticoagulants and describes new anticoagulants now being evaluated for use in VTE treatment and prevention.

II. Treatment of VTE: Thrombus Progression with UH

The ultimate goal of treatment of VTE is to eliminate the risk of fatal PE. Today, death from PE is sufficiently rare in adequately treated VTE patients that the surrogate goals of reduced clinical recurrence and rate of thrombus regression have become the main endpoints in clinical trials of anticoagulants.

In the United States, UH, given by intravenous infusion or large subcutaneous doses, remains the mainstay of acute treatment of VTE. LMWH has achieved increasing use in treatment during the last decade, but the majority of patients with acute VTE still receive UH by IV infusion with monitoring and dose adjustment. Meta-analyses of VTE treatment trials comparing UH and LMWH show that LMWH therapy results in slightly less recurrent VTE, less major bleeding, and a slightly lower all-cause mortality over the ensuing 3 months (21,22). These results are analogous to outcomes in VTE prophylaxis in orthopedic surgery patients in that LMWH seems to perform slightly better than UH.

The relative ineffectiveness of UH in reducing the rate of proximal deep vein thrombosis (DVT) following major orthopedic surgery (see Chap. 4) suggests a limitation in the ability of UH to prevent thrombus progression. Although prophylaxis trials in orthopedic surgery provide no direct data to evaluate this putative limitation of UH, inferences about the relative efficacy of LMWH and UH can be drawn from treatment studies in which an objective measure of thrombus progression is available.

Serial venography or duplex ultrasound scanning for the quantitative assessment of thrombus growth reveals that 10–28% of patients receiving UH for treatment of acute DVT show propagation of thrombus (23–25). Quantitative venography, using a scoring system that specifies a 30% reduction in thrombus size as an objective endpoint for evidence of thrombus regression has shown a 32% incidence of improvement with UH and a 42% improvement incidence with the LMWH certoparin (26). This finding suggests that certoparin may limit thrombus growth better than UH. A recent study comparing reduction in thrombus extension between certoparin and UH for initial treatment of acute DVT found a significant benefit in favor of certoparin (27). In a study utilizing repeated venography, the LMWH reviparin was significantly more effective than UH in promoting thrombus regression (53 vs 40%) in patients with documented DVT (28). A meta-analysis of thrombus progression as an efficacy measure of UH versus LMWH for initial therapy (29) showed significantly less thrombus progression in favor of LMWH with a common odds ratio of 0.51.

These clinical studies provide direct evidence that UH therapy allows thrombus progression in a sizable number of patients with DVT. The findings suggest a rationale for why fixed-dose UH is suboptimal for VTE prophylaxis in high-risk surgery. Although it remains unclear that early thrombus progression always results in clinical DVT or PE (23–25, 29), larger studies with careful patient follow-up strongly support this association (23,24,27,28).

III.   Theoretical Basis for Failure of UH to Arrest Thrombus Growth

Possible explanations for the phenomenon of failure of UH to Arrest Thrombus growth include the failure of UH to inhibit clot-bound thrombin and the frequent failure of heparin injections or infusions to achieve and maintain a therapeutic level.

Both thrombin and factor Xa bind to fibrin and retain their catalytic activities on this "solid phase," resulting in continuous local conversion of fibrinogen to fibrin and continuous local activation of prothrombin to thrombin (30,31). Direct thrombin inhibitors such as hirugen, L-propyl-p-phenyladanyl-chloromethylketone (PPACK), and hirudin effectively limit the activity of clot-bound thrombin (30,32). Unfractionated heparin is relatively ineffective toward clot-bound thrombin, which is consistent with steric interference imposed by the larger heparin-AT complex (30). Other studies have characterized the procoagulant activity of bound factor Xa and compared the relative effect of direct and indirect factor Xa inhibitors on this activity using both in vitro and in vivo experimental systems. The direct factor Xa inhibitors, tick anticoagulant peptide (TAP) and DX-9065a, each exhibited potent inhibition of clot-associated factor Xa procoagulant activity (33,34). Findings for fondaparinux, an indirect (AT-dependent) factor Xa inhibitor, are conflicting. In one study, equipotent inhibitory activity toward clot-bound factor Xa, relative to DX-9065 (34), was observed, whereas another study reported no enhancement of AT-mediated factor Xa inhibition compared to the inhibitory effect of trypsinogen-activating peptide (33).

Therapy with UH, whether given intravenously or subcutaneously, often fails to achieve an acceptable prolongation of the activated partial thromboplastin time (aPTT) (28,35,36). Some studies indicate that early failure to achieve adequate anticoagulation results in a higher rate of VTE recurrence over the following 3 months of therapy. For example, subtherapeutic doses of heparin were found to predict the onset of VTE events based on findings indicating a 23.3% frequency of VTE when aPTTs were not reached within 24 h compared to a frequency of 4–6% when the times were therapeutic or supratherapeutic (37). Another VTE treatment study using UH suggested that a subtherapeutic aPTT response within the first 48 hr was not associated with an increased risk of VTE recurrence (38). The use of heparin nomograms (35) has aided the management of heparin therapy by increasing the likelihood that therapeutic aPTT levels will be achieved within the first 24–48 hrs. Despite the use of treatment nomograms for UH and increased awareness of the unpredictability of the UH dose response, audits continue to show that approximately 25% of patients treated with UH do not achieve adequate anticoagulation within the first 24–48 hrs (28,35–37).

The difficulty and unpredictability in achieving optimum therapeutic levels stem from low bioavailability and rapid clearance of UH. The drug's high degree of nonspecific binding to a variety of plasma and cellular proteins reduces its effective bioavailability to 30–40% when given subcutaneously in a low dose, which includes regimens typically recommended for prophylactic heparin use (5000 U two or three times daily) (4,39,40). Intrinsic quantitative differences in levels of heparin-binding proteins among individuals lead to wide interindividual variation in antithrombotic response and, as a result, the unpredictability of UH therapy that necessitates frequent monitoring and dose adjustment for optimum antithrombotic activity.

Even when administered IV, the unfavorable pharmacodynamic profile of UH means it must be monitored and dose adjusted to achieve and sustain a therapeutic effect. Compounding the effect of heparin's limited bioavailability is its short half- life of 30–60 mins (40,41). Complex dosing schemes have been developed, but they still do not achieve the desired effect in a considerable number of patients.

IV.   Alternatives to UH: Beyond LMWH

The last decade has seen the development of new anticoagulants that have the potential to replace UH and even LMWH for a variety of different thrombotic indications, including VTE prevention and treatment. Most of these new anticoagulants specifically target individual components of the coagulation system, a theoretical advantage compared to the multitargeted mechanism of action of UF and, albeit to a lesser extent, of LMWH as well (Fig. 2). New drug development began with LMWH but has now expanded to include heparinoids, DTIs, direct and indirect factor Xa inhibitors, activated protein C (APC), tissue factor pathway inhibitor (TFPI), and nematode anticoagulant peptide c2 (NAPc2). Additional new drug development has focused on derivatizations of unfractionated heparin, LMWH, and DTIs that are suitable for oral administration.

The following section briefly describes agents that are being studied for the prevention and treatment of VTE. Some of these drugs may overcome many of the limitations associated with UH and LMWH.

A.   Direct Thrombin Inhibitors

In contrast to all heparin-based products, which act indirectly via AT to inhibit both thrombin and factor Xa, DTIs bind to thrombin specifically and inhibit its catalytic activity without involvement of AT. Smaller DTIs theoretically offer the advantage of inhibition of both free and bound thrombin. In this way, DTIs may provide more effective inhibition of thrombus progression than agents such as UH and LMWH that inhibit free thrombin only.

Development of DTIs began with the isolation of hirudin from the medicinal leech (*Hirudo medicinalis*). Drugs approved by the American Food and Drug Administration (FDA) now include recombinant hirudin (lepirudin), a semisynthetic DTI (bivalirudin), and a small synthetic arginine analogue (argatroban) that inhibits thrombin's active site by ionic binding. All of

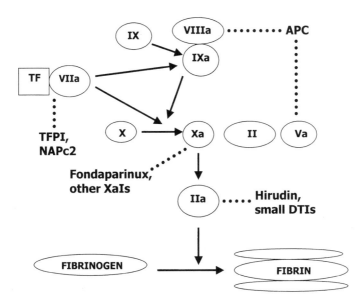

Figure 2 New anticoagulants are shown in black (see Table 3). Of these agents, TFPI, NAPc2, and various direct Xa inhibitors (XaIs) are not yet approved. New anticoagulants feature single or dual sites of inhibition as contrasted to the multiple sites of inhibition (IIa, Xa, IXa, XIa) exhibited by UH and SNAC heparin.

these drugs are given intravenously and are monitored with the aPTT or activated coagulation time in the same way as UH. Other agents in this new class of antithrombotics include desirudin, a recombinant desulfato-hirudin, hirulog, a C-terminal hirudin derivative, and the dipeptide melagatran, a DTI with reversible binding. Small DTIs have been derivatized for oral administration. Furthest along in development is ximelagatran, a prodrug given orally and rapidly metabolized to form melagatran, its active metabolite (Table 1). Ximelagatran is administered twice daily and appears to require no monitoring or dose adjustment.

Excess bleeding seen with hirudin is probably attributable to its irreversible binding to thrombin. DTIs that feature more reversible binding, such as argatroban, bivalirudin, and melagatran, may be associated with less bleeding than seen with hirudin.

Among these DTIs, recombinant hirudin (42,43), hirulog (44), and ximelagatran, alone (45,46) or in combination with melagatran (47,48), have been evaluated in clinical trials of VTE prophylaxis in hip and knee arthroplasty. For the most part, these were open-label dose-finding studies or randomized controlled trials in which efficacy and safety were compared

Table 1 Venographic DVT Rates (at 5–11 d) After Hip or Knee Surgery

Operation	Prophylaxis	No. trials/No. patients	% With proximal DVT	% With any DVT
THR	Placebo[a]/no treatment	13/947	25.0	49.0
	Aspirin	6/473	11.4	40.2
	UH	11/1016	19.3	30.1
	Warfarin	13/1828	5.2	22.1
	LMWH	30/6216	5.9	16.1
	Fondaparinux[b]	2/1689	1.2	4.4
TKR	Placebo/no treatment	6/199	15.3	64.3
	Aspirin	6/443	8.9	56.0
	UH	13/1740	11.4	43.2
	Warfarin	9/1294	10.0	46.8
	LMWH	13/1740	5.6	30.6
	Fondaparinux	1/526	2.4	12.5
HFS	Placebo/no treatment	9/381		48.0
	Aspirin	3/171		34.0
	UH	2/59		27.0
	Warfarin	5/239		24.0
	LMWH/heparinoids	6/1268		14.5
	Fondaparinux	1/831	0.9	7.9

THR = total hip replacement; TKR = total knee replacement; HFS = hip fracture surgery; UH = unfractionated heparin; LMWH = low molecular weight heparin.
[a] Rates for placebo, aspirin, UH, warfarin, and LMWH are from meta-analyses be Geerts et al. (29) and Freedman et al. (30).
[b] Rates for fondaparinux are from four clinical trials (15,16,88,89).

to UH or LMWHs or to warfarin (45,47). These DTIs appeared to be as safe and effective as their respective comparator drug, with proximal DVT and/ or PE incidences of 2–10% being reported. Larger phase III clinical trial results for oral DTI ximelagatran failed to show any clear superiority to warfarin or enoxaparin in knee surgery and hip surgery patients, respectively (46,47). These disappointing findings call into question the concept that small direct inhibitors will inactivate bound thrombin more effectively than AT-dependent drugs like UH and LMWH. Nevertheless, a twice-daily oral drug that needs no monitoring and has risk-benefit similar to LMWH and warfarin is very attractive.

B. Direct Factor Xa Inhibitors

Unlike the heparins, the direct factor Xa inhibitors exert their anticoagulant activity by Xa inhibition via an AT-independent mechanism of action (49).

Similar to the smaller DTIs, direct Xa inhibitors are theoretically capable of inhibiting circulating factor Xa as well as clot-bound forms associated with the prothrombinase complex or with fibrin.

Several direct factor Xa inhibitors are under development. These include synthetic molecules such as YM-60828 (50) and DX-9065a (51) as well as the natural inhibitors antistasin (52) and TAP (53), both of which have been produced by recombinant techniques.

As a class, the direct factor Xa inhibitors are not yet being intensively pursued in clinical studies, with most either in preclinical development or withdrawn because of undesirable properties.

C. Fondaparinux

Fondaparinux is a small, totally synthetic molecule that enhances AT-mediated inhibitory activity against factor Xa (54–57). By selectively inactivating factor Xa, fondaparinux inhibits thrombin generation without any direct effect on thrombin activity. Unlike the direct factor Xa inhibitors, the antithrombotic activity of fondaparinux is absolutely dependent on AT.

Fondaparinux binds specifically to AT and within its therapeutic range exhibits no nonspecific binding to plasma and cellular proteins (58). The lack of nonspecific binding and the molecule's 100% bioavailability result in a predictable dose-response effect and should result in less heparin-induced thrombocytopenia (HIT) and osteoporosis than is seen with UH (59–60). Recent pharmacokinetic studies have demonstrated that fondaparinux is rapidly absorbed following subcutaneous administration, reaching its maximal plasma concentration within approximately 2 hr and exhibiting a terminal half-life of 13–21 hr (61). The drug's pharmacokinetics show little interindividual variation and are independent of age and gender and are only minimally influenced by body weight. Renal insufficiency is the only clinically important condition that prolongs clearance. Fondaparinux is contraindicated in patients with severe renal impairment, but no dose adjustment or laboratory monitoring is required in patients with moderate renal dysfunction. These features allow for once-daily subcutaneous dosing with rapid onset of action and predictable duration of effect. The drug, therefore, requires no dose adjustment or monitoring in the great majority of patients.

Fondaparinux, among all the new antithrombotic agents, has shown the greatest potential for prevention of venographically demonstrated DVT associated with major hip and knee surgery. The drug recently received American and European approval for VTE prevention in hip and knee replacement and after hip fracture surgery. Phase II trials in hip replacement surgery (16) and Phase III trials in hip replacement (17,18), hip fracture (19), and major knee surgery (20) have demonstrated fondaparinux's superiority, relative to the LMWH enoxaparin, in reducing VTE risk following major orthopedic surgery. A recent meta-analysis of these Phase II trials indicates an overall significant 55.2% reduction in VTE risk ($P < .001$), in favor of fondaparinux, with no difference in clinically relevant bleeding complications at the dosing regimens employed (62). Most of this difference was accounted for by a reduction in venographically demonstrated DVT. There were no significant differences in death or clinically relevant bleeding between the two agents. There were trends for more hemoglobin decreases and blood transfusion in the fondaparinux-treated groups. This trend was statistically significant in the knee surgery study (20). Fondaparinux was given about 6 hrs after surgery compared to enoxaparin's administration at 12–24 hr after surgery. This difference in timing may have contributed both to increased efficacy and slightly increased blood loss associated with fondaparinux.

Fondaparinux demonstrated significantly greater efficacy than enoxaparin in reducing the incidence of venographically demonstrated proximal DVT in two of the four trials, one in hip replacement and the other in hip fracture surgery, with a trend toward significance demonstrated for the trial in major knee surgery. The incidence of confirmed symptomatic PE events was similarly low for both drugs. Fatal PE occurred in 0.1% of patients in both treatment groups.

The superior efficacy demonstrated by fondaparinux in reducing the rate of proximal venographically demonstrated DVT strongly implies that the drug can effectively limit thrombus progression. A Phase II dose-finding study comparing the efficacy and safety of fondaparinux to dalteparin in treatment of acute DVT provides further objective evidence for this. Positive outcomes, measured as an improvement in thrombus burden detected by follow-up ultrasonography and perfusion lung scanning, were observed across the wide range of fondaparinux doses tested (63). Results are awaited from a completed Phase III study comparing fondaparinux with enoxaparin for treatment of DVT and another Phase III study comparing fondaparinux with UH for treatment of PE. These trials will provide essential information on this drug's treatment efficacy in VTE treatment.

Based on available data, fondaparinux acting with AT as a specific Xa inhibitor appears to challenge the hypothesis that agents that inhibit circulating and clot-bound thrombin will be most effective in preventing thrombus extension. Inhibition of thrombin generation, as a consequence of factor Xa inhibition, may accomplish the same end by inhibiting feedback loops within the coagulation cascade through which thrombin activity is regulated.

An interesting finding in the Phase III studies of fondaparinux was that enoxaparin prophylaxis was more effective on the venographic endpoint than had been seen previously with this drug. Similar observations were made with enoxaparin and warfarin as the active comparators in recent trials of the prophylactic efficacy of ximelagatran. It does appear that the rate of venographic DVT is falling over time in postoperative patients. Improved surgical technique and rapid postoperative mobilization of patients probably explain this finding.

D. Other New Anticoagulants

Nematode anticoagulation peptide c2 (NAPc2) was first isolated from the blood-feeding canine hookworm but is now available as a recombinant product. It combines with factors X and Xa to inhibit the TF-VIIa complex (64,65). NAPc2 is administered subcutaneously every 2 days, and is currently being evaluated for VTE prophylaxis after elective hip replacement surgery.

Whereas UH and LMWHs are poorly absorbed in the gut and cannot be given orally, derivatization of UH to sodium N-(8(2-hydroxylbenzoyl)-amino) caprylate heparin (SNAC/heparin) facilitates oral administration (66). When this drug is administered, demonstrable prolongation of the aPTT occurs, although the duration of anticoagulant effect is similar to

Table 2 Confirmed Clinical VTE Rates at 3 Mos After Hip or Knee Surgery

Operation	VTE Prophylaxis	No. patients	% With DVT	% With nonfatal PE	% With fatal PE
Historical Rates (1960–1980)					
THR	None (31)	1172	NR	15.2	2.3
	None (32)	62	NR	5.2	3.4
TKR	None (32)	152	NR	2.0	0.7
HFS	None (33,34)	729	NR	3.7	7.5
Modern Era with VTE Prophylaxis					
THR	Warfarin (35)	1495	2.9	0.8	0.1
	Enoxaparin	1516	2.6	1.0	0.1
TKR	Cohort study (36)[a]	24,059	1.4	0.8	NR
	Cohort study (37)[b]	842	2.7	0.8	0.4
HFS	Aspirin[c] (38)	6679	1.0	0.4	0.3
	Placebo[a]	6677	1.4	0.6	0.6

THR = total hip replacement; TKR = total knee replacement; HFS = hip fracture surgery; NR = not reported.

[a] Patients had mixed prophylaxis, mostly IPC or warfarin.

[b] All patients received LMWH.

[c] Patients had additional prophylaxis, including heparin, LMWH, or ES; rates at 35 days.

Table 3 New Anticoagulants

Drug	Action	Indication or study area
Approved		
Danaparoid	Xa inhibitor	VTE prevention in THR
Lepirudin	DTI	HITTS
Argatroban	DTI	HITTS
Bivalirudin	DTI	ACS with PCI
Fondaparinux	Xa inhibitor	VTE prevention in THR, TKR, and HFS
APC	Cleaves Va and VIIIa	Severe sepsis
Phase III		
Ximelagatrin	Oral DTI	VTE, chronic AF
NAPc2	TF-VIIa inhibitor	VTE
TFPI	TF-VIIa inhibitor	Severe sepsis
SNAC heparin	Oral heparin	VTE

ACS, acute coronary syndrome; AF, atrial fibrillation; APC, activated protein C; DTI, direct thrombin inhibitor; HFS, hip fracture surgery; NAPc2, nematode anticoagulant peptide c2; PCI, percutaneous coronary intervention; TF, tissue factor; TFPI, tissue factor pathway inhibitor; THR, total hip replacement; TKR, total knee replacement.

bolus IV dosing of UH. The rapid clearance of SNAC/heparin will likely require that it be dosed frequently, especially in treatment protocols. The drug is being evaluated for VTE prophylaxis after elective hip and knee replacement. Derivatives of various LMWHs are being pursued, which may allow oral dosing of these drugs once or twice daily.

Many new anticoagulants exhibit potentially superior properties to UH, including improved pharmacodynamic profiles and targeted activity at single points in the coagulation cascade. Other favorable properties include-once- or twice-daily dosing without monitoring or dose adjustment, and in

Table 4 An Improved Anticoagulant

Multiple indications with high efficacy/risk
Oral administration, once daily
Rapid onset of action
Predictable PK/PD (even with renal/hepatic dysfunction)
Low risk of HIT, osteopenia, and other toxicities
Effective antidote available
Affordable

HIT, heparin-induced thrombocytopenia; PD, pharmacodynamic; PK, pharmacokinetic.

the case of ximelagatran, oral administration. None of these new agents will likely replace UH totally, but each drug offers advantages that require consideration as progress continues toward development of better anticoagulants (Table 2).

References

1. Barritt DW, Jordan SC. Anticoagulant drugs in the treatment of pulmonary embolism: a controlled clinical trial. Lancet 1960; 1:1309–1312.
2. Kakkar VV, Corrigan TP, Fossard DP, et al. Prevention of fatal postoperative pulmonary embolism by low doses of heparin: an international multicentre trial. Lancet 1975; 2:45–251.
3. Salzman EW, Deykin D, Shapiro RM, et al. Management of heparin therapy: controlled prospective trial. N Engl J Med 1975; 292:1046–1050.
4. Gallus AS, Jackaman J, Tillett J, et al. Safety and efficacy of warfarin started early after submassive venous thrombosis or pulmonary embolism. Lancet 1986; 2:1293–1296.
5. Hull RD, Raskob GE, Rosenbloom D, et al. Heparin for 5 days as compared with 10 days in the initial treatment of proximal venous thrombosis. N Engl J Med 1990; 322:1260–1264.
6. Monreal M, Lafoz E, Navarro A, et al. A prospective double-blind trial of a low molecular weight heparin once daily compared with conventional low-dose heparin three times daily to prevent pulmonary embolism and venous thrombosis in patients with hip fracture. J Trauma 1980; 29:873–875.
7. The European Fraxiparin Study (EFS) Group. Comparison of a low molecular weight heparin and unfractionated heparin for the prevention of deep vein thrombosis in patients undergoing abdominal surgery. Br J Surg 1988; 75:1058–1063.
8. Hull RD, Raskob GE, Pineo GF, et al. Subcutaneous low-molecular-weight heparin compared with continuous intravenous heparin in the treatment of proximal-vein thrombosis. N Engl J Med 1992; 326:975–982.
9. Prandoni P, Lensing AWA, Büller HR, et al. Comparison of subcutaneous low molecular weight heparin with intravenous standard heparin in proximal vein thrombosis. Lancet 1992; 339:441–445.
10. Hull R, Raskob G, Pineo G, et al. A comparison of subcutaneous low-molecular-weight heparin with warfarin sodium for prophylaxis against deep-vein thrombosis after hip or knee implantation. N Engl J Med 1993; 329: 1370–1376.
11. Levine MN, Hirsh J, Gent M, et al. Prevention of deep vein thrombosis after elective hip surgery. A randomized trial comparing low molecular weight heparin with standard unfractionated heparin. Ann Intern Med 1991; 114:545–551.
12. Vandermeulen EP, Van Aken H, Vermylen J. Anticoagulants and spinal-epidural anesthesia. Anesth Analg 1994; 79:1165–1177.
13. Levine M, Gent M, Hirsh J, et al. A comparison of low- molecular-weight

heparin administered primarily at home with unfractionated heparin administered in the hospital for proximal-vein thrombosis. N Engl J Med 1996; 334: 677–768.

14. Koopman MMW, Prandoni WP, Piovella P, et al. Treatment of venous thrombosis with intravenous unfractionated heparin administered in the hospital as compared with subcutaneous low-molecular-weight heparin administered at home. N Engl J Med 1996; 334:682–687.

15. Warkentin TE, Chong BH, Greinacher A. Heparin-induced thrombocytopenia: towards consensus. Thromb Haemost 1998; 79:1–7.

16. Turpie AGG, Gallus AS, Hoek JA, for the Pentasaccharide Investigators. A synthetic pentasaccharide for the prevention of deep-vein thrombosis after total hip replacement. N Engl J Med 2001; 344:619–625.

17. Turpie AGG, Bauer KA, Eriksson BI, Lassen MR. A randomised double-blind comparison of pentasaccharide with enoxaparin for the prevention of venous thromboembolism after elective hip replacement surgery. Lancet 2002; 359: 1721–1726.

18. Lassen MR, Bauer KA, Eriksson BI, Lensing AWA, Turpie AGG. Pentasaccharide versus enoxaparin for the prevention of venous thromboembolism in elective hip replacement surgery. A randomised double-blind comparison. Lancet 2002; 359:1715–1720.

19. Eriksson BI, Bauer KA, Lassen MR, et al. Fondaparinux compared with enoxaparin for the prevention of venous thromboembolism after hip-fracture surgery. N Engl J Med 2001; 345:1298–1304.

20. Bauer KA, Eriksson BI, Lassen MR, et al. Fondaparinux compared with enoxaparin for the prevention of venous thromboembolism after elective major knee surgery. N Engl J Med 2001; 345:1303–1310.

21. Gould MK, Dembitzer AD, Sanders GD, et al. Low-molecular-weight heparins compared with unfractionated heparin for treatment of acute deep venous thrombosis: a cost-effectiveness analysis. Ann Intern Med 1999; 130:789–799.

22. Dolovich LR, Ginsberg JS, Douketis JD, et al. A meta-analysis comparing low-molecular weight heparins with unfractionated heparin in the treatment of venous thrombo-embolism. Arch Intern Med 2000; 160:181–188.

23. Krupski WC, Bass A, Dilley RB, Bernstein EF, Otis SM. Propagation of deep venous thrombosis identified by duplex ultrasonography. J Vasc Surg 1990; 12:467–474.

24. van Ramshorst B, van Bemmelen PS, Hoeneveld H, Faber JA, Eikelboom BC. Thrombus regression in deep venous thrombosis. Quantification of spontaneous thrombolysis with duplex scanning. Circulation 1992; 86:414–419.

25. Marder VJ, Soulen RL, Atichartakarn V, et al. Quantitative venographic assessment of deep vein thrombosis in the evaluation of streptokinase and heparin therapy. J Lab Clin Med 1977; 89:1018–1029.

26. Kirchmaier CM, Wolf H, Schäfer H, Ehlers B, Breddin HK, for the Certoparin-Study group. Efficacy of a low molecular weight heparin administered intravenously or subcutaneously in comparison with intravenous unfractionated heparin in the treatment of deep venous thrombosis. Int Angiol 1998; 17:135–145.

27. Harenberg J, Huisman MV, Tolle AR, Breddin HK, Kirchmaier CM. Reduction in thrombus extension and clinical end points in patients after initial treatment for deep vein thrombosis with the fixed-dose body weight-independent low molecular weight heparin certoparin. Semin Thromb Hemost 2001; 27:513–518.

28. Breddin HK, Hach-Wunderle V, Nakov R, Kakkar VV. Effects of a low molecular-weight heparin on thrombus regression and recurrent thromboembolism in patients with deep-vein thrombosis. N Engl J Med 2001; 344:626–631.

29. Leizorovicz A. Comparison of the efficacy and safety of low molecular weight heparins and unfractionated heparin in the initial treatment of deep venous thrombosis. An updated meta-analysis. Drug 1996; 52(suppl 7):30–37.

30. Weitz JI, Hudoba M, Massel D, Maraganore J, Hirsh J. Clot-bound thrombin is protected from inhibition by heparin–antithrombin III but is susceptible to inactivation by antithrombin III–independent inhibitors. J Clin Invest 1990; 86:385–391.

31. Iino M, Takeya H, Takemitsu T, Nakagaki T, Gabazza EC, Suzuki K. Characterization of the binding of factor Xa to fibrinogen/fibrin derivatives and localization of the factor Xa binding site on fibrinogen. Eur J Biochem 1995; 232:90–97.

32. Prager NA, Abendschein DR, McKenzie CR, Eisenberg PR. Role of thrombin compared with factor Xa in the procoagulant activity of whole blood clots. Circulation 1995; 92:962–967.

33. Eisenberg PR, Siegel JE, Abendschein DR, Miletich JP. Importance of factor Xa in determining the procoagulant activity of whole-blood clots. J Clin Invest 1993; 91:1877–1883.

34. Hérault JP, Bernat A, Pflieger AM, Lormeau JC, Herbert JM. Comparative effects of two direct and indirect factor Xa inhibitors on free and clot-bound prothrombinase. J Pharmacol Exp Ther 1997; 283:16–22.

35. Raschke RA, Reilly BM, Guidry JR, Fontana JR, Srinivas S. The weight-based heparin dosing nomogram compared with a "standard care" nomogram. A randomized controlled trial. Ann Intern Med 1993; 119:874–881.

36. Hull Rd, Raskob GE, Hirsh J, et al. Continuous intravenous heparin compared with intermittent subcutaneous heparin in the initial treatment of proximal-vein thrombosis. N Engl J Med 1986; 315:1109–1114.

37. Hull RD, Raskob GE, Brant RF, Pineo GF, Valentine KA. Relation between the time to achieve the lower limit of the APTT therapeutic range and recurrent venous thromboembolism during heparin treatment for deep vein thrombosis. Arch Intern Med 1997; 157:2562–2568.

38. Anand SS, Bates S, Ginsberg JS, et al. Recurrent venous thrombosis and heparin therapy. Arch Intern Med 1999; 159:2029–2032.

39. Boneu B, Caranobe C, Sie P. Pharmacokinetics of heparin and low molecular weight heparin. Baillieres Clin Haematol 1990; 3:531–544.

40. Hirsh J, Warkentin TE, Shaughnessy SG, et al. Heparin and low-molecular-weight heparin: mechanisms of action, pharmacokinetics, dosing, monitoring, efficacy, and safety. Chest 2001; 119:64S–94S.

41. Frydman A. Low-molecular-weight heparins: an overview of their pharmaco-dynamics, pharmacokinetics and metabolism in humans. Haemostasis 1996; 26(suppl 2):24–38.

42. Eriksson BI, Ekman S, Lindbratt S, et al. Prevention of thromboembolism with use of recombinant hirudin. Results of a double-blind, multicenter trial comparing the efficacy of desirudin (Revasc) with that of unfractionated heparin in patients having a total hip replacement. J Bone Joint Surg Am 1997; 79-A: 326–333.

43. Eriksson BI, Wille-Jorgensen P, Kalebo P, et al. A comparison of recombinant hirudin with a low-molecular-weight heparin to prevent thromboembolic complications after total hip replacement. N Engl J Med 1997; 337:1329–1335.

44. Ginsberg JS, Nurmohamed MT, Gent M, et al. Use of Hirulog in the prevention of venous thrombosis after major hip or knee surgery. Circulation 1994; 90:2385–2389.

45. Heit JA, Colwell CW, Francis CW, et al. Comparison of the oral direct thrombin inhibitor ximelagatran with enoxaparin as prophylaxis against venous thromboembolism after total knee replacement. A phase 2 dose-finding study. Arch Intern Med 2001; 161:2215–2221.

46. Francis CW, Davisdon BL, Berkowitz SD, Lotke PA, Ginsberg JS, Lieberman JR, et al. Randomized, double-blind, comparative study of Ximelagatran (pINN, formerly H 376/95), an oral direct thrombin inhibitor, and warfarin to prevent venous thromboembolism (VTE) after total knee arthroplasty (TKA) [abstract OC44]. J Thromb Haemost, July 2001 (suppl). CD-ROM published by Excerpta Medica Medical Communications.

47. Eriksson BI, Ögren M, Agnelli G, Cohen A, Dahl OE, Mouret P, Rosencher N, Eskilson C, Nylander I, Frison L. The oral direct thrombin inhibitor ximelagatran (pINN, formerly H 376/95) and its subcutaneous form melagatran compared with enoxaparin as thromboprophylaxis after total hip or total knee replacement [abstract OC1638]. Thromb Haemost, July 2001 (suppl). CD-ROM published by Excerpta Medica Medical Communications.

48. Eriksson BI, Arfwidsson A-C, Frison L, et al. A dose-ranging study of the oral direct thrombin inhibitor, Ximelagatran, and its subcutaneous form, Melagatran, compared with Dalteparin in the prophylaxis of thromboembolism after hip or knee replacement: METHRO I. Thromb Haemost 2002; 87:231–237.

49. Samama MM, Walenga JM, Kaiser B, Fareed J. Specific factor Xa inhibitors. In: Verstraete M, Fuster V, Topol EJ, eds. Cardiovascular Thrombosis: Thrombocardiology and Thromboneurology. 2d ed. Philadelphia: Lippincott-Raven, 1998:173–188.

50. Sato K, Kawasaki T, Taniuchi Y, Hirayama F, Koshio H, Matsumoto Y. YM-60828, a novel factor Xa inhibitor: separation of its antithrombotic effects from its prolongation of bleeding time. Eur J Pharmacol 1997; 339:141–146.

51. Murayama N, Tanaka M, Kunitada S, et al. Tolerability, pharmacokinetics, and pharmacodynamics of DX-9065a, a new synthetic potent anticoagulant and specific factor Xa inhibitor, in healthy male volunteers. Clin Pharmacol Ther 1999; 66:258–264.

52. Tuszynski GP, Gasic TB, Gasic GJ. Isolation and characterization of antistasin. An inhibitor of metastasis and coagulation. J Biol Chem 1987; 262:9718–9723.
53. Vlasuk GP. Structural and functional characterization of tick anticoagulant peptide (TAP): a potent and selective inhibitor of blood coagulation factor Xa. Thromb Haemost 1993; 70:212–216.
54. Choay J, Petitou M, Lormeau JC, Sinaÿ P, Casu B, Gatti G. Structure-activity relationship in heparin: a synthetic pentasaccharide with high affinity for antithrombin III and eliciting high anti-factor Xa activity. Biochem Biophys Res Commun 1983; 116:492–499.
55. Sinay P, Jacquinet J-C, Petitou M, et al. Total synthesis of a heparin pentasaccharide fragment having high affinity for antithrombin III. Carbohydr Res 1984; 132:C5–C9.
56. van Boeckel CAA, Beetz T, Vos JN, et al. Synthesis of a pentasaccharide corresponding to the antithrombin III binding fragment of heparin. J Carbohydr Chem 1985; 4:293–321.
57. van Boeckel CAA, Petitou M. The unique antithrombin III binding domain of heparin: a lead to new synthetic antithrombotics. Angew Chem Int Ed Engl 1993; 32:1671–1690.
58. Paolucci F, Clavies M, Donat F, Necciari J. In vitro protein binding of Org31540/SR90107A in human plasma and purified antithrombin III [abstract P3095]. Thromb Haemost, July 2001 (suppl). Available on CD-ROM published by Excerpta Medica Medical Communications.
59. Warkentin TE. Heparin-induced thrombocytopenia: a clinicopathologic syndrome. Thromb Haemost 1999; 82:439–447.
60. Monreal M, Viñas L, Monreal L, Lavin S, Lafoz E, Angles AM. Heparin-related osteoporosis in rats. A comparative study between unfractionated heparin and a low-molecular-weight heparin. Haemostasis 1990; 20:204–207.
61. Donat F, Duret JP, Santoni A, Cariou R, Necciari J, Magnani H, de Greef R. Pharmacokinetics of Org31540/SR90107A in young and elderly healthy subjects: a highly favorable pharmacokinetic profile [abstract P3094]. Thromb Haemost, July 2001 (suppl). Available on CD-ROM published by Excerpta Medica Medical Communications.
62. Turpie AGG. Overview of the clinical results of pentasaccharide in major orthopedic surgery. Haematologica 2001; 86(suppl 11):59–62.
63. The Rembrandt Investigators. Treatment of proximal deep vein thrombosis with a novel synthetic compound (SR90107A/ORG31540) with pure anti-factor Xa activity: a phase II evaluation. Circulation 2000; 102:2726–2731.
64. Duggan BM, Dyson HJ, Wright PE. Inherent flexibility in a potent inhibitor of blood coagulation, recombinant nematode anticoagulant protein c2. Eur J Biochem 1999; 265:539–548.
65. Weitz JI, Hirsh J. New anticoagulant drugs. Chest 2001; 19(suppl):95S–107S.
66. Rivera TM, Leone-Bay A, Paton DR, Leipold HR, Baughman RA. Oral delivery of heparin in combination with sodium N-[8-(2-hydroxybenzoyl)-amino]caprylate: pharmacological considerations. Pharm Res 1997; 14:1830–1834.

12

Thrombolytic Therapy in Acute Pulmonary Embolism

PAUL D. STEIN

St. Joseph Mercy Oakland Hospital
Pontiac, Michigan, U.S.A.

JAMES E. DALEN

University of Arizona College of Medicine
Tucson, Arizona, U.S.A.

I. History

Streptokinase, the first thrombolytic agent to be discovered, was reported by Tillett in 1933 (1). Experimental studies demonstrated that it could quickly induce a fibrinolytic state capable of dissolving experimentally induced thrombi. Early clinical investigations uncovered two problems: pyrogenicity and inactivation of streptokinase by preexisting antibodies. The first clinical report of its use in patients with pulmonary embolism was that of Browse and James in 1964 (2). They reported the results of the infusion of streptokinase in four patients with a clinical diagnosis of acute pulmonary embolism. All four patients, including two with hypotension, recovered and were discharged.

Urokinase derived from human urine was found to have thrombolytic capability. The first clinical report of its use in patients with a variety of thromboembolic disorders, including six patients with venous thromboembolism, was by Hansen et al. in 1961 (3).

II. Administration of Thrombolytic Agents

A. U.S. Food and Drug Administration (USFDA)–Approved and –Unapproved Regimens

Regimens for the intravenous infusion of thrombolytic agents are rt-PA 100 mg administered over 2 hrs, streptokinase administered over 24 hrs and urokinase administered over 12–24 hrs (4) (Table 1). Shorter infusions of streptokinase and of urokinase have been used, as well as other thrombolytic agents (5). These regimens, not approved by the USFDA, are also shown in Table 1. Urokinase had been withdrawn from the market because of issues related to assurance of viral inactivation in the manufacturing process (6), but it has now been approved again by the USFDA.

B. Infusion Directly into the Pulmonary Artery

Standard Doses Infused into the Pulmonary Artery

We are aware of only one investigation in which an infusion of thrombolytic agent directly into the pulmonary artery was compared with an intravenous infusion of the same thrombolytic agent (7). An infusion of rt-PA 50 mg over 2 hrs directly into the pulmonary artery (19 patients) was not more effective than an intravenous injection of rt-PA 50 mg (15 patients) (7). The respective changes in the angiographic severity score were −9 and −10. Some of the patients received a repeat dose of 50 mg rt-PA over 5 hrs.

One randomized trial compared an infusion of streptokinase into the main pulmonary artery with a heparin infusion into the main pulmonary

Table 1 Thrombolytic Regimens

USFDA Approved[a]
t-PA 100mg/2h
Streptokinase   250,000 U/30 min
100,000 U/hr × 24 hr
Urokinase   4,400 U/kg/10 min
4,400 U/kg/hr × 12–24 hr
Not USFDA Approved[b]
Urokinase[b] 3,000,000 U/2 hr
Streptokinase 1,500,000 U/1–2 hr
Reteplase 10 U, repeat 10 U in 30 min
Saruplase 80 mg/30 min
Staphylokinase 20 mg/30 min

[a] *Source*: Ref. 4.
[b] *Source*: Ref. 5.

artery (8). Streptokinase was infused as a loading dose of 600,000 U over 30 mins followed by 100,000 U/hr for 72 hr. The mean angiographic score decreased by 13.3 in the streptokinase arm and it decreased by 2.8 in the heparin arm ($P < .001$) (Table 2).

Low Doses Infused into the Pulmonary Artery

Several case series evaluated an infusion of low doses of a lytic agent directly into the pulmonary artery, but there was no comparison with other routes of administration or other drugs (9–13). In a case series by Leeper and associates, in which streptokinase in low doses was infused into the pulmonary artery in combination with heparin, the perfused lung showed a reduction of the angiographic severity index score (9). Even though the dose of streptokinase was only 5–9% of the USFDA-approved dose for systemic use, severe bleeding occurred in two of seven patients (28.6%). In a case series by Gallus and associates, low doses of streptokinase infused into the pulmonary artery showed considerable lysis in all seven patients who had posttreatment angiograms (10). Severe bleeding occurred in 2 of 13 patients (15.4%) (10). Vujic and associates, in three patients, used even lower doses of streptokinase (5500–10,000 U in combination with heparin infused over 16–30 hrs (11). There was significant angiographic improvement and no major bleeding. Others also showed improvement in most and no bleeding following an intrapulmonary artery infusion of low doses of urokinase (13) or streptokinase (12).

Table 2   Rate of Resolution: Lytic Agents Versus Heparin

Lytic agent	No. patients		Time after start lytic (hr)	Resolution		Reference
	Lytic	Heparin		Lytic	Heparin	
UK	64	62	24	24.1%	8.3%[a]	14
SK (IP)	11	12	72	−13.3	−2.8[b]	8
SK	14	10	72	−11.3	−3.4[c]	16
rt-PA	9	4	24	10%	0%[d]	17
rt-PA	33	25	24	34.4%	12.0%[e]	20
rt-PA	20	16	2	−3.5	−0.1[c]	18
rt-PA	46	55	24	14.6%	1.5%[f]	19

UK, urokinase; SK, streptokinase; IP, intrapulmonary artery.
[a] Mean percentage of resolution in scan deficit (significant).
[b] Change in pulmonary angiogram ($P < .01$ to $P < .001$).
[c] Change in pulmonary angiographic severity score ($P < .01$).
[d] Percentage of improvement in mismatched scan deficit (NS).
[e] Percentage of patients showing $> 50\%$ improvement of perfusion scan ($P = .026$).
[f] Proportion of lung showing improved perfusion ($P < .0001$).

III. Rate and Extent of Resolution of Pulmonary Embolism

A. Resolution with Urokinase

Thrombolytic therapy causes a more rapid rate of resolution of pulmonary embolism (PE) than occurs with natural processes or with heparin. This was demonstrated in the Urokinase Pulmonary Embolism Trial (UPET)(14). Patients with pulmonary embolism documented by pulmonary angiography were randomized to a 12-hr infusion of urokinase or to intravenous heparin. Eighty-two patients received urokinase (2000 U/lb loading dose over 10–15 min followed by 2000 U/lb/hr for 12 hr) and 78 patients received heparin alone. Mean percentage resolution on perfusion lung scans 24 hrs after starting urokinase was 24.1% compared with 8.3% among patients who received heparin alone. By day 14, mean percentage resolution was comparable in both groups (55.4 vs 56.2%). At the end of 1 year, mean percentage resolution remained comparable in both groups (78.8 vs 77.2%). Among patients with no prior cardiopulmonary disease, 88% of patients treated with urokinase showed more than 90% resolution of the perfusion lung scan versus 91% of those treated only with anticoagulants. Among patients with prior cardiopulmonary disease, the percentage of patients who showed more than 90% resolution of the perfusion lung scan was 77% with urokinase and 72% with anticoagulants.

B. Resolution with Streptokinase

In the Urokinase-Streptokinase Embolism Trial, a second phase of the UPET, 167 patients with angiographically documented pulmonary embolism were randomized to treatment with 12 hrs of urokinase as in the Phase I trials, or 24 hrs of urokinase, or 24 hrs of streptokinase (15). Angiographic follow-up showed no significant differences among the three regimens. Perfusion lung scans, however, showed that 24-hour urokinase resulted in significantly more resolution than 24 hrs of streptokinase. All three regimens were more effective in accelerating resolution of PE than heparin alone was in the Phase I trial (15).

C. Comparisons of Rate of Resolution with Heparin

We are aware of seven randomized trials in which the rate of resolution of PE with thrombolytic agents was compared with heparin. Three of these were with streptokinase or urokinase (8,14,16) and 4 were with rt-PA (17–20) (see Table 2). Different methods were used for comparing resolution of the angiogram or perfusion lung scan. Thrombolytic agents in all investigations in which there were 10 or more patients in each arm showed a more rapid rate of resolution of PE than with heparin alone.

D. Comparisons of Resolution with rt-PA, Urokinase, and Streptokinase

We found five investigations comparing the rate of resolution of PE following treatment with rt-PA with the rate of resolution following urokinase or streptokinase (21–25) (Table 3). The rt-PA was given in a dose of 100 mg over 2 hrs. At 2 hrs, resolution was greater with rt-PA than with streptokinase or urokinase administered over 12–24 hrs (21,23,24). However, resolution at the time of completion of the infusion of urokinase or streptokinase (12–24 hrs) was comparable with rt-PA (21,23,24). When streptokinase or urokinase was administered over 2 hrs, resolution at 2 hrs was comparable with rt-PA (22,25).

E. Resolution of Functional Abnormalities

Although residual perfusion defects in the UPET were comparable after 1 year among patients treated with thrombolytic agents and patients treated with anticoagulants alone, in small numbers of patients the pulmonary

Table 3 Resolution Rate: rt-PA 100 mg/2 hr Versus Other Thrombolytic Agents

Dose other thrombolytic agent	No. patients		Resolution		Reference
	rt-PA	Other	rt-PA	Other	
Urokinase 2,000 U/lb bolus 2,000 U/lb/h for 24 h	22	23	Angiographic improvement at 2 hr 82%	48% ($P = .008$) Lung scan perfusion at 24 hr Both groups equal (NS)	21
Urokinase 4,400 U/kg bolus 4,400 U/kg/h for 12 h	34	29	TPR change at 2 hr −42%	−21% ($P < 0.0001$) Angiographic severity score at 12 hr −7.5 (NS)	23
			−5.9		
Streptokinase 250,000 U/15 min 1,200,000 U/12 h	25	25	TPR change at 2 hr −42%	−13% ($P < .001$) TPR change at 12 h −40% (NS)	24
			−48%		
Urokinase 1,000,000 U/10 min 2,000,000 U/110 min	42	45	Patients showing angiographic improvement at 2 hr 79%	67% (NS)	22
Streptokinase 1,500,000 U/2	23	43	TPR change at 2 hr −38%	−31% (NS)	25

TPR, total pulmonary resistance.
rt-PA dose was 100 mg/2 hr in all investigations.

diffusing capacity (DLCO) after 1 year was higher among patients who received thrombolytic therapy (26). Among 21 patients treated with anticoagulants compared with 19 patients treated with thrombolytic agents, the DLCO was 72% predicted versus 93% predicted, respectively (26).

Follow-up a mean of 7.4 years later of 12 patients treated with urokinase or streptokinase and 11 patients treated with heparin showed that mean pulmonary artery pressure was higher in the heparin group (22 versus 17 mmHg) as was pulmonary vascular resistance (351 dyne sec cm^{-5} versus 171 dyne sec cm^{-5}) (27). Exercise increased the pulmonary artery mean pressure and pulmonary vascular resistance in the heparin group, but not in the thrombolytic therapy group. Among patients treated with urokinase or streptokinase, 8 of 12 (67%) were New York Heart Association (NYHA) Class 0 to I compared with 3 of 11 (27%) in the heparin therapy arm.

IV. Mortality with Thrombolytic Therapy

A. Mortality of Patients Not in Shock

Among symptomatic patients with acute PE who were not in shock, the mortality with heparin was comparable to the mortality with thrombolytic therapy irrespective of whether treatment was with urokinase administered over 12 hrs, urokinase 12 hrs/day for 3 days, or rt-PA (14,17–20,28,29) (Table 4). The largest trial, the UPET, showed a 2-week mortality of 2 of 73 (2.7%) patients treated with urokinase and 6 of 73 (8.2%) patients treated with heparin (NS) (14). Regarding more recent trials, pooled data from five randomized trials that compared rt-PA with heparin showed a mortality of 8 of 226 (3.5%) among patients treated with rt-PA and 6 of 238 (2.5%) among

Table 4 Mortality of Patients Not in Shock: Thrombolytic Agents Versus Heparin

Lytic agent	No. patients		Mortality		Reference
	Lytic	Heparin	Lytic n (%)	Heparin n (%)	
Urokinase	73	73	2 (2.7)	6 (8.2)	14
Urokinase	20	10	0 (0)	0 (0)	28
rt-PA	9	4	1 (11.1)	0 (0)	17
rt-PA	33	25	1 (3.0)	0 (0)	20
rt-PA	20	16	2 (10.0)	1 (6.3)	18
rt-PA	46	55	0	2 (3.6)	19
rt-PA	118	138	4 (3.4)	3 (2.2)	29
Total	319	321	10 (3.1)	12 (3.7)[a]	

[a] All differences, lytic vs heparin, not significant.

patients treated with heparin (NS) (17–20,29) (Table 4). Among all trials, mortality with thrombolytic therapy was 10 of 319 (3.1%) versus 12 of 321 (3.7%) in patients treated with heparin alone (NS).

B. Mortality of Patients in Shock

Among patients in shock from acute PE, data comparing thrombolytic therapy with heparin are sparse. Among patients in shock in the UPET, there was a comparable 2-week mortality among those treated with urokinase and those treated with anticoagulants: 4 of 9 (44%) versus 1 of 5 (20%) patients, respectively (NS) (14).

In a trial of patients with massive PE, all of whom were in shock, four of four randomized to streptokinase 1,500,000 U in 1 hr improved within the first hour after treatment and all survived (30). Among four patients randomized to heparin alone, none survived ($P = .02$). The likelihood of obtaining such comparative data in the future is remote.

C. Mortality in Patients with Right Ventricular Dilatation or Dysfunction

Among stable patients with baseline right ventricular hypokinesis, the mortality was 0 of 18 (0%) among patients randomized to rt-PA compared with 2 of 18 (11.1%) randomized to heparin alone (NS) (19) (Table 5). In a retrospective investigation of 64 patients with right ventricular dysfunction who received thrombolytic therapy compared with 64 who received heparin alone, the mortality was also comparable in both groups (31) (Table 5).

Konstantinides et al. reported the clinical course of stable patients with submassive acute PE who were treated either with rt-PA plus heparin or heparin alone (29). Right ventricular dysfunction was present in 31% of

Table 5 Recurrent PE and Mortality in Patients with Right Ventricular Dysfunction or Dilatation and Not in Shock: Thrombolytic Agents Versus Heparin

| Lytic agent | No. patients | | Recurrent PE | | Mortality | | Reference |
	Lytic	Heparin	Lytic n (%)	Heparin n (%)	Lytic n (%)	Heparin n (%)	
rt-PA	18	18	0 (0)	5 (27.8)[a]	0 (0)	2 (11.1)	19
rt-PA, urokinase, saruplase	64	64	3 (4.7)	3 (4.7)	4 (6.3)	0 (0)	31

[a] $p < .02$.

patients in both treatment arms. Mortality was comparable in both groups (see Table 4). "Rescue thrombolysis" was required in 23% of the patients in the heparin arm (29).

V. Recurrent PE with Thrombolytic Therapy

A. Recurrent PE with Urokinase

In the UPET, recurrent PE by 14 days was comparable in both arms of the study (14). Recurrent PE documented by both clinical evidence and perfusion lung scan was observed in 5 of 82 (6.1%) patients in the urokinase arm and in 7 of 78 (9.0%) patients in the heparin arm. After a mean of 7.4 years, recurrent PE occurred in 2 of 19 (10.5%) patients in the thrombolytic therapy arm and 4 of 21 (19.0%) patients in the heparin arm ($P < .05$) (27).

B. Recurrent PE with rt-PA

Recurrent PE in randomized trials in which rt-PA was compared with heparin is shown in Table 6. Recurrent PE confirmed by lung scan, pulmonary angiogram, or contrast-enhanced spiral computed tomography (CT), based on pooled data, was shown in 5 of 217 (2.3%) patients treated with rt-PA and in 6 of 234 (2.6%) patients treated with heparin alone (NS) (18–20,29).

C. Recurrent PE with Right Ventricular Dysfunction or Dilatation

The suggestion that thrombolytic therapy may be indicated in patients with right ventricular dysfunction was proposed by Goldhaber and associates (19). Among stable patients with baseline right ventricular hypokinesis, 18 patients had been randomized to rt-PA followed by heparin and 18 patients had been randomized to heparin alone. In this subgroup of patients with

Table 6 Recurrent PE rt-Pa Versus Heparin: Randomized Trials

No. patients		Recurrent PE objective test		
rt-PA	HEP	rt-PA n (%)	HEP n (%)	Reference
33	25	0 (0)	0 (0)	20
20	16	1 (5)	0 (0)	18
46	55	0 (0)	2 (3.6)	19
118	138	4 (3.4)	4 (2.9)	29
217	234	5 (2.3)	6 (2.6)[a]	Total

[a] Not significant.

right ventricular dysfunction, there was no recurrent PE among patients treated with rt-PA, but 5 of 18 (27.8%) treated with heparin alone suffered clinical or objective evidence of recurrent PE ($p < .02$) (see Table 5). In two of those with suspected recurrent PE, the diagnosis of recurrent PE was confirmed by a perfusion lung scan.

In a retrospective investigation of 64 patients with right ventricular dysfunction who received thrombolytic therapy, compared with 64 patients who received heparin alone, the rate of recurrent PE was the same in both groups: 3 of 64 patients (4.7%) (31) (see Table 5).

VI. Major Bleeding with Thrombolytic Therapy

A. Overview

The overwhelming necessity for a cautious and prudent use of thrombolytic therapy in patients with PE is the risk of major bleeding. Narrow indications of the recommendations for thrombolytic therapy in patients with PE are based on high rates of bleeding. Over three decades of experience have shown that high rates of bleeding occur with thrombolytic therapy for PE in spite of modifications of the type of thrombolytic agent, the dose, the rate of administration, and care in avoiding arterial punctures and venipunctures in patients.

B. Definition of Major Bleeding

We define major bleeding as bleeding associated with a reduction of hemoglobin ≥ 2 g/dL, blood transfusion ≥ 2 U, intracerebral bleed, retroperitoneal bleed, pericardial bleed, bleeding that required a surgical intervention, bleeding into a major joint, or bleeding into the eye (32). We also define a reduction of hematocrit >10 points as major bleeding.

C. Major Bleeding Among Patients in Registries

Among 169 stable patients with PE (19% diagnosed by pulmonary angiography) who received thrombolytic therapy in a multicenter registry, major bleeding occurred in 21.9% (33) (Table 7). Intracranial hemorrhage occurred in 1.2%. Death from complications of diagnostic procedures or from therapy occurred in 0.6% In another multicenter registry, the International Cooperative Pulmonary Embolism Registry, major bleeding was reported in 21.7% of patients who received thrombolytic therapy and intracranial hemorrhage occurred in 3.0% (34). In a review of seven investigations with t-PA or urokinase, in which high-risk patients were excluded, major bleeding occurred in 61 of 312 patients (19.6%) (35). Bleeding at the site of catheter-

Table 7   Major Bleeding with Various Thrombolytic Agents in Treatment of PE[a]

Patients	No.	Angiography n (%)	Major bleed n (%)	Major Catheter site bleed n (%)	Lytic agent	Reference
Registry Hemodynamically Stable	169	32 (19)	37 (21.9)	?	Any	33
Registry Major PE	304	58 (19)	66 (21.7)	?	Any	34
Registry RV Dilation, Dysfunction	64	?	10 (15.6)	?	t-PA Urokinase Saruplase	31
Randomized	23	23 (100)	11 (47.8)	?	Urokinase	21
Randomized	46	46 (100)	6 (13.0)	?	Urokinase	22
Randomized	20	20 (100)	1 (5.0)	0	Urokinase	28
Randomized	129	129 (100)	16 (12.4)	2 (1.6)	Urokinase	39
Randomized	29	29 (100)	8 (27.6)	2 (6.9)	Urokinase	23
Randomized	43	43 (100)	3 (7.0)	2 (4.7)	Streptokinase	25
Randomized	4	0 (0)	0 (0)	0	Streptokinase	30
Randomized	25	25 (100)	3 (12.0)	2 (8.0)	Streptokinase	24

[a] Only investigations since the 1980s are included.

ization occurred in 34 patients (10.9%). Intracranial hemorrhage occurred in five patients (1.6%).

D.   Major Bleeding with rt-PA

Among patients in randomized trials who received rt-PA, 63 of 430 patients (14.7%) suffered major bleeding (7,17–25,36,37) (Table 8). Among those who received rt-PA not accompanied by simultaneous heparin, pooled data showed major bleeding in 54 of 362 patients (14.9%) (18–23,25,36,37). In those who received simultaneous heparin, the rate of major bleeding was not higher, 9 of 68 patients (13.2%) (7,17,24). The criteria for major bleeding were the criteria described above. Patients with a high risk of bleeding were excluded. Among those who had pulmonary angiograms, major bleeding at the insertion site occurred in 20 of 286 patients (7%) (7,17–20,23–25,36,37) (Table 8).

In a review of patients in randomized trials that used rt-PA and in whom the diagnosis of PE was made by pulmonary angiography, Levine found major bleeding in only 19 of 227 patients (8.4%) (38). The definition of major bleeding that he used did not include a 10-point drop in hematocrit

Table 8 Major Bleeding with rt-PA in Randomized Trials of Treatment of PE[a,b]

No.	Angiography n (%)	Major bleed n (%)	Major Catheter site bleed n (%)	With heparin	Reference
34[c]	34 (100)	4 (11.8)	0 (0)	Yes	7
9	9 (100)	1 (11.1)	1 (11.1)[d]	Yes	17
20	20 (100)	3 (15.0)	0 (0)	No	18
22	22 (100)	4 (18.2)	?	No	21
44	44 (100)	9 (20.5)	?	No	22
46	6 (13)	4 (8.7)	1 (16.7)	No	19
33	22 (67)	0 (0)	0 (0)	No	20
34	34 (100)	7 (20.6)	2 (5.9)	No	23
87	60 (69)	14 (16.1)	4 (6.7)	No	37
23	23 (100)	5 (21.7)	4 (17.4)	No	25
25	25 (100)	4 (16.0)	3 (12.0)	Yes	24
53	53 (100)	8 (15.1)	5 (9.4)	No	36

[a] In all trials, only patients at low risk of bleeding were included.
[b] Investigations were excluded if we could not determine the rate of major bleeding according to our definition.
[c] Intrapulmonary and intravenous.
[d] Many sites including site of catheter insertion.

or a transfusion of 2 U of blood. Konstantinides and associates reported major bleeding with rt-PA in only 1 of 118 patients (0.8%) (29). They defined major bleeding as fatal bleeding, hemorrhagic stroke, or a drop in the hemoglobin concentration of at least 4 g/dL.

Among patients who received urokinase in randomized trials in the 1980s or more recently, the rate of major bleeding based on pooled data was 42 of 247 patients (17%) (21–23,28,39) (see Table 7). The criteria for major bleeding were the criteria described above. Patients with a high risk of bleeding were excluded. All patients had pulmonary angiograms.

Pooled data from randomized trials showed comparable rates of major bleeding among patients treated with rt-PA (14.7%) (7, 17–25,36,37) (see Table 8) and patients treated with urokinase (17.0%) (21–23,28,39) (see Table 7). Only sparse data are available in recent trials of patients treated with streptokinase (24,25,30) (see Table 7).

E. Major Bleeding at the Site of Catheter Insertion

Among all patients in randomized trials since the 1980s, irrespective of whether treatment was with rt-PA, urokinase, or streptokinase, major bleed-

Table 9 Intracranial Hemorrhage with Thrombolytic Agents in Treatment of PE

Patients	No.	ICH n (%)	Fatal ICH n (%)	Lytic agent	References
Major PE hemodynamically stable registry	169	2 (1.2)	1 (0.6)	Any	33
Major PE registry	304	9 (3.0)	-	Any	34
PE trials pooled	312	6 (1.9)	2 (0.6)	rt-PA, urokinase	41
PE trials pooled	559	12 (2.1)	9 (1.6)	rt-PA	40

ICH, intracranial hemorrhage.

ing at the site of catheter insertion was reported in 28 of 532 patients (5.3%) (7,17–20,23–25,28,30,36,37,39) (see Tables 7 and 8). Major bleeding at the site of catheter insertion among patients treated with rt-PA was 20 of 286 patients (7%) (7,17–20,23–25,36,37) (see Table 8). In the Urokinase Pulmonary Embolism Trial, severe bleeding from the venous cutdown site among patients treated with urokinase occurred in 8 of 82 patients (9.8%) (14). Isolated bleeding at the site of the arterial puncture "was rare." Severe bleeding unrelated to the venous cutdown in the Urokinase Pulmonary Embolism Trial occurred in 14 of 82 patients (17.1%).

F. Intracranial Hemorrhage

Dalen and associates, based on pooled data in 559 patients, showed an incidence of intracranial hemorrhage of 2.1% among patients treated with rt-PA for acute PE (40) (Table 9). The incidence of fatal intracranial hemorrhage with rt-PA was 1.6%. Others, based on data from registries or pooled data, showed a comparable rate of intracranial hemorrhage with various thrombolytic agents (33,34,41) (Table 9).

VII. Diagnostic Tests Before Thrombolytic Therapy

The risks of serious and perhaps fatal bleeding are so great that some have recommended a pulmonary angiogram to confirm the diagnosis of PE in all patients prior to thrombolytic therapy (42). This would result in bleeding in some patients at the site of insertion of the catheter. If contrast-enhanced spiral CT or gadolinium-enhanced MRI is confirmed to be sufficiently accurate and practical, these tests may minimize the need for pulmonary angiography in such patients. Some believe that if there is a high probability ventilation-perfusion lung scan in a patient in whom the clinical suspicion is also high, this combination is sufficient to allow the administration of thrombolytic therapy (42).

VIII. Categories of Patients in Whom Thrombolytic Therapy Has Been Considered

Thrombolytic therapy has been considered for four categories of patients with PE: (1) all patients with PE, (2) those who are stable with right ventricular dysfunction, (3) those who are hemodynamically unstable, and (4) those with massive PE who are undergoing resuscitation for cardiopulmonary arrest.

A. Thrombolytic Therapy for All Patients with PE

The possibility that all patients with PE should receive thrombolytic therapy at one time had been suggested on the basis of physiological follow-up evaluation of patients who had been enrolled in the Urokinase Pulmonary Embolism Trial (26). Subsequent investigation by the same group of investigators showed a physiological and clinical benefit of thrombolytic therapy in many of these patients after 7 years (27). Even so, thrombolytic therapy for all patients with PE is not recommended because the bleeding rate is high, and the mortality among patients treated with heparin alone is very low (43).

B. Thrombolytic Therapy for Stable Patients with PE and Right Ventricular Dysfunction

At one major university center, thrombolytic therapy is given to all patients with PE who have right ventricular dysfunction unless contraindicated in spite of sparse data as to its efficacy (44). The need for a randomized trial in such patients, however, is recognized (31,44). In our opinion, data are insufficient to recommend thrombolytic therapy in such patients; the risk of bleeding would seem to exceed the benefits.

C. Patients with PE Who Are Hemodynamically Unstable

Hemodynamic instability is a generally accepted indication for the administration of thrombolytic therapy (43). Intuitively, the indication seems valid. There are, however, no definitive trials to prove the validity of thrombolytic therapy in PE even for unstable patients. One randomized controlled trial was halted for ethical reasons after four desperately ill patients with PE who received thrombolytic therapy survived, whereas four treated only with heparin died (30). Our opinion is that thrombolytic therapy is indicated in patients who are hemodynamically unstable provided there are no contraindications even though the effectiveness has not been established by randomized controlled trials.

D. Thrombolytic Therapy for Patients with Massive PE Who Are Being Resuscitated from Cardiopulmonary Arrest

Several case reports and case series have shown survival among patients with cardiopulmonary arrest who received thrombolytic therapy during the resuscitative effort (45). This is a heroic measure that may benefit some patients. A Consensus Committee on Pulmonary Embolism in 1996 cautioned that there should be some objective evidence of PE, such as right ventricular dysfunction on an echocardiogram, or a positive noninvasive leg test (42). Others on the committee felt that the risks of a misdiagnosis are so great that a definitive diagnosis by pulmonary angiography (or now perhaps contrast-enhanced spiral CT) is mandatory (42). Our opinion is that if there is no contraindication, thrombolytic therapy is indicated in patients in cardiopulmonary arrest in whom the diagnosis appears to be PE.

References

1. Tillett WS, Garner RL. The fibrinolytic activity of hemolytic streptococci. J Exp Med 1933; 58:485–502.
2. Browse NL, Brist MD, James DCO. Streptokinase and pulmonary embolism. Lancet 1964; 2:1039–1043.
3. Hansen PF, Jorgensen M, Kjeldgaard NO, Ploug J. Urokinase an activator of plasminogen from human urine. Experiences with intravenous application on twenty-two patients. Angiology 1961; 12:367–371.
4. Goldhaber SZ. The current role of thrombolytic therapy for pulmonary embolism. Semin Vasc Surg 2000; 13:217–220.
5. Goldhaber SZ. Pulmonary embolism thrombolysis: do we need another agent? Am Heart J 1999; 138:1–2.
6. Zoon KC. Important drug warning: safety information regarding the use of Abbokinase (urokinase). http://www.fda.gov/cber/1tr/abb012599.htm.
7. Verstraete M, Miller GAH, Bounameaux H, Charbonnier B, Colle JP, Lecorf G, Marbet GA, Mombaerts P, Olsson CG. Intravenous and intrapulmonary recombinant tissue-type plasminogen activator in the treatment of acute massive pulmonary embolism. Circulation 1988; 77:353–360.
8. Tibbutt DA, Davies JA, Anderson JA, Fletcher EWL, Hamill J, Holt JM, Thomas ML, Lee G de J, Miller GAH, Sharp AA, Sutton GC. Comparison by controlled clinical trial of streptokinase and heparin in treatment of life-threatening pulmonary embolism. BMJ 1974; 1:343–347.
9. Leeper KV, Popovich J, Lesser BA, Adams D, Froelich JW, Burke MW, Shetty PC, Thrall JH, Stein PD. Treatment of massive acute pulmonary embolism.

The use of low doses of intrapulmonary arterial streptokinase combined with full doses of systemic heparin. Chest 1988; 93:234–240.

10. Gallus AS, Hirsch J, Cade JF, Turpie AGG, Walker IR, Gent M. Thrombolysis with a combination of small doses of streptokinase and full doses of heparin. Semin Thromb Hemostasis 1975; 2:14–32.

11. Vujic I, Young JWR, Gobien RP, Dawson WT, Liebscher L, Shelley BE Jr. Massive pulmonary embolism: treatment with full heparinization and topical low-dose streptokinase. Radiology 1983; 148:671–675.

12. Ambrose JE, Venditto M, Dickerson WH. Local fibrinolysis for the treatment of massive pulmonary embolism: efficacy of streptokinase infusion through pulmonary arterial catheter. J Am Osteopath Assoc 1985; 85:97–101.

13. Edwards IR, MacLean KS, Dow JD. Low-dose urokinase in major pulmonary embolism. Lancet 1973; 2:409–413.

14. A National Cooperative Study. The urokinase pulmonary embolism trial. Circulation (suppl 2) 1973; 47(suppl 2):II-1–II-108.

15. A Cooperative Study. Urokinase-streptokinase embolism trial, Phase 2 results. JAMA 1974; 229:1606–1613.

16. Ly B, Arnesen H, Eie H, Hol R. A controlled clinical trial of streptokinase and heparin in the treatment of major pulmonary embolism. Acta Med Scand 1978; 203:465–470.

17. PIOPED Investigators. Tissue plasminogen activator for the treatment of acute pulmonary embolism. Chest 1990; 97:528–533.

18. Dalla-Volta S, Palla A, Santolicandro A, Giuntini C, Pengo V, Visioli O, Zonzin P, Zanuttini D, Barbaresi F, Agnelli G, Morpurgo M, Marini MG, Visani L. PAIMS 2: alteplase combined with heparin versus heparin in the treatment of acute pulmonary embolism. Plasminogen activator Italian multicenter study 2. J Am Coll Cardiol 1992; 20:520–526.

19. Goldhaber SZ, Haire WD, Feldstein ML, Miller M, Toltzis R, Smith JL, Da Silva AMT, Come PC, Lee RT, Parker JA, Mogtader A, McDonough TJ, Braunwald E. Alteplase versus heparin in acute pulmonary embolism: randomized trial assessing right-ventricular function and pulmonary perfusion. Lancet 1993; 341:507–511.

20. Levine M, Hirsh J, Weitz J, Cruickshank M, Neemeh J, Turpie AG, Gent M. A randomized trial of a single bolus dosage regimen of recombinant tissue plasminogen activator in patients with acute pulmonary embolism. Chest 1990; 98:1473–1479.

21. Goldhaber SZ, Heit J, Sharma GVRK, Nagel JS, Kim D, Parker JA, Drum D, Reagan K, Anderson J, Kessler CM, Markis J, Dawley D, Meyerovitz M, Vaughan DE, Tumeh SS, Loscalzo J, Selwyn AP, Braunwald E. Randomized controlled trial of recombinant tissue plasminogen activator versus urokinase in the treatment of acute pulmonary embolism. Lancet 1988; 2:293–298.

22. Goldlhaber SZ, Kessler CM, Heit JA, Elliott CG, Friedenberg WR, Heiselman DE, Wilson DB, Parker JA, Bennett D, Feldstein ML, Selwyn AP, Kim D, Sharma GVRK, Nagel JS, Meyerovitz MF. Recombinant tissue-type plasminogen activator versus a novel dosing regimen of urokinase in acute pulmonary

embolism: a randomized controlled multicenter trial. J Am Coll Cardiol 1992; 20:24–30.

23. Meyer G, Sors H, Charbonnier B, Kasper W, Bassand J-P, Kerr IH, Lesaffre E, Vanhove P, Verstraete M. Effects of intravenous urokinase versus alteplase on total pulmonary resistance in acute massive pulmonary embolism: a European multicenter double-blind trial. J Am Coll Cardiol 1992; 19:239–245.

24. Meneveau N, Schiele F, Vuillemenot A, Valette B, Grollier G, Bernard Y, Bassand J-P. Streptokinase vs alteplase in massive pulmonary embolism. A randomized trial assessing right heart haemodynamics and pulmonary vascular obstruction. Eur Heart J 1997; 18:1141–1148.

25. Meneveau N, Schiele F, Metz D, Valette B, Attali P, Vuillemenot A, Grollier G, Elaerts J, Mossard J-M, Viel J-F, Bassand J-P. Comparative efficacy of a two-hour regimen of streptokinase versus alteplase in acute massive pulmonary embolism: immediate clinical and hemodynamic outcome and one-year follow-up. J Am Coll Cardiol 1998; 31:1057–1063.

26. Sharma GVRK, Burleson VA, Sasahara AA. Effect of thrombolytic therapy on pulmonary-capillary blood volume in patients with pulmonary embolism. N Engl J Med 1980; 303:842–845.

27. Sharma GVRK, Folland ED, McIntyre KM, Sasahara AA. Long-term benefit of thrombolytic therapy in patients with pulmonary embolism. Vasc Med 2000; 5:91–95.

28. Marini C, Di Ricco G, Rossi G, Rindi M, Palla R, Giuntini C. Fibrinolytic effects of urokinase and heparin in acute pulmonary embolism: a randomized clinical trial. Respiration 1988; 54:162–173.

29. Konstantinides S, Geibel A, Heusel G, Heinrich F, Kasper W. for the Management Strategies and Prognosis of Pulmonary Embolism-3 Trial Investigators. Heparin plus alteplase compared with heparin alone in patients with submassive pulmonary embolism. N Engl J Med 2002; 347:1143–1150.

30. Jerjes-Sanchez C, Ramirez-Rivera A, Garcia M de L, Arriaga-Nava R, Valencia S, Rosado-Buzzo A, Pierzo JA, Rosas E. Streptokinase and heparin versus heparin alone in massive pulmonary embolism: a randomized controlled trial. J Thromb Thrombolysis 1995; 2:227–229.

31. Hamel E, Pacouret G, Vincentelli D, Forissier JF, Peycher P, Pottier JM, Charbonnier B. Thrombolysis or heparin therapy in massive pulmonary embolism with right ventricular dilation. Results from a 128-patient mono-center registry. Chest 2001; 120:120–125.

32. Stein PD, Hull RD, Raskob G. Risks for major bleeding from thrombolytic therapy in patients with acute pulmonary embolism. Consideration of noninvasive management. Ann Intern Med 1994; 121:313–317.

33. Konstantinides S, Geibel A, Olschewski M, Heinrich F, Grosser K, Rauber K, Iversen S, Redecker M, Kienast J, Just H, Kasper W. Association between thrombolytic treatment and the prognosis of hemodynamically stable patients with major pulmonary embolism. Results of a multicenter registry. Circulation 1997; 96:882–888.

34. Goldhaber SZ, Visani L, De Rosa M for ICOPER. Acute pulmonary embolism:

clinical outcomes in the International Cooperative Pulmonary Embolism Registry (ICOPER). Lancet 1999; 353:1386–1389.

35. Mikkola KM, Patel SR, Parker JA, Grodstein F, Goldhaber SZ. Increasing age is a major risk factor for hemorrhagic complications after pulmonary embolism thrombolysis. Am Heart J 1997; 134:69–72.

36. Sors H, Pacouret G, Azarian R, Meyer G, Charbonnier B, Simmonneau G. Hemodynamic effects of bolus vs 2-h infusion of alteplase in acute massive pulmonary embolism. A randomized controlled multicenter trial. Chest 1994; 106:712–717.

37. Goldhaber SZ, Agnelli G, Levine MN. Reduced dose bolus alteplase vs conventional alteplase infusion for pulmonary embolism thrombolysis. An international multicenter randomized trial. Chest 1994; 106:718–724.

38. Levine MN. Thrombolytic therapy for venous thromboembolism: complications and contraindications. Clin Chest Med 1995; 16:321–328.

39. UKEP Study Research Group. The UKEP study: multicentre clinical trial on two local regimens of urokinase in massive pulmonary embolism. Eur Heart J 1987; 8:2–10.

40. Dalen JE, Alpert JS, Hirsh J. Thrombolytic therapy for pulmonary embolism: Is it effective? Is it safe? When is it indicated? Arch Intern Med 1997; 157: 2550–2556.

41. Kanter DS, Mikkola KM, Patel SR, Parker JA, Goldhaber SZ. Thrombolytic therapy for pulmonary embolism. Frequency of intracranial hemorrhage and associated risk factors. Chest 1997; 111:1241–1245.

42. ACCP Consensus Committee on Pulmonary Embolism. Opinions regarding the diagnosis and management of venous thromboembolic disease. Chest 1996; 109:233–237.

43. Hyers TM, Agnelli G, Hull RD, Morris TA, Samama M, Tapson V, Weg JG. Antithrombotic therapy for venous thromboembolic disease. Chest 2001; 119 (suppl):176S–193S.

44. Goldhaber SZ. Thrombolysis in pulmonary embolism. A large-scale clinical trial is overdue. Circulation 2001; 104:2876–2878.

45. Bailen MR, Cuadra JAR, de Hoyos EA. Thrombolysis during cardiopulmonary resuscitation in fulminant pulmonary embolism: a review. Crit Care Med 2001; 29:2211–2219.

13

Vena Cava Interruption

BRUCE E. JARRELL and WILLIAM R. FLINN

University of Maryland
Baltimore, Maryland, U.S.A.

I. Introduction

Venous thromboembolism remains a challenging problem for practitioners in virtually all specialties who care for adult, hospitalized patients. The risk factors for development of deep venous thrombosis (DVT) are well known, and patients at high risk for DVT and pulmonary embolism (PE) have been well defined. There are validated pharmacological and physiomechanical techniques of prophylaxis to reduce the incidence of DVT and PE in high-risk patient groups (see Chap. 2 for risk factors). Nevertheless, it has been estimated that over 500,000 pulmonary emboli occur annually in the United States each year, and more than 100,000 deaths result from PE (1) (see Chap. 4 for prevention of venous thromboembolism). Despite our sophisticated appreciation of the problem of venous thromboembolism, PE remains a major cause of death among hospitalized patients, and many physicians consider PE to be the single most preventable cause of death among adult patients. This is of particular concern among patients who would otherwise be expected to survive following their illness, surgery, or injury.

Therapeutic interventions for venous thromboembolism include both prevention and treatment. When DVT prophylaxis effectively prevents

DVT, it translates directly into a lower risk of PE. When established DVT is accurately diagnosed and treated, there is a proven reduction in the rate of PE. A reduced rate of PE clearly saves lives, since about 10% of PEs will be fatal. In addition, if PE is recognized and treated, there is a reduction in mortality from 30% in untreated PE to less than 5% with treated PE. Therefore, in any discussion of venous thromboembolism, the primary endpoint ultimately is the prevention of fatal PE. From a purely practical standpoint, the prevention of fatal PE may necessitate one or more of several strategies:

- Prevent the formation of DVT
- Diagnose and effectively treat DVT before it embolizes and causes death
- Prevent the migration of extremity DVT by venous interruption

Obviously, the latter is the topic of this discussion, but to understand the current therapeutic role of venous interruption, we must first understand the clinical situations in which the former strategies fail to be effective.

- *Prevent DVT.* Proximal DVT can be prevented using the pharma-cological and mechanical techniques that have been shown to be effective. However, in some cases, DVT prophylaxis cannot be used, and in others, even the most "effective" prophylaxis does not result in a clinically relevant reduction in the risk of subsequent fatal PE. For example, consensus studies (2) have defined "very high risk" patient groups as those having a > 8% incidence of proximal DVT that is associated with a 1–5% incidence of fatal PE. The study of Geerts et al. (3) observed that proximal DVT occurred in 18% of multitrauma patients when no DVT prophylaxis was used. Given the consensus figures noted above, these patients would clearly have a very high risk for fatal PE. The use of "effective" DVT prophylaxis in such a patient group might reduce the incidence of proximal DVT by 50%, a "statistically significant" reduction in DVT. However, even with effective DVT prophylaxis, this patient group would theoretically be left with a 9% incidence of proximal DVT which would still be very high risk for fatal PE! Despite an aggressive use of all effective methods of DVT prophylaxis, fatal PE remains a critical problem in multitrauma patients. This becomes particularly dis-turbing since many of these (typically younger) trauma patients would have a normal life expectancy if they recover from their traumatic injuries. It is logical and necessary in these cases to seek alternative strategies for prevention of fatal pulmonary embolism.
- *Detect and treat proximal DVT before embolization.* When DVT or PE has been accurately diagnosed, treatment with anticoagulant

therapy has been shown to reduce the risk of subsequent fatal pulmonary embolism (5,6). However, some patients at high risk for venous thromboembolism, such as postoperative patients or those suffering major trauma, may be inappropriate candidates for anticoagulation. In other patients, standard anticoagulation may have caused hemorrhagic or other complications; or failed to control the thromboembolic phenomena. Additionally, studies using serial ultrasound scans have observed propagation of thrombus in 30% of cases (7) even with the use of heparin therapy. In the only randomized prospective comparison of inferior vena cava (IVC) filters to anticoagulant therapy (8), the overall mortality was the same for the two groups (filter vs anticoagulation alone), but no patients receiving IVC filters died of PE, whereas 80% of the early deaths in the medically treated patients were due to PE. Thus, accurate diagnosis and treatment with medical therapy alone did not prevent fatal PE in that study. Venous interruption did not prevent all patient deaths, but it appeared to eliminate fatal PE. In other studies, venous duplex ultrasound scanning has been used for interval DVT surveillance in high-risk patient groups. In a large prospective study of DVT surveillance in a high-risk neurosurgical population (4), this strategy· was effective in nearly eliminating fatal PE. Despite the use of DVT prophylaxis, proximal DVT was diagnosed by surveillance duplex scan in 5% of cases (still in the high-risk level for fatal PE), and 80% of proximal DVT were asymptomatic at the time of diagnosis. Waiting for high-risk patients to become symptomatic before testing will result in an unacceptable number of undiagnosed in situ proximal DVTs, and clearly explains the well-recognized clinical scenario of sudden death due to PE in patients who seem to be recovering uneventfully. Earlier diagnosis of these proximal DVTs by surveillance duplex scan allowed placement of IVC filters, and fatal PE occurred in only 0.07% of more than 2500 patients studied. Ultrasound scan surveillance combined wih venous interruption in these cases had the clinical effect of shifting a high risk for proximal DVT to a low risk (or essentially no risk) for fatal PE.

II. History of Venous Interruption

Homans (9), in 1934, first popularized femoral venous ligation for the prevention of PE before the routine use of heparin treatment for DVT. Since the iliac veins above the site of venous interruption remained at risk for thrombus formation, it is not surprising that a 5–8% rate of fatal recurrent PE was observed following these procedures (8) and led ultimately to their abandonment. Interruption of the IVC by ligation, popular in the mid 1960s, addressed the problem of embolization from the iliac veins, but IVC ligation was associated with an operative mortality rate of up to 14% (10).This resulted from the combination of the necessary laparotomy, the sudden decrease in cardiac preload, and the already unstable cardiopulmonary status of patients who had already suffered PEs. Additionally, among the survivors, IVC occlusion led to chronic lower limb venous dysfunction in up to one-third of patients (11). Later, IVC suture plication and partitioning techniques or the placement of external, partially occluding clips (e.g., Moretz, Miles, Adams-DeWeese clips (12–14) were used in attempts to prevent PE but maintain caval patency. These techniques generally proved to be as effective as IVC ligation for the prevention of PE, but ultimately resulted in a 40–50% rate of IVC occlusion. Additionally, they all still required a major open surgical procedure to be performed in patients who were often critically ill.

This evolving surgical experience with IVC interruption began to clarify the desirable features of an "ideal" technique:

- *Prevent pulmonary embolism.* Partially occluding devices will not prevent the migration of small thrombi that may occur through the interstices; that is, not all PE will be prevented. However, fatal PEs are much more likely to arise from larger thrombi, particularly in the iliac veins, so the "burden of thrombus" clearly impacts upon the clinical outcome. Ultimately it is the prevention of *fatal* PE that is the measure of success for these techniques.
- *Maintain IVC patency.* Patients who had IVC ligation or who developed IVC thrombosis following partial interruption had a much higher rate of late venous dysfunction with the classic sequelae of leg edema, hyperpigmentation, and ulceration. Acute IVC occlusion has led to phlegmasia cerulea dolens in some patients and even to venous gangrene. However, caval occlusion following IVC interruption in some cases may represent the successful trapping of a massive embolus that was a lifesaving event.
- *Evolution to a less invasive procedure.* The need for a major intracavitary surgical procedure to perform caval interruption obviously contributed to increased morbidity and mortality for these patients.

A. Types of Intracaval Devices

Mobin-Uddin Umbrella

Transvenous placement of an intracaval device for IVC interruption was first popularized in the late 1960s with the introduction of the Mobin-Uddin umbrella (15). Placement of the device still required a surgical procedure, but it was simple exposure of the jugular vein in the neck rather than a laparotomy. The morbidity of insertion was significantly reduced, but the Mobin-Uddin umbrella was still associated with a high rate of IVC occlusion, and detachment with migration and massive thromboembolism was observed in some cases.

Greenfield Vena Cava Filter

The Greenfield vena cava filter was introduced in 1973 and over the past quarter century has become the clinical benchmark for comparison among transvenous intracaval IVC interruption devices. The Greenfield filter introduced the unique conical design that allowed thrombus to be trapped and fill 70–80% of the filter's depth without reducing flow through the IVC. This design resulted in a significant improvement in IVC patency rates compared to all previous techniques. A prospective study using ultrasound scanning observed an 86.7% IVC patency rate for patients receiving Greenfield filters (16). In late follow-up among survivors, a 98% IVC patency rate has been observed for the Greenfield filter (17). Recurrent PE has been observed in only 4–5% of cases, and fatal pulmonary embolism following successful placement of the Greenfield filter is rare.

Initially, placement of a Greenfield filter still required direct surgical exposure of the internal jugular vein (or with subsequent designs, the femoral vein) since the original stainless steel filter used a 24F diameter (8 mm) insertion device. The expanding experience with catheter-based interventions in the mid 1980s, coupled with miniaturization of catheter components, led ultimately to a smaller, percutaneous insertion system that could be used routinely and eliminated the need for any surgical exposure in these cases.

Other Devices

Understandably, the boom in endovascular interventions has led to the development of a wide array of devices similar (and in some cases, dissimilar) to the original Greenfield filter. These have included the Venatech filter (18), the Nitinol filter (19), and the TrapEase filter (20) with structural configurations similar to the Greenfield filter. Another device, the bird's nest filter, is unique in its design. The bird's nest filter is constructed of four stainless steel wires shaped with nonmatching bends that fill the IVC in a random cluster. The bird's nest filter was felt to be ideal for venae cavae with large diameters (so called "mega-cava") where the fixed diameter of the strut configuration in conical filters (28 mm for the Greenfield filter) might prevent hook fixation to the wall of the IVC with possible cephalad

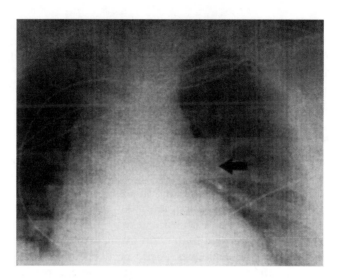

Figure 1   A Greenfield filter is shown in the left pulmonary artery.

migration of the filter into the right heart or pulmonary artery (Fig. 1). All these devices have been shown to offer successful prevention of fatal PE.

There have been reports that suggested a higher incidence of angulation, migration, and IVC thrombosis in devices other than the Greenfield filter. However, the only prospective comparison showed no higher incidence of IVC thrombosis (16) for nitinol and bird's nest filters compared to Greenfield filters. It should also be noted that the original stainless steel Greenfield filter has undergone several significant structural design and material changes over the years. A titanium Greenfield filter with a smaller carrier was initially developed to allow percutaneous insertion. Clinical experience with that device led to concerns about filter angulation and asymmetry of the struts following placement. This has now been largely replaced by a lower profile stainless steel filter that is closer to the original design.

Overall, no device clinically available has been observed to be superior to the Greenfield filter; however, there has never been a randomized prospective comparison of the different devices and their complications.

III.   Indications for IVC Filter Insertion

The past decade has seen a dramatic expansion of less invasive, catheter-based "endovascular" technologies in all realms of vascular diagnosis and treatments. This has been coupled with increasingly sophisticated, more portable, and noninvasive imaging modalities. Combined with the conversion of virtually all IVC filters to percutaneous insertion systems, this has led clinically to a liberalization in the indications for IVC filter insertion. As noted previously, the traditional indications for filter insertion included:

- *A contraindication to anticoagulant therapy.* This most often is a history of, an ongoing, or an unacceptable risk of developing a bleeding diathesis. This may also include a known previous adverse reaction to heparin such as heparin-induced thrombotic thrombocytopenia (HIT).
- *A complication of heparin therapy.* This is most often a hemorrhagic complication, but might also be HIT syndrome. However, today patients with HIT may be treated with alternative antithrombins such as lepirudin or argatroban.
- *A failure of standard anticoagulant therapy.* Recurrent or worsening venous thromboembolism while receiving therapeutic levels of standard anticoagulant therapy obviously dictate the use of an alternative strategy to prevent fatal embolism.

These "standard" indications are expanded in clinical practice today to often include:

- *"Free-floating" or major clots in the iliac veins or vena cava.* Fatal PE is more likely to arise from major proximal thrombi (21). Coupled with the observation that anticoagulant therapy alone may not halt the propagation of thrombus (7), an argument for the placement of an IVC filter becomes clinically reasonable in patients with free-floating thrombus in the iliac veins or vena cava, particularly in patients expected to make a full recovery from associated illness or injury. The single randomized prospective comparison of IVC filters to anticoagulant therapy (8) had similar numbers of cases of iliac and IVC thrombi in the two treatment groups. However, the outcomes from specific anatomical groups were not individually reported. Overall in that study though, death due to PE occurred only in patients treated without IVC filters.
- *Critically ill and/or multitrauma patients.* Owing to the extent or location of their injuries, many trauma patients cannot receive anticoagulants as therapy or prophylaxis. Patient with extremity injuries may not be candidates for mechanical devices for DVT prophylaxis. As noted previously, even with the ongoing use of aggressive, effective DVT prophylaxis, multitrauma patients often remain in the high risk, or very high risk groups for fatal PE. Fatal PE remains a compelling problem in trauma patients, since many of these (typically

younger) patients would have a normal life expectancy if they recovered from their injuries. This has led some trauma specialists to advocate the prophylactic placement of IVC filters in selected cases at high risk for PE (22–25) even in the absence of documented DVT or PE. Although the rationale for the placement of prophylactic IVC filters would appear to be clinically reasonable, there has not been uniform agreement concerning this issue among trauma specialists. In addition to questions about the therapeutic efficacy in these cases (26), there has been significant concern about the costs of this strategy (approximately $5000 per filter) (27). Additionally, there remain concerns about the long-term fate of these devices, particularly in younger patients, since other late complications of IVC filters have been reported. A scientifically valid randomized prospective study of these questions is hampered by both the heterogeneity of trauma patients and the well-documented difficulties with late follow-up in the trauma patient population.

- *Patients "in extremis" from pulmonary embolus.* Patients who have a massive PE resulting in sustained hypotension, right heart failure, and hypoxemia are candidates for IVC filters based upon the concept that they would not tolerate an additional embolic insult. This concept could also be applied to patients requiring pulmonary embolectomy for massive PE. Typically, these are emboli that impact the bifurcation of the pulmonary artery (saddle embolus) or cause near total obstruction of both pulmonary arteries. There are no large experience with this type of patient, because most patients with PE either die very quickly or recover very quickly. It is the unusual patient who gets to this point of severity for a long enough time to undergo a procedure. Thus, it will be difficult to validate this strategy, but it seems to be a logical approach.

B. Insertion Techniques

The placement of IVC filters in selected patients has also been facilitated by simplification of the overall insertion process. Traditionally, patients requiring IVC filters have required transport to the operating room or an interventional suite for filter placement under fluoroscopic guidance. Multitrauma patients may have neurospinal injuries requiring immobilization or complex pelvic or long bone fractures, and many (during their high-risk period) require inotropic or ventilatory support. Transportation of these patients out of critical care areas to the operating room or the interventional suite often requires additional medical, nursing, and paramedical staff. Transport in these cases is always cumbersome and can be hazardous. In many of these patients, filter insertion can be accomplished at the bedside using duplex ultrasound scan guidance (28) or intravascular ultrasound (IVUS) (29). These techniques for insertion also avoid contrast and radiation exposure, and may significantly reduce both the cost and complexity of this procedure. Bedside insertion requires familiarity with ultrasonic techniques and equipment, but may be highly beneficial in selected cases.

C. Complications

The clinical enthusiasm for IVC filter placement is tempered by concerns about the past and potential future complications of these devices.

Misplacement/Migration

Since most PE originate from DVT in the lower extremities, ideal placement of an IVC filter is in the IVC just below the level of the renal veins. As noted previously, earlier techniques for IVC interruption had a high rate of caval thrombosis. It was felt that if the device was too low in the IVC, thrombus could form above it in the cul-de-sac of static flow below the renal veins (but above the device) and serve as a source of recurrent PE. If the device was placed too high and caval thrombosis occurred, renal vein thrombosis might lead to renal dysfunction. With today's cone-shaped filters, the device should ideally be symmetrically aligned with the long axis of the IVC and fully expanded to be maximally effective. Misplacement of IVC filters has been reported in almost every imaginable axial portion of the venous system that is accessible with the insertion devices (17,30–32). Misplacement occurs most often into the iliac veins, the right renal vein, or the gonadal veins. Since the thrombosis rates of modern filters is significantly lower, these misplacements generally do not require any specific treatment. However, it is usually necessary to place a second filter in the IVC to confer adequate protection from PE. Vena cava filters have been misplaced into the suprarenal IVC, but since thrombosis is rare, these require no further treatment. Suprarenal filter placement has been documented to be acceptably safe and has been used successfully for the management of complex cases of embolization from thrombus above a previously placed infrarenal filter (33). Filters have been misplaced in the hepatic veins, the superior vena cava and the heart (31,34–36). These latter cases are, of course, more serious and have often required surgical removal. Misplacement into the retroperitoneum outside the vena cava has even been observed (37) (Fig. 2). Misplacement of filters may occur because of inadequate or inaccurate imaging of venous anatomy, or due to premature release of the device from its delivery

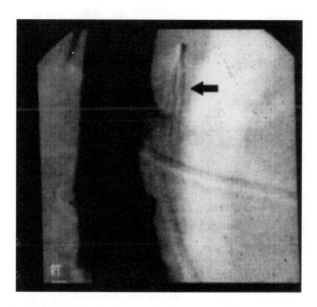

Figure 2   A Greenfield filter is shown outside the IVC.

system. Misplacement may also occur secondarily if the device fails to expand properly upon release or fails satisfactorily to engage the wall of the IVC for fixation. In these cases, the device may migrate cephalad in an unpredictable fashion and the filter itself may embolize into the right heart or pulmonary artery. Even if fixation on the caval wall occurs, if the device does not expand properly, adequate protection from PE is not provided, and placement of a second filter is performed. In some cases, conical filters placed at an appropriate level may be tilted or skewed, or the struts asymmetrically aligned. Since the clot trapping function of these filters is directly related to their design configuration, this too represents an undesirable placement. Temporary, removable filters (38–40) have been developed recently, but migration has been a concern with all these devices, since they are designed not to achieve fixation to the wall of the vena cava. No removable IVC filter is currently approved for use in the United. Late migration of permanent filters that were apropriately placed may also occur (41). Movement, both cephalad and caudad, of up to 1 cm. may be observed in up to one-third of cases studied rigorously, but these rarely require intervention. However, some cases of more extensive late migration have required more complex treatments (42). Overall, the true incidence of misplacement and migration of IVC filters is not known, since most cases are not reported or recorded.

Thrombotic Complications

Thrombotic complications are generally categorized as those that occur related to the insertion of the IVC filter, and those that are observed during later follow-up of these patients, although the complications and the ultimate consequences may be quite similar. Early thrombotic complications include thrombosis at the catheter insertion site used for placement and IVC thrombosis.

- *Insertion site thrombosis.* Insertion site thrombosis IST is the most common complication of IVC filter insertion in the modern era, and has been reported in 4–41% of cases (16,41,43). It was observed in 24.7% of cases in a prospective study using ultrasound scanning. IST occurred with equivalent frequency in both the jugular and femoral veins (16), so the site of insertion appeared not to have an effect on this complication, which seems to be a direct mechanical result of the insertion procedure. The clinical impact of thrombosis at the insertion site remains poorly defined, and the majority of patients were asymptomatic at the time of diagnosis. However, thrombosis of the common femoral vein may produce venous valvular dysfunction or venous obstruction that may contribute to the later development of chronic venous dysfunction. This would be of particular clinical importance in patients having prophylactic IVC filters, since these patients do not have DVT prior to filter placement. In the prospective study of Aswad et al. (16), IST was observed in 14% of patients having prophylactic filter placement.
- *Vena cava thrombosis.* IVC thrombosis may also occur following placement of an IVC filter. As noted previously, the precise etiology of this complication is open to varied interpretation. The placement of a partially occlusive foreign body in the vena cava of a patient with known risks for thrombotic events may induce spontaneous IVC thrombosis. Alternatively, trapping of massive thrombus migrating from the lower extremities is the precise function of these devices, but when this occurs, IVC thrombosis may follow. Regardless of its precise etiology, however, when IVC thrombosis occurs in these patients, the overall prognosis is compromised compared to those with a patent vena cava. Acute IVC thrombosis may predispose to the development of phlegmasia cerulea dolens with the risk of venous gangrene (44). In most cases of IVC thrombosis though, there is simply a significantly increased risk of the development of chronic venous dysfunction with chronic edema. hyperpigmentation, or eventual ulceration that has been observed in 6–45% of cases in late follow-up (41). Overall, controlling the risks

of the development of IVC thrombosis has been confounded by at least two major clinical variables. First, in more than half the cases where IVC filter placement is required, there is a contraindication to, or has been a complication of, anticoagulant therapy, whereas in the other cases, heparin and/or warfarin can be used after filter placement. In the prospective study of Aswad et al. (16), IVC thrombosis was diagnosed by ultrasound scan in 12% of cases, but this study, like most reports, was not controlled for the use of postprocedural anticoagulant therapy. In the prospective randomized study of Decousus et al. (8), all patients having IVC filters received either heparin or low molecular weight heparin, and no patients were reported to have acute IVC thrombosis. However, 37 patients who received IVC filters suffered late recurrent PE, and IVC thrombosis was observed in 9% (16 cases), most of whom had completed their course of anticoagulant therapy. It would be reasonable to presume that patients who are treated with anticoagulant therapy after filter placement will have a lower rate of IVC thrombosis, but no truly reliable data exist.

The other confounding variable is the compromise of late follow-up in most series. The relatively high mortality rate for groups of patients receiving IVC filters is understandable considering the overall complexity of the clinical situations that lead to filter placement. As noted above, Aswad et al. (16) detected IVC thrombosis in 12% of cases, but 19.5% of patients in that series died before leaving the hospital, and the late impact of these thrombotic complications was not known. Greenfield (41), in a report of a 20-year clinical experience, observed IVC thrombosis in only 4% of patients in late follow-up. However, 15% of patients having Greenfield filters died before discharge, another 14% of patients died within the next 12 months, and of those surviving, information was available in only 54% of cases. Early mortality after filter placement was only 2.5% in the study of Decousus et al. (8), but patients with a "short life expectancy" were excluded from that study. Nevertheless, 22% of patients with IVC filters died within the 2-year period of follow-up. As noted above, IVC thrombosis was observed 9% of late survivors in that prospective series, but only 37 symptomatic patients were evaluated, so the true incidence of IVC thrombosis in this study was unknown. Past reports have suggested that devices such as the nitinol filter, the Venatech filter, and the bird's nest filter have a higher incidence of IVC thrombosis than the Greenfield filter (45–47). However, the prospective study of Aswad et al. (16) observed no significant difference in the rate of IVC thrombosis for the different filters (nitinol, bird's nest, Greenfield) used. Encouragingly though, in that study, no patient having a prophylactic IVC filter experienced IVC thrombosis.

Overall, there is no consistent, reliable, and/or comparative data for different devices regarding the true incidence of IVC thrombosis following placement of an IVC filter or the subsequent late clinical consequences of this complication.

• *Recurrent PE.* The primary therapeutic goal of an IVC filter is to prevent (fatal) PE. The single prospective randomized comparison of IVC filter to conventional anticoagulant therapy (8) confirmed that patients receiving IVC filters had a significantly lower risk of early PE (1.1 vs 4.8% for anticoagulant therapy alone, $P = .03$). Filter placement in that study also eliminated fatal PE within the first 12 days, which caused 80% of early deaths in the patients treated with anticoagulant therapy alone. After the placement of a permanent. Indwelling IVC filter, this protection from (fatal) PE would ideally continue thereafter for patients. However, after 2 years, Decousus et al. (8) reported late PE in 3.4% of patients having an IVC filter, which was not significantly lower than the 6.3% incidence of late PE in patients treated with anticoaglant therapy. Additionally, one fatal PE occurred late in each treatment group (filter vs anticoagulant). Greenfield (41) reported late PE in 9% of patients with an IVC filter who had survived more than 1 year after placement. The late PEs occurring in that study were fatal in three cases (1.2%), but follow-up information was available in only 54% of cases overall. Late or recurrent PE after filter placement may occur as a result of propagation of thrombus above the filter (48,49), which appears to be more likely when IVC thrombosis has occurred or when there is malposition or angulation of the device (50). Prevention of further PEs in these cases has been successfully managed by the placement of a second, suprarenal filter (33). Late PE in some cases may also originate from the upper extremities or the right heart; events that would be unrelated to the function of the IVC filter. However, it is clear that the placement of an IVC filter does not confer indefinite protection from (fatal) PE. Similar to acute IVC thrombosis, the compromised survival and incomplete late follow-up prevent us from knowing the true incidence of this complication. Late lower extremity deep venous thrombosis ocurred significantly more frequently in patients with an IVC filter (20.8%) compared to those initially receiving anticoagulant therapy (11.6%, $P = .02$) in the prospective randomized comparison reported by Decousus et al. (8). However, these events were not controlled for the status of the anticoagulant therapy at the time of the new thrombotic event. These investigators concluded that the initial beneficial effect of the IVC filter for the prevention of PE was counterbalanced by this higher risk of late deep venous thrombosis.

Other late complications of IVC filters are rare, but would be of particular concern in cases where prophylactic filters are placed in the absence of established venous thromboembolism, as has been the case in many multitrauma patients who face a lifetime of risk with these indwelling devices if they recover from their critical injuries. Late complications have included structural failure of the devices (51–53), late hemorrhage (54), ureteral injury (55), and bowel obstruction (56,57). The true incidence of these complications is unknown, but considering that approximately 30,000–40,000 IVC filters are placed each year in the United States (58), the rarity of reports such as these suggest that it is likely that these complications will remain isolated instances and effect few patients.

D. New Developments—Temporary Filters

The discussions above concerning early and late thrombotic and non-thrombotic complications of permanent intracaval devices suggest the clinical utility of temporary IVC interruption devices. Such filters can be placed during period of highest risk and then removed when that period has passed or when alternative therapies can be safely employed. This strategy would obviously eliminate concerns about the long-term fate of permanent filters in younger patients. The availability of a temporary IVC filter might also further liberalize the indications for usage, so short-term efficacy and safety is of critical importance.

Nonpermanent IVC filters in use today can be classified as temporary and retrievable. Temporary filters are not currently approved for use in the United States, but those that have been used elsewhere have included the Gunther filter (38,39,59), the Antheor filter (39,59), and the Prolyser filter (59). Temporary filters are designed to be removed after a fixed period of time; usually less than 14 days. Endothelialization of the filter may occur during longer periods of implantation and cause damage to the wall of the vena cava during explantation (60). It is known that in many cases where a temporary filter would be most desirable (e.g., younger trauma patients), the period of high risk often extends well beyond a 2-week period, although some patients may be able to be safely converted to standard anticoagulant therapy by that time. At present, temporary filters have been used most often in cases of iliocaval thrombosis being treated with catheter-directed thromblytic therapy. In those cases, thrombus may be destabilized by ongoing clot lysis and pose a serious risk of PE, which would be prevented by the filter, but the treatment period is usually only several days. Temporary filters must also remain affixed to an external guide wire or catheter during implantation which, like any central venous catheter, has a risk of infection with longer periods of implantation. As noted previously, since these devices intentionally avoid fixation to the caval wall, filter migration has been a problem with temporary devices. Lorch et al. (39) reported a multi-institutional experience with temporary IVC filters in 188 patients and observed filter dislocation in 4.8% of cases, filter thrombosis is 16%, and fatal PE in 2.1% of patients. No prospective trials of theses devices have been reported.

Retrieveable filters may be removed after a short period, but have the option of remaining permanently in place if clinically indicated. The Amplatz retrievable filter was the first described device (61), but it has been withdrawn because of its high rate of IVC thrombosis and the complexity of removal. Millward et al. (62) have reported experience in nine cases with retrieval of a Gunther tulip filter after a mean insertion period of 8.6 days with no caval wall damage or IVC thrombosis. Abbott (20) described successful retrieval of this same device after a mean implantation period of over 22 days. This preliminary experience appears encouraging, and the concept of a retrievable filter would have useful clinical applications. However, a much broader experience will be necessary to clarify the role of these and other retrievable IVC filters that may be developed.

IV. Conclusions

The past decade has seen a near elimination of the need for surgical venous interruption in the management of venous thromboembolism. The explosion of endovascular technologies has made transvenous placement of IVC filters routine, being performed even at the bedside in some cases. These technological advancements have made filter insertion simpler and safer, but with this has come a liberalization in the clinical indications for filter placement. Published data on this topic would suggest that some of this practice has not been suitably validated, but it is clinically very real and clearly suggest the need for additional study. These same technological advancements have also resulted in the introduction of an increasing variety of IVC filter devices. Even the clinical "standard," the Greenfield filter, has undergone at least two major modifications. Overall there is little reliable information regarding the comparative performance or safety of these devices. The information reviewed in this chapter would suggest the following conclusions:

1. In patients with established proximal lower limb DVT or PE originating from the lower extremities, IVC filter placement offers

superior protection from subsequent early PE compared to medical therapy alone. There is considerably more clinical experience with the Greenfield IVC filter, but there is no evidence that this device is superior to other approved devices for the prevention of PE.

2. Traditionally effective strategies for prevention of fatal PE may be inadequate in very high-risk patients groups like multitrauma patients. Prophylactic placement of an IVC filter may reduce the risk of fatal PE in selected patients. Further prospective study of the potentially beneficial effect (and its overall risks and costs) is indicated.

3. Vena cava filters must be appropriately positioned and anchored in the IVC to provide the full measure of protection from pulmonary embolism. Percutaneous transvenous insertion is possible in virtually all cases. Filters may be placed appropriately using fluoroscopic or ultrasonic guidance.

4. Vena cava thrombosis occurs following IVC filter insertion in between 2 and 12% of cases. Vena cava thrombosis after filter insertion will result in a higher incidence of chronic venous dysfunction among surviving patients. There is considerably more clinical experience with the Greenfield filter, and no other device has demonstrated a reduced rate of IVC thrombosis compared to the Greenfield filter. However, there is no reliable evidence that the Greenfield filter is truly superior to other devices in this regard. Overall, the true early and late incidence of IVC thrombosis is not known. Patients treated with anticoagulant therapy after IVC filter placement may have a lower risk of acute IVC thrombosis. The risk of IVC thrombosis in patients having prophylactic filters appears to be lower than that in patients with established venous thromboembolism, but no reliable data are available. Further study of this question is warranted considering the increasing number of devices and insertions and the late morbidity of IVC thrombosis.

5. Late PE occurs in 3–6% of patients after IVC filter and late fatal PE occurs in 1–2% of cases. Late PE has not been proven to be less likely in patients with IVC filter than in those who had been initially treated with anticoagulant therapy alone. The effect of the duration of anticoagulant therapy on late PE has not been demonstrated. The accuracy of data regarding late PE in patients receiving IVC filters is compromised by their relatively high mortality rates (primarily due to underlying comorbidities) and the small percentage of patients having reliable follow-up. Further prospective study of late thromboembolic complications in patients with IVC filters is warranted.

6. Late DVT occurs in 10–20% of cases with IVC filters. Late DVT is significantly more likely in patients having IVC filters than those treated initially with anticoagulant therapy. The relationship of these events to ongoing anticoagulant therapy in these cases remains unclear. The late morbidity from these events is uncertain. Further study is warranted to determine more precisely the etiological relationship of IVC filters combined with the duration of anticoagulant therapy to all recurrent thromboembolic events.

7. The role of anticoagulation following insertion of IVC filter is undefined but is a significant question relative to Conclusions 2, 4, 5, and 6 stated above.

8. Late serious, nonthrombotic complications of IVC filters are rare. The true incidence of these complications is unknown, but more accurate information would be of particular interest in a clinical assessment of the risks and benefits of prophylactic filter placement in very high-risk patient groups.

9. Temporary, or retrievable, IVC filters may be useful in patients with proximal iliocaval thrombosis receiving catheter-directed thrombolytic therapy or in other patients with clinically limited period of risk for PE; ideally less than 14 days. Temporary filters have as yet unsolved problems with migration and filter thrombosis. Retrievable filters may be a preferable strategy, since they can be left in permanently if clinically indicated. No reliable comparative data exist concerning these devices.

V. Opportunities for Further Clinical Information

It is obvious from the above analysis that most of our knowledge about IVC interruption is based upon incomplete information and limited results from single-institution trials. Significant information would be gained from a uniform reporting system for all IVC filters inserted, especially if data relating to the long-term performance of the device were included. This is particularly compelling relative to the high interest in patient safety and the paucity of knowledge comparing the long-term problems with these devices. We would propose the following system:

1. The adoption of the Society of Vascular Surgery/American Association for Vascular Surgery Recommended Reporting Standards for vena caval filter insertion and patient follow-up (64).

2. The inclusion of additional data relating to the
   a. Indication for insertion, especially related to prophylactic insertion

   b. Complete data regarding the manufacturer and model of device
   c. Imaging method used to guide the insertion
   d. Long-term imaging results relative to technical complications and related clinical complications
   e. Long-term clinical outcome
3. A recommendation from an expert panel describing the appropriate follow-up in terms of
   a. Type of imaging
   b. Frequency of imaging
   c. Type of clinical follow-up
   d. Qualifications of physicians performing the clinical follow-up; that is, should it be a vascular expert
   e. Indications for the use of anticoagulation following IVC insertion
4. Definite inclusion into the reporting system of new or investigational devices, with particular inclusion of removable devices with their long-term effects and complications.

References

1. Hirsch J, Hoak J. Management of deep vein thrombosis and pulmonary embolism. A statement for healthcare professionals. Circulation 1996; 93:2212–2245.
2. Clagett GP, Anderson FA, Levine MN, Saltzman EW, Wheeler HB. Prevention of venous thromboembolism. Chest 1992; 102:391S–401S.
3. Geerts WH, Code KI, Jay RM, Chen E, Szalai JP. A prospective study of venous thromboembolism after major trauma. N Engl J Med 1994; 331:1601–1606.
4. Flinn WR, Sandager GP, Silva MB, Benjamin ME, Cerullo LJ, Taylor M. Prospective surveillance for perioperative venous thombosis. Experience in 2643 patients. Arch Surg 1996; 131:472–480.
5. Coon WW, Willis PW, Symons MJ. Assesment of anticoagulant treatment of venous thromboembolism. Ann Surg 1969; 170:559–568.
6. Barritt DW, Jordan SC. Anticoagulant drugs in the treatment of pulmonary embolism: a controlled trial. Lancet 1960; 1:1309–1312.
7. Meissner MH, Caps MT, Bergelin RO, Manzo RA, Strandness DE. Propagation, rethrombosis and new thrombus formation after acute deep venous thrombosis. J Vasc Surg 1995; 22:558–567.
8. Decousus H, Leizorovicz A, Parent F, et al. A clinical trial of vena caval filters in the prevention of pulmonary embolism in patients with proximal deep vein thrombosis. N Engl J Med 1998; 338:409–415.
9. Homans J. Thrombosis of the deep veins of the legs causing pulmonary embolism. N Engl J Med 1934; 211:993–997.

10. Bernstein EF. The place of venous interruption in the treatment of pulmonary embolism. In: Moser KM, Stein M, eds. Pulmonary Thromboembolism. St Louis: Mosby-Year Book, 1973:312–323.

11. Piccone VA, Vida E, Yarnoz M, Glass BS, Leveen HH. The late results of caval ligation. Surgery 1970; 68:980–988.

12. Moretz WH, Rhode CM, Shepard MH. Prevention of pulmonary emboli by partial occlusion of the inferior vena cava. Am Surgeon 1959; 25:617–626.

13. Miles RM. Clinical evaluation of the serrated vena caval clip. Surg Gynecol Obstet 1971; 132:581–587.

14. Adams JT, DeWeese JA. Experimental and clinical evaluation of partial vein interruption in the prevention of pulmonary emboli. Surgery 1965; 57:82–102.

15. Mobin-Uddin KM, McClean R, Jude JR. A new catheter technique for interruption of the inferior vena cava for prevention of pulmonary embolism. Am Surg 1969; 35:889–894.

16. Aswad MA, Sandager GP, Pais SO, Malloy PC, Killewich LA, Lilly MP, Flinn WR. Early duplex scan evaluation of four vena caval interruption devices. J Vasc Surg 1996; 24:809–818.

17. Greenfield LJ, Michna BA. Twelve year clinical experience with the Greenfield vena cava filter. Surgery 1988; 104:706–712.

18. Ricco JB, Crochet D, Sebilotte B, et al. Percutaneous transvenous caval interruption with the 'LGM' filter: early resutls of a multicenter trial. Ann Vasc Surg 1988; 3:242–247.

19. Dorfman GS. Percutaneous inferior vena caval filters. Radiology 1990; 174: 987–992.

20. Decousus H, Leizorovicz A, Parent F, et al. A clinical trial of vena caval filters in the prevention of pulmonary embolism in patients with proximal deep-vein thrombosis. N Engl J Med 1998; 338(7):409–416.

21. Berry RE, George JE, Shaver WA. Free-floating deep venous thrombosis: a retrospective analysis. Ann Surg 1990; 211:719–723.

22. Wilson JT, Rogers FB, Wald SL, Shackford SR, Ricci MA. Propylactic vena cava filter insertion in patients with traumatic spinal cord injury: preliminary results. Neurosurgery 1994; 35:234–239.

23. Rodriguez JL, Lopez JM, Proctor MC, et al. Early placement of prophylactic vena caval filters in injured patients at high risk for pulmonary embolism. J Trauma 1996; 40:797–804.

24. Rogers FB, Shackford SR, Ricci MA, Wilson JT. Routine prophylactic vena cava filter insertion in severely injured trauma patients decreases the incidence of pulmonary embolism. J Am Coll Surg 1995; 180:641–647.

25. Carlin AM, Tyburski JG, Wilson RF, Steffes C. Prophylactic and therapeutic inferior vena cava filters to prevent pulmonary emboli in trauma patients. Arch Surg 2002; 137:521–527.

26. McMurtry AL, Owings JT, Anderson JT, Battistella FD, Gosselin R. Increased use of prophylactic vena cava filter in trauma patients failed to decrease overall incidence of pulmonary embolism. J Am Coll Surg 1999; 189:314–320.

27. Maxwell RA, Chavarria-Aguilar M, Cockerham WT, et al. Routine pro-

phylactic vena cava filtration is not indicated after acute spinal injury. J Trauma 2002; 52:902–906.

28. Benjamin ME, Sandager GP, Cohn JE, et al. Duplex ultrasound insertion of inferior vena cava filters in multitrauma patients. Am J Surg 1999; 178:92–97.

29. Ebaugh JL, Chiou AC, Morasch MD, Matsumura JS, Pearce WH. Bedside vena cava filter placement guided with intravascular ultrasound. J Vasc Surg 2001; 34:21–26.

30. Vesely TM. Technical problems and complications associated with inferior vena cava filters. Semin Interv Radiol 1994; 11:121–133.

31. Kaufman JA, Geller SC, Rivitz M, Waltman AC. Operator errors during percutanous placement of vena cava filters. Am J Roentgenol 1995; 165:1281–1287.

32. Carabasi RA, Moritz MJ, Jarrell BE. Complications encountered with the use of the Greenfield filter. Am J Surg 1984; 154:163–168.

33. Stewart JR, Peyton JWR, Crute SL, Greenfield LJ. Clinical results of suprarenal placement of the Greenfield vena cava filter. Surgery 1982; 92:1–4.

34. Gelbish GA, Ascer E. Intracardiac and intrapulmonary Greenfield filters: a long-term follow-up. J Vasc Surg 1991; 14:614–617.

35. Lahey SJ, Meyer LP, Karchmer AW, et al. Misplaced caval filter and subsequent pericardial tamponade. Ann Thorc Surg 1991; 51:299–301.

36. Hirsch SB, Harrington EB, Miller CM, Estioko MR, Haimov M. Accidental placement of the Greenfield filter in the heart: report of two cases. J Vasc Surg 1987; 6:609–610.

37. Adye BA, Raabe RD, Zobell RL. Errant percutaneous Greenfield filter placement into the retroperitoneum. J Vasc Surg 1990; 12:60–61.

38. Millward SF. Temporary and retrievable inferior vena cava filters: current status. J Vasc Interv Radiol 1988; 9:381–387.

39. Lorch H, Welger D, Wagner V, et al. Current practice of temporary vena cava filter insertion: a multicenter registry. J Vasc Interven Radiol 2000; 11:83–88.

40. Watanabe S, Shimokawa S, Moriyama Y, et al. Clinical experience with temporary vena cava filters. Vasc Surg 2001; 34:285–291.

41. Greenfield LJ, Proctor MC. Twenty-year clinical experience with the Greenfield filter. Cardiovasc Surg 1995; 3:199–205.

42. Sidawy AN, Menzoian JO. Distal migration and deformation of the Greenfield vena cava filter. Surgery 1986; 99:369–372.

43. Kantor A, Glanz S, Gordon DH, Sclafini SJ. Percutaneous insertion of the Kimray-Greenfield filter: incidence of femoral vein thrombosis. Am J Roentgenol 1987; 149:1065–1066.

44. Feinman LJ, Meltzer AJ. Phlegmasia cerulea dolens as a complication of percutaneous insertion of a vena caval filter. J Am Osteopath Assoc 1989; 89:63–68.

45. Dorfman GS. Percutaneous inferior vena caval filters. Radiology 1990; 174: 987–992.

46. Murphy TP, Dorfman G, Yedlicka JW, et al. LGM vena cava filter: objective evaluation of early results. J Vasc Interv Radiol 1991; 2:107–115.

47. Mohan CR, Hoballah JJ, Sharp WJ, Kresowik TF, et al. Comparative efficacy and complications of vena caval filters. J Vasc Surg 1995; 21:235–246.

48. Geisinger MA, Zelch MG, Risius B. Recurrent pulmonary embolism after Greenfield filter placement. Radiology 1987; 165:383–384.

49. Richenbacher WE, Atnip RG, Campbell DB, Waldhausen JA. Recurrent pulmonary embolism after inferior vena caval interruption with a Greenfield filter. World J Surg 1989; 13:623–627.

50. McCauley CE, Webster MW, Jarrett F, Hirsch SA, Steed DL. The Greenfield intracaval filter as a source of recurrent pulmonary thromboembolism. Surgery 1984; 96:574–578.

51. Awh MH, Taylor FC, Lu CT. Spontaneous fracture of a Vena-tech inferior vena caval filter. Am J Roentgenol 1991; 157:177–178.

52. Plaus WJ, Hermann G. Structural failure of a Greenfield filter. Surgery 1988; 103:662–664.

53. Taheri SA, Kulaylat MN, Johnson E, Hoover E. A complication of the Greenfield filter: fracture and distal migration of two struts—a case report. J Vasc Surg 1992; 16:96–99.

54. Howerton RM, Watkins M, Feldman L. Late arterial hemorrhage secondary to a Greenfield filter requiring operative intervention. Surgery 1991; 109:265–268.

55. Goldman HB, Hanna K, Dmochowski RR. Ureteral injury secondary to an inferior vena cava filter. J Urol 1996; 156:1763.

56. Kupferschmid JP, Dickson CS, Townsend RN, Diamond DL. Small-bowel obstruction from an extruded Greenfield filter strut: an unusual late complication. J Vasc Surg 1992; 16:113–115.

57. Lok SY, Adkins J, Asch M. Caval perforation by a Greenfield filter resulting in small-bowel volvulus. J Vasc Interv Radiol 1996; 7:95–97.

58. Magnant JG, Walsh DB, Juravsky LI, Cronenwett JL, Barson JA. Current use of inferior vena cava filters in the Medicare population. J Vasc Surg 1992; 16:701–706.

59. Zwaan M, Lorch H, Kulke C, et al. Clinical experience with temporary vena caval filters. J Vasc Interv Radiol 1998; 9:594–601.

60. Burbridge BE, Walker DR, Millward SF. Incorporation of the Gunther temporary inferior vena cava filter into the caval wall. J Vasc Interv Radiol 1996; 7:289–290.

61. Epstein DH, Darcy MD, Hunter DW, et al. Experience with the Amplatz retrievable vena cava filter. Radiology 1989; 172:105–110.

62. Millward SF, Bhargava A, Aquino J, et al. Gunther tulip filter: preliminary clinical experience with retrieval. J Vasc Interv Radiol 2000; 11:75–82.

63. Abbott GT. Prophylactic use of temporary IVC filters for prevention of pulmonary thromboembolization in a district general hospital. J Vasc Interven Radiol 1999; 10(S):288.

64. Bonn J, Cho KJ, Cipolle M, and the participants in the Vena Caval Filter Consensus Conference. Recommended reporting standards for vena caval filter placement and patient follow-up. J Vasc Surg 1999; 30:573–579.

14

Pulmonary Embolectomy

JAMES E. DALEN and JOSEPH S. ALPERT

University of Arizona College of Medicine
Tucson, Arizona, U.S.A.

I. Introduction

Pulmonary embolectomy, first described by Trendelenburg in 1908 (1), consists of emergency thoracotomy, and then, while occluding the main pulmonary artery and aorta, emboli are removed through an incision in the pulmonary artery. After developing this procedure in the animal laboratory, Trendelenburg noted that most patients who die of massive pulmonary embolish (PE) survive for at least 15 min; therefore, he said, "Within a hospital there will often be sufficient time for the operation to be undertaken, provided that the instruments are always kept ready" (2). He undertook this procedure in three patients; none survived. This heroic procedure was attempted in patients in extremis based on a clinical diagnosis and unaided by chest radiography, electrocardiogram, lung scan, pulmonary angiogram echocardiogram, or chest computed tomography!

The first successful pulmonary embolectomy was performed in 1924 by one of Trendelenburg's trainees, Kirschner (2). Crafoord of Sweden described two dramatic successful embolectomies in 1928 (3). His first operation "took about eight minutes," both patients were without a pulse at the onset of the operation (3). The first successful embolectomy in the United

States was performed at the Peter Bent Brigham hospital in Boston by Steenburg and Warren in 1958 (4).

Pulmonary embolectomy was the first definitive therapy for PE, and it was the only available therapy until the introduction of venous ligation by Homans in 1934 (5) and heparin by Murray and Best in 1938 (6) and Crafoord in 1939 (7). Given the difficulty of making an accurate diagnosis of PE and then rapidly proceeding to emergency thoracotomy in a patient in extremis, pulmonary embolectomy was very infrequent until the 1960s.

The feasibility of pulmonary embolectomy was greatly increased after the introduction of pulmonary angiography, which permitted accurate preoperative diagnosis. Stoney et al. (8) and Sautter et al. (9) in 1963 were the first to report successful pulmonary embolectomy in patients in whom the diagnosis was established by pulmonary angiography. The use of cardiopulmonary bypass also increased the feasibility of embolectomy. Cooley et al. (10) were the first to report successful pulmonary embolectomy utilizing cardiopulmonary bypass.

The availability of pulmonary angiography and cardiopulmonary bypass led to a significant increase in the number of patients undergoing pulmonary embolectomy in the 1960s, 1970s, and 1980s. In 1985, Del Campo (11) reviewed 651 reports of pulmonary embolectomy. The total mortality was 42%; 50% in cases done without bypass and 40% in those done with cardiopulmonary bypass.

The largest series of patients undergoing embolectomy at one hospital was reported by Meyer et al. in 1991 (12). During a 20-year period, 96 (3%) of the 3000 PE patients referred to the Laennec Hospital in Paris underwent embolectomy. The preoperative diagnosis was confirmed by selective pulmonary angiography in 92 of the 96 patients. Shock was present in 81% of the patients, and 25% of the patients had suffered cardiac arrest prior to surgery. The overall operative mortality was 37.5%. Three factors were predictors of mortality: the presence of shock, preoperative cardiac arrest, and coexisting cardiopulmonary disease. The mortality of those in shock was 42% compared to 17% without shock. Those with preoperative cardiac arrest had a 58% mortality compared to 31% in those without arrest. Patients with associated heart or lung disease had a 64% mortality compared to 34% in patients without heart or lung disease (12).

The primary cause of death in the postoperative period for those who survive embolectomy is recurrent PE. Meyer et al. (12), Greenfield (13), and more recently Aklog et al. (14) have stressed the need for IVC interruption at the time of surgery.

The primary indication for pulmonary embolectomy is the presence of massive PE complicated by shock requiring catecholamine support, which occurs in approximately 10% of patients in whom PE is diagnosed (15).

The results of embolectomy in patients with massive PE complicated by shock in three series (16–18), in addition to the report by Meyer et al. (12), are shown in Table 1. The overall mortality in these 167 patients averaged 35%. More than a third of these patients had a cardiac arrest prior to embolectomy. In addition to the report by Meyer et al. (12) of the increased mortality of embolectomy in patients with cardiac arrest, Ullmann et al. (18) have reported similar results. They reported a 63% mortality in 19 patients with preoperative cardiac arrest compared to 10% in 21 patients without arrest (18).

Embolectomy in patients without shock or preoperative cardiac arrest carries a much lower operative risk. Aklog et al. (14) have reported the results of embolectomy in patients in whom the indication was moderate to severe right ventricular dysfunction despite preserved systemic arterial pressure. Of 29 patients undergoing embolectomy, only three patients had hypotension, and one patient had preoperative cardiac arrest. The mortality for the total group was 11%. Mortality in the 25 patients without shock or cardiac arrest was 8% (14). They advocate their "liberalized" criteria for acute pulmonary embolectomy; the presence of right ventricular dysfunction in patients who are not in shock (14). Since nearly half of all patients with PE have right ventricular dysfunction (19), this liberalized approach would result in an extraordinary increase in the number of patients undergoing pulmonary embolectomy.

Aside from the report by Aklog et al. (14), embolectomy is rarely performed in patients without shock and in only a fraction of the patients who do have massive PE complicated by shock. In a registry of patients treated for PE at 204 hospitals in Germany in 1993 and 1994, there were 594 patients with shock and/or cardiac arrest (20). Only 1% underwent embolectomy. In a series of 2454 patients diagnosed with PE at 52 hospitals in seven countries in Europe and North America in 1995 and 1996 (19), only 15 patients underwent pulmonary embolectomy.

Table 1 Results of Pulmonary Embolectomy in Patients with Massive PE with Shock

Report (Reference)	Years of surgery	No. of patients	% Preop CPR	% Mortality
Meyer et al. (12)	1968–1988	78	25	42
Doerge et al. (16)	1979–1994	36	39	25
Gulba et al. (17)	1988–1994	13	69	23
Ullmann et al. (18)	1989–1997	40	52	35
Total		167	37	35

There are many reasons why only a minority of patients with PE complicated by shock undergo embolectomy. Many hospitals do not have facilities for cardiac surgery, and in hospitals that do, the patient may die before the diagnosis is confirmed or before the procedure can be performed, since approximately 70% of patients who die of massive PE die within 1 hr of the onset of symptoms (21). In other cases, the presence of associated heart or lung disease, other life-threatening disease, or advanced age may be relative contraindications.

Thrombolytic therapy has emerged as an alternative therapy for PE patients with shock, as discussed in Chapter 12. Meyer et al. (12), in their 1991 report of 96 embolectomies, concluded that they would reserve embolectomy for patients with contraindications to thrombolytic therapy and for "patients so severely affected that the time required for an attempt of medical treatment is thought to be unacceptable." In the report by Kasper et al. (20), 52% of 594 PE patients with shock and/or cardiac arrest were treated with thrombolytic therapy in 1993 and 1994.

It must be noted that there is no evidence that pulmonary embolectomy or thrombolytic therapy is more effective than heparin in patients with PE complicated by shock (15). In addition, there have been no randomized clinical trials comparing thrombolytic therapy to pulmonary embolectomy in these patients. Gulba et al. (17) compared the outcome of thrombolytic therapy in 24 patients with the results of embolectomy in 13 patients in a nonrandomized series. The mortality was nearly the same in the two groups; 23% in patients undergoing embolectomy and 33% in those receiving thrombolytic therapy (17).

II. Catheter Embolectomy

An alternative to pulmonary embolectomy by means of a thoracotomy and cardiopulmonary bypass is embolectomy by means of a specially devised catheter. This technique, performed with local anesthesia, was first described by Greenfield in 1969 (23). It involves the introduction of a cardiac catheter with a suction device at its tip into a jugular or femoral vein. After localizing the pulmonary emboli via pulmonary angiography, the catheter is passed to the site of the emboli where suction is applied to remove the emboli. Greenfield et al. (13) summarized their experience with this technique in 46 patients during a 22-year period (1970–1992). The indication for catheter embolectomy was hypotension despite inotropic support in 42 patients and respirator dependence in 4. Emboli were successfully removed in 76%. The hospital mortality for the total group was 30%. Mortality was 17% in those patients in whom the emboli were extracted (13). Timsit et al. (24) reported a similar (28%) mortality with catheter embolectomy in a series of 18 patients in whom "fibrinolysis and surgery were impossible." Despite these reports of successful catheter embolectomy, there have been few additional reports. The apparatus necessary for the procedure is bulky, and manipulation of the suction catheter requires special training. More attention has been directed at techniques to use catheters to fragment emboli (25–27).

III. Fragmentation of Emboli

Stein et al. (28) demonstrated that a specially designed catheter could be used to fragment PEs that had been induced in dogs by injecting autologous blood clot into a jugular vein. The catheter with a rotating tip (Kensey catheter) was able to fragment emboli in 6 of 11 dogs. Successful fragmentation of emboli in three patients with massive PE was reported by Brady et al (25) in 1991. They used conventional catheters to break up the emboli and disperse the fragments distally. Cardiac output was rapidly restored in all three patients (25).

Fragmentation of emboli with conventional angiographic catheters and angioplastic balloons and intrapulmonary thrombolysis was used to treat massive PE in 16 patients by Fava et al. (27). They reported significant decreases in mean pulmonary artery pressure and increases in systemic pressure after fragmentation. Urokinase was infused directly into the pulmonary emboli, before or after fragmentation, for 18–24 hrs. Fourteen (87.5%) of the patients survived. Murphy et al. (29) and Wong et al. (30) have also reported the use of catheter fragmentation of emboli combined with intrapulmonary thrombolysis in patients with massive PE.

The most extensive experience with catheter fragmentation of emboli has been reported by Schmitz-Rode and colleagues (26,31–33). They tested a variety of sophisticated catheters with high-speed rotating tips and encapsulated impellers in a glass model of the pulmonary arterial tree (31,32). They concluded that a modified standard pigtail catheter was the most effective and the safest for emboli fragmentation (26). The modified pigtail catheter has an additional oval side hole proximal to the pigtail tip. Passage of a guide wire through this hole allows rotation of the coiled catheter tip (26).

They tested the pigtail rotation catheter in 10 patients with angiographic evidence of more than 50% occlusion of the pulmonary circulation and involvement of the central (main and/or lobar) pulmonary arteries (26). Fragmentation was successful in 7 of the 10 patients, in whom vascular obstruction decreased by 36% ($\pm$ 10.0%) after fragmentation. Eight of the 10 patients also received thrombolytic therapy. The mean total procedure time was 41 min and the mean fragmentation time was 17 min. The overall mortality was 20% (26). They suggested that catheter fragmentation combined with thrombolytic therapy is an alternative to surgical embolectomy.

Schmidt-Rode and colleagues (33) then tested the pigtail rotation catheter in a multicenter clinical trial. Twenty patients with massive (>50% obstruction) were studied. The average degree of pulmonary vascular obstruction was 67%. Seventeen of the 20 patients were receiving high-dose catecholamines, and 14 required mechanical ventilation. Catheter fragmentation was successful in 16 patients, resulting in a 33% reduction in pulmonary vascular obstruction. Fifteen patients also received thrombolytic therapy after fragmentation. Sixteen of the 20 patients survived (20% mortality). Three of the four deaths occurred in patients who had undergone prolonged cardiac resuscitation prior to catheter fragmentation of their emboli (33).

The results of catheter fragmentation of emboli (26,27,33) seem comparable to the reported results of surgical pulmonary embolectomy (12,16–18).

At the present time, the vast majority of patients with massive PE are treated with heparin or thrombolytic therapy. The relative efficacy of these two treatments in patients with massive PE has not been assessed by a randomized clinical trial (22,34).

Furthermore, the efficacy of surgical embolectomy, catheter embolectomy, or catheter fragmentation has not been compared to heparin or thrombolytic therapy (15).

Until the various therapies for massive PE are compared in randomized clinical trials, the role of pulmonary embolectomy will remain uncertain. Many believe that pulmonary embolectomy should be reserved for patients with massive PE with shock in whom thrombolytic therapy is contraindicated or has failed (12,16) or in patients with severe hemodynamic distress (12). At the other extreme, Aklog et al. (14) believe that the indication for pulmonary embolectomy should be "liberalized" to include all patients with evidence of right ventricular dysfunction with or without shock.

If the promising results of catheter fragmentation of emboli are confirmed, this procedure may replace pulmonary embolectomy, and catheter fragmentation with or without thrombolytic therapy could become the treatment of choice for massive PE complicated by shock.

References

1. Trendelenburg F. Ueber die operative behandlung der embolie der lungenarterie. Arch Klin Chir 1908; 86:686–700.
2. Meyer JA. Friedrich Trendelenburg and the surgical approach to massive pulmonary embolism. Arch Surg 1990; 125:1202–1205.
3. Crafoord C. Two cases of obstructive pulmonary embolism successfully operated on. Acta Chir Scand 1928; 114:172–186.

4. Steenburg RW, Warren R, Wilson RE, et al. A new look at pulmonary embolectomy. Surg Gynecol Obstet 1958; 107:214.

5. Homans J. Thrombosis of the deep veins of the lower leg, causing pulmonary embolism. N Engl J Med 1934; 211:993–997.

6. Murray GDW, Best CH. Heparin and thrombosis: the present situation. JAMA 1938; 110:118–122.

7. Crafoord C. Heparin and post-operative thrombosis. Acta Chir Scand 1939; 82:319–335.

8. Stoney WS, Jacobs JK, Collins HA. Pulmonary embolism and embolectomy. Surg Gynecol Obstet 1963; 116:292–296.

9. Sautter RD, Lawton BR, Magin OE, et al. Pulmonary embolectomy: report of a case with preoperative and postoperative angiograms. N Engl J Med 1963; 269:997–999.

10. Cooley DA. Acute massive pulmonary embolism. JAMA 1961; 177:283.

11. Del Campo CD. Pulmonary embolectomy: a review. Can J Surg 1985; 28:111–113.

12. Meyer G, Tamisier D, Sors H, et al. Pulmonary embolectomy: a 20-year experience at one center. Ann Thorac Surg 1991; 51:232–236.

13. Greenfield LJ, Proctor MC, Williams DM, et al. Long-term experience with transvenous catheter pulmonary embolectomy. J Vasc Surg 1993; 18:450–457.

14. Aklog L, Williams CS, Byrne JG, Goldhaber SZ. Acute pulmonary embolectomy: a contemporary approach. Circulation 2002; 105:1415–1419.

15. Dalen JE. Pulmonary embolism: what have we learned since Virchow? 2: Treatment and prevention. Chest 2002; 122:1440–1456.

16. Doerge HC, Schoendube FA, Loeser H, Walter M, Messmer BJ. Pulmonary embolectomy: review of a 15-year experience and role in the age of thrombolytic therapy. Eur J Cardiothorac Surg 1996; 10(11):952.

17. Gulba DC, Schmid C, Borst HG, et al. Medical compared with surgical treatment for massive pulmonary embolism. Lancet 1994; 343:576–577.

18. Ullmann M, Hemmer W, Hannekum A. The urgent pulmonary embolectomy: mechanical resuscitation in the operating theatre determines the outcome. Thorac Cardiovasc Surg 1999; 47(1):5–8.

19. Goldhaber SZ, Visani L, De Rosa M. Acute pulmonary embolism: clinical outcomes in the international cooperative pulmonary embolism registry (ICOPER). Lancet 1999; 353:1386–1389.

20. Kasper W, Stavros K, Geibel A, Olschewshi, et al. Management strategies and determinants of outcome in acute major pulmonary embolism: results in a multicenter registry. J Am Coll Cardiol 1997; 30:1165–1171.

21. Dalen JE, Alpert JS. Natural history of pulmonary embolism. Progr Cardiovasc Dis 1975; 17:259–270.

22. Dalen JE. The uncertain role of thrombolytic therapy in the treatment of pulmonary embolism. Arch Int Med 2002; 162:2521–2523.

23. Greenfield LJ, Kimmell GO, McCurdy WC. Transvenous removal of pulmonary emboli by vacuum-cup catheter technique. J Surg Res 1969; 9:347–352.

24. Timsit JF, Reynauld P, Meyer G, Sors H. Pulmonary embolectomy by catheter device in massive pulmonary embolism. Chest 1991; 100:655–658.
25. Brady AJ, Crake T, Oakley CM. Percutaneous catheter fragmentation and distal dispersion of proximal pulmonary embolus. Lancet 1991; 338(8776): 1186–1189.
26. Schmitz-Rode T, Janssens U, Schild HH, Basche S, Hanrath P, Gunther RW. Fragmentation of massive pulmonary embolism using a pigtail rotation catheter. Chest 1998; 114(5):1237–1238.
27. Fava M, Soledad L, Flores P, Huete I. Mechanical fragmentation and pharmacologic thrombolysis in massive pulmonary embolism. J Vasc Intern Radiol 1997; 8:261–266.
28. Stein PD, Sabbah HN, Basha MA, Popovich J Jr, Kensey KR, Nash JE. Mechanical disruption of pulmonary emboli in dogs with a flexible rotating-tic catheter (Kensey catheter). Chest 1990; 98(4):994–998.
29. Murphy JM, Mulvihill N, Mulcahy D, Foley B, Smiddy P, Molloy MP. Percutaneous catheter and guide wire fragmentation with local administration of recombinant tissue plasminogen activator as a treatment for massive pulmonary embolism. Eur Radiol 1999; 9(5):959–964.
30. Wong PS, Singh SP, Watson RD, Lip GY. Management of pulmonary thromboembolism using catheter manipulation: a report of four cases and a review of literature. Postgrad J Med 1999; 75(890):737–741.
31. Schmitz-Rode T, Gunther RW. Percutaneous mechanical thrombolysis. A comparative study of various rotational catheter systems. Invest Radiol 1991; 26(6):557–563.
32. Schmitz-Rode T, Gunther RW. New device for percutaneous fragmentation of pulmonary emboli. Radiology 1991; 180(1):135–137.
33. Schmitz-Rode T, Janssens U, Duda S, Erley CM, Gunther RW. Massive pulmonary embolism: percutaneous emergency treatment by pigtail rotation catheter. J Am Coll Cardiol 2000; 36:375–379.
34. Dalen JE, Alpert JS, Hirsh J. Thrombolytic therapy for pulmonary embolism. Arch Intern Med 1997; 157:2530–2556.

15

Chronic Thromboembolic Pulmonary Hypertension

RICHARD N. CHANNICK and PETER F. FEDULLO

University of California San Diego Medical Center
La Jolla, California, U.S.A.

I. Introduction

Chronic thromboembolic pulmonary hypertension is a potential long-term consequence of nonresolved acute pulmonary emboli. Depending on the location and extent of the thromboembolic obstruction, its duration, and secondary remodeling at the level of the distal pulmonary vasculature, the resulting decrease in cross-sectional area of the pulmonary vascular bed may result in pulmonary hypertension, cor pulmonale, and death.

Since its initial recognition, the perception of this disease entity has evolved from that of an autopsy curiosity to a recognized and potentially correctable form of pulmonary hypertension (1–6). In 1984, the only 85 operated patients were reported, with a perioperative mortality rate of 22%. Approximately 1500 thromboendarterectomy procedures have now been performed worldwide (Table 1), the majority at the University of California, San Diego Medical Center (UCSDMC) (Fig. 1). Accompanying this increased experience, mortality rates reported by established programs with experience in the evaluation and management of patients with this disease process have fallen to the range of 6–8% (7).

Table 1 Published Results for Pulmonary Thromboendarterectomy Since 1996

Year	Author	Location	Patients (n)	Preoperative PVR[a]	Postoperative PVR[a]	Mortality (%)
1997	Nakajima	Japan	30	937 ± 45	299 ± 16	13.3
1997	Mayer	Germany	32	967 ± 238	301 ± 151	9.3
1998	Gilbert	Baltimore	17	~700 ± 200[b]	~170 ± 80[b]	23.5
1998	Miller	Philadelphia	25	?	?	24
1999	Dartevelle	France	68	1174 ± 416	519 ± 250	13.2
1999	Ando	Japan	24	1066 ± 250	268 ± 141	20.8
2000	Jamieson	San Diego	457	877 ± 452	267 ± 192[c]	7
2000	Mares	Austria	33	1478 ± 107[c]	975 ± 93[b]	9.1
2000	Mares	Austria	14	1334 ± 135[c]	759 ± 99[c]	21.4
2000	Rubens	Canada	21	765 ± 372	208 ± 92	4.8
2000	D'Armini	Italy	33	1056 ± 344	196 ± 39[d]	9.1

[a] Pulmonary vascular resistance in dynes-sec-cm^{-5}.
[b] Estimate derived from graph.
[c] Results expressed as pulmonary vascular resistance index.
[d] Data in 23 patients at 3-month follow-up.

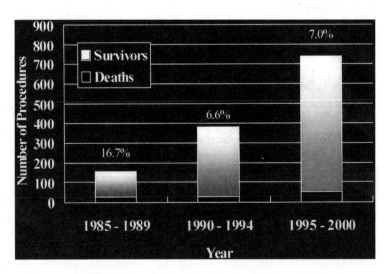

Figure 1 Number of operated cases and mortality rates in 1140 patients undergoing thromboendarterectomy at UCSDMC between 1985 and 1999.

This chapter will review the history of nonresolved pulmonary thromboembolism, proposed pathogenesis of chronic thromboembolic pulmonary hypertension (CTEPH), clinical evaluation of these patients, and treatment.

II. Natural History

Any discussion of the natural history of chronic thromboembolic pulmonary hypertension must take into consideration the natural history of acute pulmonary embolism. Although the embolic basis of chronic thromboembolic disease has been questioned, extensive clinical experience with this patient population would suggest that failure of thromboembolic resolution following a single or multiple embolic events is present in the majority of patients with the disease (8,9). What is not subject to controversy is the natural history of the disease in the absence of definitive intervention. Once established, the pulmonary hypertension appears to be progressive, albeit perhaps at a slower rate than that encountered in primary pulmonary hypertension, and, in the absence of definitive intervention, eventually leads to right ventricular failure and death (10–12).

The precise incidence of nonresolved pulmonary emboli is not known. It is estimated that 250,000–500,000 episodes of acute pulmonary embolism occur each year in the United States that result in 50,000–100,000 deaths (13). Despite the magnitude of the disease and extensive investigative efforts into its pathogenesis, diagnosis and therapy over the last four decades, the late natural history of those who survive an embolic event has not been well characterized (14). Clinically, the vast majority of patients have resolution of the signs and symptoms of acute thromboemblism with return to normal or near-normal function. However, how often residua are present and how often these residua lead to pulmonary hypertension are not precisely known.

Recent investigations, however, have begun to offer insights into the natural history and the long-term consequences of acute venous thromboembolism. First, it has become increasingly apparent that the perception of venous thromboembolism as an acute, self-limited disease is erroneous, especially in patients who present with spontaneous thromboembolism (15). Over the past decade, an increasing number of inherited and acquired thrombotic predispositions, beyond those conferred by clinical circumstances alone, have been identified (16). These predispositions include deficiencies of protein C, protein S, and antithrombin III, the recently described factor V Leiden and the G20210A prothrombin gene mutations, the lupus anticoagulant and antiphospholipid antibodies, and elevated levels of factor VIII and homocysteine (16,17). It has also become increasingly evident that the clinical presentation of venous thrombosis and pulmonary embolism may be subtle or imperceptible and easily confused with a number of other diagnostic alternatives (18–20). As a result, it is reasonable to suggest that a considerable number of thromboembolic events go unrecognized and therefore untreated.

There are recent data suggesting that incomplete anatomical resolution of an acute embolic event may be more common than is generally believed. In a recent review of 157 patients with symptomatic, acute pulmonary embolism from the THESEE study, 104 patients (66%) had residual perfusion defects 3 months after the acute event (21). Of these, 21 patients (20%) had residual pulmonary vascular obstruction of at least 40% as determined by perfusion scanning. Perfusion scanning has been demonstrated to understate the actual extent of angiographic obstruction in chronic thromboembolic disease (22). It is possible, therefore, that these figures also understate the degree of residual thromboembolic obstruction in patients recovering from an acute embolic event. In fact, experience with pulmonary angioscopy at UCSDMC supports this possibility. Evidence of web formation, recannalization, and luminal narrowing can be encountered in areas of vascular distribution associated with normal perfusion scan findings. These organized partially obstructing residuals may contribute to abnormal pulmonary hemodynamics at rest or with exercise.

Previous published experience suggested that residual pulmonary hypertension following single or even recurrent episodes of pulmonary embolism was uncommon (12). However, the number of patients studied was small. Recent data suggest that partial thromboembolic resolution associated with mild degrees of pulmonary hypertension may be more common than previously suspected (23). In one study, 1-year echocardiographic follow-up and 5-year clinical follow-up of 78 patients hospitalized with acute pulmonary embolism were reported (24). An early dynamic phase followed by a protracted stable phase of pulmonary artery pressure decline after an acute thromboembolic event was identified. The time to achieve the stable phase was 38 days and was independent of whether the therapeutic intervention was thrombolytic therapy or heparin. In patients with a pulmonary artery *systolic* pressure >50 mm Hg at the time of diagnosis of the acute episode, the risk for persistent pulmonary hypertension increased threefold; four patients (5.1%) developed chronic pulmonary hypertension and three subsequently underwent successful pulmonary thromboendarterectomy.

Hemodynamically, it is important to note that acute pulmonary embolism should not lead to elevation in mean pulmonary arterial pressure >40 mm Hg due to inability of a nonhypertrophied right ventricle to "deal" with such pressures (25). However, chronically, in the setting of incomplete thromboembolic resolution of sufficient magnitude to increase right ventricular afterload, right ventricular hypertrophy and other compensatory mechanisms occur, cardiac output is restored, and pulmonary hypertension develops (26).

Despite intensive efforts, a specific or unique abnormality of the coagulation or thrombolytic systems has not been identified in patients suffering from chronic thromboembolic pulmonary hypertension other than the presence of an anticardiolipin antibody in approximately 10–20% of patients (27,28). Chronic thromboembolic disease should be viewed as a failure of clot lysis rather than hypercoagulability. Chronic thromboembolic pulmonary hypertension, therefore, may represent part of the normal spectrum of disease associated with pulmonary embolism: complete hemodynamic and anatomical resolution in a minority of patients, partial resolution associated with a normal symptomatic status in most, and progression to pulmonary hypertension in the remaining few.

Although exact incidence figures are not available, it is probable, based on the number of embolic survivors and the number of patients referred for pulmonary thromboendarterectomy, that chronic thromboembolic pulmonary hypertension of sufficient severity to require surgical intervention occurs in no more than 0.1% of patients who experience an embolic event.

Because the majority of patients present with established, fixed pulmonary hypertension, the hemodynamic evolution of the disease has not been well established. The symptomatic history provided by patients with this disease process can provide certain insight. In patients with a documented venous thromboembolic event, symptomatic recovery occurs, although often not to a level equivalent to that prior to the acute event. In patients without a documented acute thromboembolic event, many can provide a history consistent with that diagnosis such as an episode of pleurisy, lower extremity muscle strain, or prolonged, atypical pneumonia. Or they may describe a hospitalization or surgical procedure from which they never fully recovered. Following a period of clinical stability, which may range from months to years, worsening exertional dyspnea, hypoxemia, and right ventricular dysfunction ultimately ensue.

This "honeymoon" period following an acute event and subsequent worsening of symptoms suggests either progression of a secondary vasculopathy, loss of right ventricular adaptive mechanisms, or both. It does not appear that the progressive worsening in most patients is due to recurrent embolic events. There is evidence, based on lung biopsy findings obtained at the time of thromboendarterectomy, that changes in the microvasculature are, in fact, quite similar to that seen in other forms of pulmonary hypertension; giving further weight to the concept of a secondary vasculopathy developing in some patients with chronic pulmonary embolism which may significantly contribute to the pulmonary hypertension and right ventricular dysfunction (29,30). Potential involvement of the distal vascular bed is further supported by an animal study of unilateral pulmonary artery ligation in which the ligated lung showed an increase in the muscular, adventitial, and intimal thickness of the pulmonary artery, an increase in size and number of bronchial arteries, and an increase in endothelin and nitric oxide synthase receptor immunoreactivity (31). As will be discussed below, the presence of secondary microvascular changes may complicate the evaluation of a patient with chronic thromboemboli for surgery.

III. Clinical Presentation

As with patients with all other forms of pulmonary hypertension, the complaint common to patients with chronic thromboembolic pulmonary hypertension is exertional dyspnea; likely due to increased dead space ventilation and limitation on cardiac output associated with the pulmonary vascular obstruction and resulting pulmonary hypertension. Additional complaints include nonproductive cough, hemoptysis, and chest pain. In more severe cases, presyncopal symptoms or true syncope may develop. Patients often complain of lightheadedness and increased dyspnea when bending from the waist; perhaps related to a transient decrease in venous return and cardiac output.

As there may be no history indicating acute venous thromboembolism, the clinical presentation may be quite nonspecific and the correct diagnosis not considered. The progressive dyspnea and exercise intolerance associated with the chronic thromboembolic pulmonary hypertension are often erroneously attributed to asthma, physical deconditioning, advancing age, interstitial lung disease, coronary artery disease, or psychogenic dyspnea.

Physical findings may also be subtle, especially early in the course of the disease, thereby contributing to diagnostic delay. Prior to the development of significant right ventricular hypertrophy or overt right ventricular failure, abnormalities can be limited to widened splitting of the second heart sound or accentuation of its pulmonic component. As the pulmonary hypertension progresses, classic findings of pulmonary hypertension develop: a right ventricular lift, accentuation of the pulmonic component of the second heart sound, widened and eventually fixed splitting of the second heart sound, a right ventricular S_4 gallop, and varying degrees of tricuspid regurgitation. In patients with overt right ventricular failure, elevated jugular venous pressure with a prominent v wave, a right-sided S_3, lower extremity edema, hepatomegaly, ascites, and cyanosis may develop. The intensity of the tricuspid regurgitant murmur may diminish as the tricuspid annulus dilates and the transvalvular pressure gradient decreases. Lower extremity edema may be the result of right heart failure or venous obstruction related to residual venous thrombosis. Findings consistent with the postphlebitic syndrome may also be present.

A notable physical finding in many patients with chronic thromboembolic disease is the presence of pulmonary flow bruits (32). These bruits, present in approximately 30% of patients with chronic thromboembolic pulmonary hypertension, and which appear to result from turbulent flow across partially obstructed pulmonary vascular segments, are high pitched and blowing in quality, audible over the anterior and posterior lung fields rather than the precordium, and are most apparent during a mid inspiratory breath-holding maneuver. These bruits are not unique to chronic thromboembolic disease; they have been described in other disease states associated with focal narrowing of large pulmonary arteries such as congenital branch stenosis and pulmonary arteritis. They have not, however, been described in primary pulmonary hypertension.

IV. Diagnostic Evaluation

Under most circumstances, the diagnostic pathway is relatively straightforward once the possibility of pulmonary hypertension has been considered. As in any other form of pulmonary hypertension, the intent of the diagnostic sequence is to quantify the degree of pulmonary hypertension (at rest and if indicated, with exercise), to establish its etiology, and, if major vessel thromboembolic disease is present, to determine whether it is accessible to surgical intervention.

Transthoracic echocardiography commonly provides the initial objective evidence that pulmonary hypertension is present and that it is not the result of primary left ventricular dysfunction or valvular disease. In addition, echocardiography is useful in estimating the severity of the pulmonary hypertension, looking for "secondary" causes such as left ventricular or left-sided valvular disease and septal defects, and examining for a patent foramen ovale (using agitated saline contrast) in CTEPH patients with significant hypoxemia. Typical findings include enlargement of the right cardiac chambers, an increased velocity of the tricuspid regurgitant envelope from which the pulmonary artery systolic pressure can be estimated, flattening or paradoxical motion of the interventricular septum, and encroachment of an enlarged right ventricle on the left ventricular cavity.

Once the presence of pulmonary hypertension has been established, distinguishing between major vessel occlusive disease and small vessel pulmonary arterial hypertension becomes the next critical step in the diagnostic sequence. Ventilation-perfusion lung scanning represents a simple, noninvasive means of achieving this end under most circumstances (33–37). In chronic thromboembolic disease, at least one (and more commonly several) segmental or larger mismatched perfusion defects are present (38,33) (Fig. 2). It is important to emphasize that small residual pulmonary emboli do not lead to pulmonary hypertension. In other words, chronic thromboembolism is not synonymous with chronic thromboembolic pulmonary hypertension. Thus, the universal presence of large perfusion defects in the latter disease. In contrast, primary pulmonary hypertension perfusion scans are either normal or exhibit a "mottled" appearance (33,37) (Fig. 3). Occasionally, the perfusion scan pattern in small vessel pulmonary hypertension demonstrates a striking basilar redistribution of flow, suggesting obstruction of the upper and middle lobe arteries. This redistribution of flow, however, is in a nonsegmental pattern, and at angiography, patent proximal vessels are present.

Despite the ventilation-perfusion scan abnormalities seen in chronic thromboembolic disease, the scans often understate, in certain cases to a

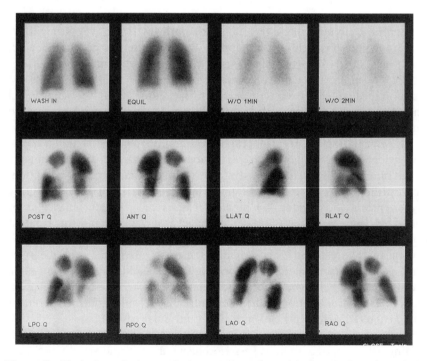

Figure 2 Typical ventilation-perfusion scan in patient with chronic thromboembolic pulmonary hypertension demonstrating multiple, mismatched segmental defects.

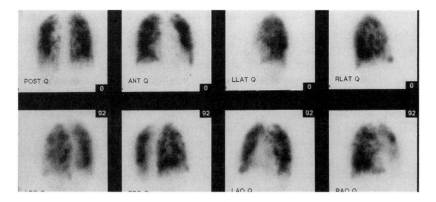

Figure 3 Perfusion scan in patient with primary pulmonary hypertension. Note presence of multiple subsegmental defects providing a mottled appearance.

remarkable degree, the actual extent of angiographic obstruction (22). In addition, "gray" areas of perfusion are common in CTEPH, indicating partially recannalized channels allowing some tracer to enter the distal vasculature. Therefore, in a patient with pulmonary hypertension, even the presence of a single, mismatched, segmental ventilation-perfusion scan defect should raise concerns regarding a potential thromboembolic basis regardless of whether this defect appears to be proportionate to the extent of the pulmonary hypertension.

It is also important to recognize that the presence of mismatched segmental defects in a patient with pulmonary hypertension does not necessarily imply the presence of thromboembolic obstruction. Other processes that result in obstruction of the central pulmonary arteries or veins such as pulmonary artery sarcoma, large vessel pulmonary vasculitides, extrinsic vascular compression by mediastinal adenopathy or fibrosis, and, on occasion, pulmonary venoocclusive disease, can yield "high-probability" ventilation-perfusion scans.

Routine hematological and blood chemistry studies are usually unremarkable. Secondary polycythemia, resulting from longstanding hypoxemia, is occasionally encountered. Mild elevations of transaminase, alkaline phosphatase, or bilirubin levels due to passive liver congestion may be present. A prolonged activate partial thromboplastin time in the absence of heparin therapy or a decreased platelet counts may suggest the possibility of a lupus anticoagulant or anticardiolipin antibody, which has been identified in 10–20% of patients with chronic thromboembolic pulmonary hypertension (27,28). As in other variants of pulmonary hypertension, elevated uric acid levels are also encountered commonly, and appear to correlate positively with the level of mean right atrial pressure and inversely with the level of the cardiac output (39,40).

Chest radiographic findings, although neither sensitive nor specific, may demonstrate one or more abnormalities consistent with the diagnosis of pulmonary hypertension on a thromboembolic basis (41,42). In chronic thromboembolic disease, asymmetry in the size of the central pulmonary arteries may be present in conjunction with areas of relative hypoperfusion and hyperperfusion. The asymmetry of the central pulmonary arteries may be so dramatic as to suggest pulmonary artery agenesis, whereas the areas of increased perfusion may suggest a focal infiltrate or interstitial disease (42). Chest radiographic abnormalities in pulmonary hypertension on a small vessel basis, when present, are characterized by enlargement of both pulmonary arteries associated with a uniform decrease in the peripheral pulmonary vasculature. In pulmonary veno-occlusive disease, signs of interstitial pulmonary edema, including Kerley B lines, may be present. There also may be parenchymal or pleural scars, which are consistent with prior infarcts (43). Enlargement of the right ventricle, given its anterior anatomical position, may be evident only on the lateral film by encroachment on the retrosternal space.

Lower extremity duplex ultrasonography will demonstrate findings consistent with prior venous thrombosis in approximately 45% of patients (9).

Pulmonary function testing, often performed as part of the evaluation of the patient's dyspnea, is often normal. Approximately 20% of patients show a mild to moderate restrictive impairment; to a large extent caused by parenchymal scarring related to prior infarcts (43). Although a mild to moderate reduction in single-breath diffusing capacity for carbon monoxide (DLCO) can be observed, a normal value does not exclude the diagnosis (44,45).

In terms of gas exchange consequences, the arterial Po_2 may be within normal limits. However, the alveolar-arterial oxygen gradient is typically widened and the majority of patients have a decrease in the arterial Po_2 with exercise (46,47). The hypoxemia appears to be the consequence of moderate ventilation-perfusion inequality and a limited cardiac output, which depresses mixed venous Po_2. Desaturation during exercise appears to be related to the inability of the right ventricle to augment cardiac output in the setting of increased demand resulting in further depression of the mixed venous Po_2. In patients with a patent foramen ovale, exercise-related hypoxemia may result from an increase in right-to-left shunting.

The role of helical computed tomographic (CT) scanning in the diagnosis of CTEPH has been debated. A variety of CT abnormalities have been described in patients with chronic thromboembolic pulmonary hypertension: right ventricular enlargement, dilated central pulmonary arteries, chronic thromboembolic material within the central pulmonary arteries, bronchial artery collateral flow, parenchymal abnormalities consistent with prior infarcts, and mosaic attenuation of the pulmonary parenchyma (48–50) (Fig. 4). None of these findings, however, is completely sensitive or specific for chronic thromboembolic pulmonary hypertension (51).

There is no question that intraluminal thrombus within the central pulmonary arteries can be demonstrated by helical tomography. However, thrombus that is well endothelialized may not be apparent. Therefore, the absence of thrombus proximal to the segmental arteries by CT does not preclude the possibility of surgical intervention. The authors have seen several patients in whom helical CT scans were read as being "negative" by experienced radiologists but conventional pulmonary angiography revealed extensive disease that was highly amenable to surgery. Furthermore, the demonstration of central thrombus does not necessarily confirm the diagnosis of surgically accessible chronic thromboembolic pulmonary hypertension. Central thrombi have been described in primary pulmonary hypertension and other forms of chronic lung disease (52,53). It is therefore the authors' strong opinions that helical CT scanning should not replace pulmonary angiograpy in the evaluation of patients for chronic thromboembolic pulmonary hypertension.

CT does, however, have a role in the diagnostic pathway in selected patients. It appears most useful in that small subset of patients with unilateral or predominantly unilateral vascular occlusion in whom the probability of other diagnostic possibilities (sarcoma, vasculitis, malignancy, mediastinal fibrosis) is increased (54). It is also useful, along with physiological testing, in helping to define the status of the pulmonary parenchyma in patients with coexisting obstructive or restrictive lung disease. Preliminary data also suggest that CT scanning, in conjunction with other diagnostic techniques, may be useful in defining the extent of the small vessel component of the disease and therefore a better predictor of postoperative hemodynamic outcome (55).

Despite concerns regarding cardiac catheterization and pulmonary angiography in patients with pulmonary hypertension, these interventions remain essential in determining the severity of pulmonary hypertension at rest and, if necessary, with exercise; in establishing the presence of chronic thromboembolic obstruction and defining its extent and proximal extension (and, therefore, surgical accessibility); and in excluding other diagnostic possibilities (56,57).

The angiographic appearance of chronic thromboembolic disease is generally very distinct from that of acute pulmonary embolism. Well-defined, intraluminal filling defects found in acute disease are not present. Instead, the angiographic patterns encountered in chronic thromboembolic disease reflect the complex patterns of organization and recanalization that occur following an acute thromboembolic event (56).

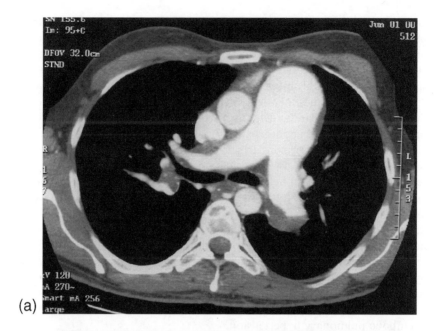

(a)

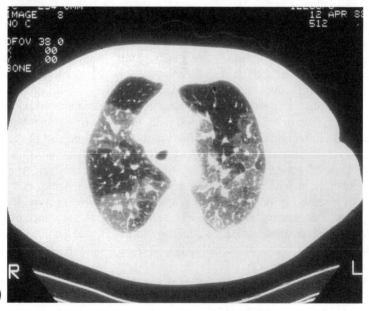

(b)

Figure 4 (a) Transverse CT angiogram in patient with chronic thromboembolic disease revealing extensive central thrombus. (b) Transverse CT angiogram in the same patient obtained with lung windows shows asymmetrical vessel size and mosaic pattern of perfusion.

Five distinct angiographic patterns have been described that correlate with the finding of chronic thromboembolic material at the time of surgery: (1) pouch defects; (2) pulmonary artery webs or bands; (3) intimal irregularities; (4) abrupt, often angular narrowing of the major pulmonary arteries; and (5) complete obstruction of main, lobar, or segmental vessels at their point of origin (4). In most patients with extensive chronic thrombembolic disease, two or more of these angiographic findings are present and the findings are present bilaterally (Figs. 5–7). In a recent review of 410 patients with suspected chronic thromboembolic disease, unilateral or predominantly unilateral thromboembolic involvement was encountered in only 22 patients (5.4%) (54).

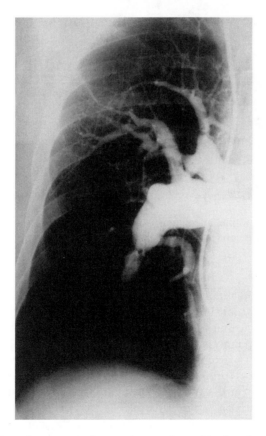

Figure 5 Right pulmonary angiogram in a patient with chronic thromboembolic disease. Note web in upper lobe artery and classic "pouch" defect in lower lobe artery.

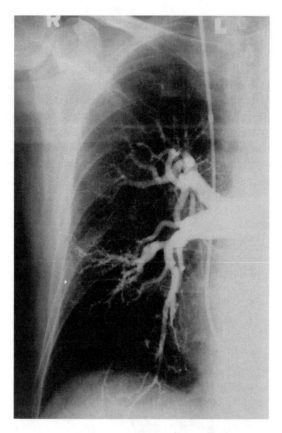

Figure 6 Right cut-film angiogram showing web in upper lobe artery, poststenotic dilatation of middle lobe artery, and several absent lower lobe branches.

Competing diagnoses exist with angiographic findings similar to those encountered in chronic thromboembolic disease (4). Bandlike narrowing can be a feature of medium or large vessel pulmonary arteritis or can be seen with congenital pulmonary artery stenosis. Total or partial obstruction of central pulmonary arteries can be the consequence of an intravascular obstructing process (primary pulmonary artery tumors) or an extravascular, compressive one (mediastinal or hilar lymphadenopathy, lung carcinoma, mediastinal fibrosis).

Several large series have documented that pulmonary angiography can be performed safely despite concerns that have been raised about performing the procedure in patients with severe pulmonary hypertension (57,58). This is

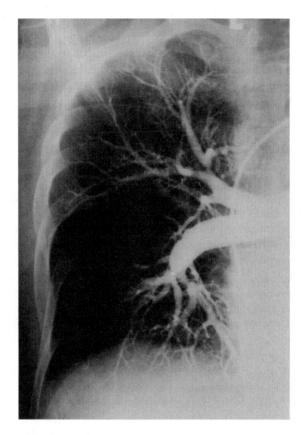

Figure 7 Right pulmonary angiogram demonstrating more subtle features of chronic thromboembolism including intimal irregularity along the lateral border of the descending pulmonary artery.

not meant to suggest that the procedure is free of potential risk. However, by modifying standard angiographic approaches and paying careful attention to patient monitoring, the procedure can be performed safely.

Precautions taken to minimize the risk of the procedure include the use of a single injection of nonionic contrast material into the right and left pulmonary arteries. There is no need for multiple, subsegmental injections, since these will not provide useful information regarding surgical accessibility. The contrast volume and infusion rate are modified based on the level of cardiac output and the mixed venous saturation, the degree of pulmonary hypertension, and the degree of central vascular filling determined by a

10-mL contrast hand injection prior to the formal study. Based on these criteria, contrast volumes range from 15 to 60 mL injected over 2.5–3.0 sec.

In terms of angiographic technique, cut-film biplane acquisition appears to provide optimal anatomical detail. On a number of occasions, the authors have encountered areas of intimal irregularity and recannalization through central pouch defects that have been obscured on digital subtraction studies. We have also found utilization of the lateral projection invaluable in providing a much more detailed view of the lobar and segmental branches and in avoiding the uncertainty resulting from dilated, overlapping vessels. This is especially true for obstruction in the lower lobe arteries below the superior segment level in which branches of the dilated right middle lobe and the superior segment artery obscure the degree of vascular obstruction in the anterior projection.

In a select group of patients, fiberoptic pulmonary angioscopy can be a useful adjunctive technique in confirming the presence of chronic thromboembolic obstruction and in determining whether it is amenable to surgical intervention (59–61). The angioscope, a fiberoptic device 120 cm in length and 3.0 mm in external diameter with distal 180-degree flexion and extension capability, is introduced through a vascular sheath, preferably using a right internal jugular approach, and passed into the pulmonary arteries under fluoroscopic guidance. Inflation of the distal balloon with carbon dioxide obstructs pulmonary artery blood flow and allows visualization of the arterial wall. The features of organized chronic emboli consist of roughening or pitting of the intimal surface, bands and webs traversing the vascular lumen, pitted masses of chronic embolic material within the lumen, and partial recannalization (Fig. 8).

At UCSDMC, angioscopy is performed in approximately 25% of patients undergoing evaluation to determine their candidacy for thromboendarterectomy. The procedure appears to be most useful under two circumstances: (1) predicting a beneficial hemodynamic outcome in patients with relatively modest levels of pulmonary hypertension in whom the angiographic images do not precisely define the proximal extent of the thromboembolic disease; and (2) confirming operability in patients with severe pulmonary hypertension who would not have been referred to surgery based on the angiographic findings alone (61).

If the patient is considered to be an operative candidate, several other interventions must be undertaken prior to surgery. Given the risk of embolic recurrence, both over the long-term and especially during the high-risk perioperative period when potential postoperative bleeding complications may contraindicate the administration of even prophylactic doses of anticoagulation, an inferior vena caval filter is routinely placed. Although recent evidence suggests that filter placement may increase the long-term risk of

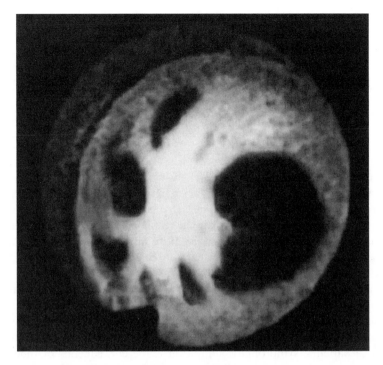

Figure 8 Angioscopic appearance of chronic thromboembolic disease. Note complex pattern of recannalization and web formation.

deep vein thrombosis (DVT), all patients undergoing thromboendarterectomy are treated with lifelong anticoagulation, thereby minimizing this potential risk (62). To avoid the development of bleeding complications at the insertion site in the postoperative period, the filter is placed several days prior to surgery preferably by a percutaneous transfemoral approach.

For those at risk of coronary artery disease, coronary angiography is routinely performed prior to surgery, usually at the time of the right heart catheterization and pulmonary angiography. Coronary artery bypass grafting, if necessary, can be performed at the time of the thromboendarterectomy. In elderly patients with evidence of atherosclerotic disease, evaluation of the carotid circulation by ultrasonography is also performed prior to surgery.

In patients with thrombocytopenia, the possible presence of heparin-induced thrombocytopenia must be considered, as patients will typically receive high doses of unfractionated heparin during cardiopulmonary bypass. In patients who do prove to have heparin-induced thrombocytopenia, thromboendarterectomy has been successfully performed using intravenous iloprost with heparin during bypass, danaparoid sodium, or recombinant hirudin (63–65). If danaparoid sodium is to be used, a platelet aggregation study should be performed with this agent because of reported cross reactivity (66). The use of danaparoid sodium is also limited by its long half-life and need for intraoperative monitoring with anti–factor Xa levels (64).

V. Surgical Selection

The central purpose of this comprehensive preoperative evaluation is to determine the need for thromboendarterectomy and to estimate the anticipated risk in the individual patient. In terms of need, the presence of pulmonary vascular obstruction should result in hemodynamic or ventilatory impairment at rest or with exercise. With rare exception, patients undergoing surgery have a resting pulmonary vascular resistance in excess of 300 dynes/sec/cm^{-5} with the majority of operated patients having a pulmonary vascular resistance in the range of 800–1000 dynes/sec/cm^{-5} (67). Patients who fall into the lower range of pulmonary hemodynamic impairment include those with involvement of one main pulmonary artery, those with unusually vigorous lifestyle expectations, and those who live at high altitude. In these patients, symptomatic limitation is the consequence of their high dead space and minute ventilatory demands as well as limitations on maximal cardiac output with exercise.

Surgery is also offered to patients with only moderate levels of pulmonary hypertension at rest but who develop significant levels of pulmonary hypertension with exercise. Based on what is known about the natural history of the disease, it is probable, although not yet fully substantiated, that these high pressures and flows over a prolonged period of time may contribute to the progressive development of a small vessel arteriopathy, thereby perpetuating the cycle of pulmonary hypertension. If the decision is made not to proceed with surgery in patients with this hemodynamic profile, either by the physician or patient, it is essential that the patient be followed carefully and serial catheterizations be performed with repeat assessment of resting and exercise hemodynamics. Symptomatic decline associated with progressive elevation in the resting or exercise pulmonary artery pressures or a decrease in cardiac output would provide an objective basis to proceed with surgery. Follow-up with serial echocardiographic studies is feasible but may lack the sensitivity to detect subtle changes in pulmonary hemodynamic findings that may occur.

The second and most absolute criterion for surgical intervention is the surgical accessibility of the thrombi as defined by angiography and, when indicated, angioscopy. Experienced surgeons can access disease starting as distally as the segmental vascular bed. However, in addition to considering the proximal extent of disease, one must determine whether the degree of pulmonary hypertension can be sufficiently "explained" by the thromboemboli present. This aspect of the evaluative process, and the one that requires the greatest experiential base to master, is determining whether the degree of pulmonary hypertension is consistent with the extent of accessible thromboembolic material and estimating the hemodynamic and symptomatic improvement that might be achieved through surgical intervention. Reestablishing blood flow to the equivalent of three or four segmental arteries might have a profound hemodynamic and symptomatic effect on a patient with relatively mild pulmonary hypertension, whereas having negligible effects in a patient with severe pulmonary hypertension. This determination is critical. Failure to remove sufficient chronic thromboembolic material to lower pulmonary vascular resistance, especially in patients with severe pulmonary hypertension and right ventricular dysfunction, is associated with significant postoperative morbidity and mortality.

As experience with this patient population has grown, it has become increasingly apparent that, at least in certain patients, the pulmonary hypertension associated with chronic thromboembolic disease has several contributing components. These include the central, surgically accessible chronic thromboembolic obstruction; the distal, surgically inaccessible obstruction; and the resistance conferred by the presence of a secondary, small vessel arteriopathy. As a result of these contributing factors, the correlation between the hemodynamic impairment and the extent of central, angiographically apparent obstruction can range from excellent to poor. A central focus of the evaluative process, therefore, involves an assimilation of the hemodynamic, angiographic, and angioscopic findings as a means of partitioning the central, surgically accessible component of the hemodynamic impairment from that which is not surgically correctable. One technique that may prove to be promising in partitioning the central from peripheral (inaccessible) components of the pulmonary hypertension is analyzing the decay of the pulmonary artery occlusion pressure waveform. Preliminary work suggests that the slope of the decay upon balloon inflation correlates with postoperative pulmonary vascular resistance (68), raising the possibility that this technique will be a valuable tool in evaluating these patients.

The third consideration in assessing surgical candidacy is the evaluation of comorbid conditions that may adversely influence perioperative mortality or morbidity as well as long-term survival. Patient management in the postoperative period may be complicated by the presence of coexisting coronary artery disease, parenchymal lung disease, renal insufficiency, or hepatic dysfunction. Patients with chronic hematological malignancies and other chronic comorbid conditions have been offered surgery if relief of the pulmonary hypertension will improve both the quality and duration of their lives. By taking due precautions, patients with sickle cell anemia have successfully undergone the procedure without cold-related sickling complications (69). Therefore, advanced age or the presence of collateral disease do not represent absolute contraindications to pulmonary thromboendarterectomy, although they do influence risk assessment which must be discussed carefully with the patient and family members prior to surgery. The one exception to this guideline is the presence of severe underlying parenchymal lung disease either obstructive or restrictive. In these patients, exercise limitations may be more due to the lung disease than the pulmonary hypertension; thus even successful thromboendarterectomy might not benefit the patient.

VI. Surgical Approach and Postoperative Course

The goal of pulmonary thromboendarterectomy is to relieve pulmonary hypertension, not simply extract thrombus. Therefore, the technique involves a true endarterectomy, not simply an embolectomy. Removal of the central, intraluminal component of the disease without subsequent dissection of the distal extensions, which are fibrotic and incorporated into the vessel wall, will result in an inadequate hemodynamic outcome (Fig. 9).

Surgical pulmonary thromboendarterectomy was first attempted in 1958 (5). Since then, several modifications in surgical technique have occurred. Details of those modifications and the current surgical approach are beyond the scope of this chapter but have been reviewed in length in several recent publications (3,6). These modifications were implemented as awareness of the unique problems encountered in the operative management of this disease entity became apparent. The need for sternotomy was clear as the bilateral nature of the disease became more appreciated. The use of cardiopulmonary bypass provided a mechanism of extracorporeal support in patients with severe hemodynamic compromise. Because bronchial back bleeding from the luxuriant bronchial circulation encountered during surgery often obscured the operative field impairing the ability to perform an optimal endarterectomy, periods of complete hypothermic circulatory arrest were initiated to provide a bloodless operative field. Modifications of the surgical approach, intended to decrease risk or improve hemodynamic outcome, continue to be explored. These include the use of intraoperative video-assisted angioscopy to increase visibility in the distal pulmonary arteries, thereby allowing surgical intervention in patients with previously inaccessible disease; division rather than retraction of the superior vena cava; and selective antegrade cerebral perfusion to decrease the risk of neurological sequelae (23,70,71).

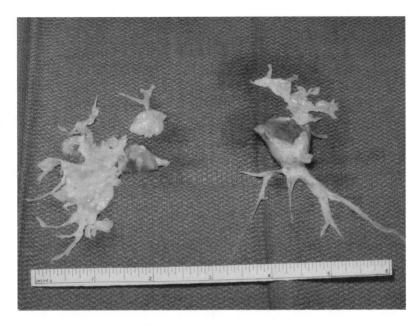

Figure 9 Surgical specimen obtained from a patient with chronic thromboembolic disease revealing fibrotic appearance and multiple segmental extensions.

Several of the problems encountered in the postoperative period such as coagulation disorders, bleeding, arrhythmias, wound infections, delirium, pleural and pericardial effusions, postcardiotomy syndrome, and atelectasis are identical to those of patients undergoing other forms of cardiac surgery (72). The postoperative care of patients undergoing pulmonary thrombo-endarterectomy is further complicated by the acute physiological changes that occur as a result of the procedure: a dramatic redistribution of pulmonary blood flow accompanied by an equally dramatic reduction in right ventricular afterload.

The temporary alteration of blood flow, termed pulmonary artery "steal," represents a redistribution of pulmonary arterial blood flow away from previously well-perfused pulmonary segments and into the newly endarterectomized segments (73). Although the basis for this redistribution remains speculative, it is probably related to the loss of normal pulmonary vasoregulatory mechanisms and the development of differential resistances in the pulmonary vascular bed. Its major importance lies in its contribution to postoperative gas exchange abnormalities. Long-term follow-up has demonstrated that this redistribution of flow is reversible in most circumstances (74).

Another consequence of both the redistribution described above and, probably, the trauma itself to the pulmonary vasculature, is reperfusion pulmonary edema. Although the exact pathophysiological basis for reperfusion pulmonary edema remains uncertain, it appears, biochemically and clinically, to represent a localized form of high-permeability, neutrophil-mediated lung injury (75,76). The disorder most commonly manifests itself in the first 24 hr after surgery but may appear up to 72 hr after surgery and is highly variable in severity, ranging from a mild form resulting in mild to moderate postoperative hypoxemia in the majority of affected patients to profound alveolar hemorrhage that may be fatal. The unique aspect of this form of lung injury is that it is limited to those areas of the lung served by pulmonary arteries from which proximal thromboembolic obstructions have been removed.

Management of patients with reperfusion pulmonary edema is generally supportive and similar to management strategies for other forms of acute lung injury, including low tidal volume ventilation, positive end-expiratory pressure (PEEP), and pressure-control ventilation. Extracorporeal membrane oxygenation has been utilized successfully in patients with reperfusion lung injury in whom aggressive, conventional support has been proven to be inadequate to maintain oxygenation. ‘

Given the neutrophil-mediated bases for the lung injury, interventions with pharmacological management have been attempted with mixed success. In a recent trial of 51 randomized patients, the intraoperative and early postoperative administration of a novel, selectin-mediated neutrophil adhesion blocking agent reduced the relative risk of reperfusion injury by 50% but had no impact on mortality, ventilator days, or days in the intensive care unit (75).

Patients posing the most difficult management problem in the postoperative period are those with persistent pulmonary hypertension, a group that encompasses approximately 10% of those undergoing the procedure. In those patients with severe levels of residual pulmonary hypertension, mortality is significant. Maximizing cardiac function with inotropic and pressor support may be useful until the already limited right ventricle recovers from the trauma of surgery. In addition, the authors have had favorable anecdotal experience with intravenous epoprostenol (Flolan) in patients with severe postoperative right ventricular failure.

VII. Outcome

The perioperative mortality rate following pulmonary thromboendarterectomy has decreased from over 16 (1985–1989) to 8% (1995–1999) (see Fig. 1).

This mortality reduction is no doubt due to improvement in patient selection, operative technique, and postoperative care. These mortality figures, supported by experience at other centers, strongly suggest that this procedure is a high-risk intervention even in experienced hands, one that requires a requisite experiential base, in terms of both total and annual number of cases, to minimize the morbid and mortal risks of the procedure (6,50,67,77–80). The commonest cause of mortality is residual pulmonary hypertension, followed by reperfusion lung injury.

In the majority of patients undergoing thromboendarterectomy, the long-term hemodynamic and symptomatic outcomes have been favorable. Dramatic reduction, and at times normalization, of the pulmonary artery pressure and pulmonary vascular resistance can be achieved (6,26,30,79). Corresponding improvements in gas exchange and exercise capacity have also been reported (79,81). The majority of patients, who were initially in NYHA class III or IV status preoperatively, return to NYHA class I or II status and are able to resume normal activities (36,79). One follow-up of 308 patients surveyed a mean of 3.3 years after surgery found that 62% of patients who were unemployed prior to thromboendarterectomy had returned to work (82).

In approximately 10% of patients undergoing thromboendarterectomy, significant levels of pulmonary hypertension persist following the procedure. This group includes patients whose disease involves a substantial component of distal, surgically inaccessible thromboemboli and patients who have developed severe, irreversible secondary pulmonary hypertensive changes in their distal pulmonary vascular bed.

What has not yet been precisely defined is the level of pulmonary artery pressure or pulmonary vascular resistance that must be achieved to assure a favorable long-term outcome or to predict an unfavorable one. The experience at UCSDMC suggests that a pulmonary vascular resistance below 300 dynes sec cm^{-5} is predictive of a favorable outcome, whereas a level above 500 dynes sec cm^{-5} is predictive of a potentially unfavorable one. Experience with this latter group of patients suggests that progression of the pulmonary hypertension may occur over the subsequent 2–5 years as the distal arteriopathy worsens. A number of these patients have subsequently undergone successful lung transplantation. What has not yet been determined in a systematic manner is whether these patients would benefit from either medical therapy (i.e., epoprostenol) or from a combined therapeutic approach: thromboendarterectomy to manage the central component of the disease and pharmacological therapy to manage the distal arteriopathy.

All patients are maintained on lifelong anticoagulation with warfarin. Thromboembolic recurrence requiring repeat thromboendarterectomy has occurred in less than 0.5% of patients undergoing the procedure. A number of these individuals suffered from inadequate management of their anti-coagulation and/or did not undergo placement of an inferior vena caval filter prior to their primary procedure. Repeat thromboendarterectomy has also been performed successfully in number of a patients who initially underwent an inadequate procedure either by a way of a thoracotomy or sternotomy approach. A second pulmonary thromboendarterectomy can be performed with comparable morbidity and mortality as the primary procedure, but the consequent improvement in hemodynamics has been less rewarding (83).

VIII. Conclusions

Chronic thromboembolic disease represents a unique and often undiagnosed sequlae of acute thromboembolism, which must be considered in a dyspneic patient with or without a history of acute thromboembolism, as it is a curable form of pulmonary hypertension. Significant advances have occurred in our understanding of the natural history, clinical features, diagnostic approach, and treatment of this disorder. Despite these advances, a great deal needs to be achieved if the morbidity and mortality of the disease process is to be further reduced.

First, the preliminary insights that have been achieved into the natural history of the disease must be further defined. The level of pulmonary hypertension encountered in the majority of patients with chronic throm-boembolic pulmonary hypertension at the time of initial clinical recognition cannot be achieved on an acute basis. Gradual hemodynamic progression, therefore, must occur over time. The basis for this progression, why it occurs in certain patients following an acute thromboembolic event and not others, and why it appears to occur over months in certain patients and over decades in others, remains entirely speculative. It is possible that the overall extent of central pulmonary vascular obstruction represents the primary pathophysio-logical determinant of disease progression. However, given the lack of correlation between the degree of central thromboembolic obstruction and hemodynamic impairment in certain patients, it is also possible that other factors, such as endothelial dysfunction, circulating vasoconstrictors, the development of a hypertensive pulmonary arteriopathy, an individual genetic predisposition to pulmonary hypertension, or the compensatory adaptations of the right ventricle, contribute to the extent and rate of disease progression.

It is also important to recognize that the development of chronic thromboembolic pulmonary hypertension often represents a failure in prevention and management follow-up surveillance in patients with acute thromboembolism. Recent insights into the recurrent nature of acute thromboembolic disease and its potential for only partial resolution in a number of afflicted individuals suggest that close follow-up including repeat ventilation-perfusion scan and echocardiogram are prudent following a significant acute pulmonary embolism, especially if discontinuation of anticoagulation is being contemplated. Further enhancement in diagnostic techniques are needed, especially to isolate the group of patients who will not significantly benefit from surgery and in whom medical therapy would be more prudent.

References

1. Carroll D. Chronic obstruction of major pulmonary arteries. Am J Med 1950; 9:175–185.
2. Chitwood WR, Lyerly HK, Sabiston DC. Surgical management of chronic pulmonary embolism. Ann Surg 1985; 201:11–26.
3. Daily PO, Dembitsky WP, Jamieson SW. The evolution and the current state of the art of pulmonary thromboendarterectomy. Semin Thorac Cardiovasc Surg 1999; 11:152–163.
4. Hollister LE, Cull VL. The syndrome of chronic thrombosis of the the major pulmonary arteries. Am J Med 1956; 21:312–320.
5. Houk VN, Hufnagel CA, McClenathan JE, et al. Chronic thrombotic obstruction of major pulmonary arteries: report of a case successfully treated by thromboendarterectomy and a review of the literature. Am J Med 1963; 35:269–282.
6. Jamieson SW, Kapelanski DP. Pulmonary endarterectomy. Curr Probl Surg 2000; 37(3):165–252.
7. Daily PO, Auger WR. Historical perspectives: surgery for chronic thromboembolic disease. Semin Thorac Cardiovasc Surg 1999; 11:143–151.
8. Egermayer P, Peacock AJ. Is pulmonary embolism a common cause of pulmonary hypertension? Limitations of the embolic hypothesis. Eur Respir J 2000; 15:440–448.
9. Fedullo PF, Rubin LJ, Kerr KM, et al. The natural history of acute and chronic thromboembolic disease: the search for the missing link. Eur Respir J 2000; 15:435–437.
10. De Soyza NB, Murphy ML. Persistent post-embolic pulmonary hypertension. Chest 1972; 62:665–668.
11. Kunieda T, Nakanishi N, Satoh T, et al. Prognoses of primary pulmonary hypertension and chronic major vessel thromboembolic pulmonary hypertension determined from cumulative survival curves. Intern Med 1999; 38:543–566.
12. Riedel M, Stanek V, Widimsky J, Prevovsky I. Longterm follow-up of patients with pulmonary thromboembolism: Late prognosis and evolution of hemodynamic and respiratory data. Chest 1982; 81:151–158.
13. Dalen JE, Alpert JS. Natural history of pulmonary embolism. Prog Cardiovasc Dis 1975; 17:259–270.

14. Peterson KL. Acute pulmonary embolism. Has its evolution been redefined. Circulation 1999; 99:1280–1283.
15. Hansson Per-Olaf, Sorbo J, Eriksson H. Recurrent venous thromboembolism after deep venous thrombosis. Arch Intern Med 2000; 160:769–774.
16. Murin S, Marelich GP, Arroliga AC, Matthay RA. Hereditary thrombophilia and venous thromboembolism. Am J Respir Crit Care Med 1998; 158:1369–1373.
17. Kyrle PA, Minar E, Hirshcl M, et al. High plasma levels of factor VIII and the risk of recurrent venous thromboembolism. N Engl J Med 2000; 343:457–462.
18. Karwinski B, Svendsen E. Comparison of clinical and postmortem diagnosis of pulmonary embolism. J Clin Pathol 1989; 42:135–139.
19. Meignan M, Rosso J, Gauthier H, et al. Systematic lung scans reveal a high frequency of silent pulmonary embolism in patients with proximal deep venous thrombosis. Arch Intern Med 2000; 160:159–164.
20. Stein PD, Terrin ML, Hales CA, et al. Clinical, laboratory, roentgenographic, and electrocardiographic findings in patients with acute pulmonary embolism and no pre-existing cardiac or pulmonary disease. Chest 1991; 100:598–603.
21. Wartski M, Collignon M-A. Incomplete recovery of lung perfusion after 3 months in patients with acute pulmonary embolism treated with antithrombotic agents. J Nucl Med 2000; 41:1043–1048.
22. Ryan KL, Fedullo PF, Davis GB, et al. Perfusion scan findings understate the severity of angiographic and hemodynamic compromise in chronic thromboembolic pulmonary hypertension. Chest 1988; 93:1180–1185.
23. Dartevelle P, Fadel E, Chapelier A, et al. Angioscopic video-assisted pulmonary endarterectomy for post-embolic pulmonary hypertension. Eur J Cardiothorac Surg 1999; 16:38–43.
24. Ribeiro A, Lindmarker P, Johnsson H, Juhlin-Dannfelt A, Jorfeldt L. Pulmonary embolism. One-year follow-up with echocardiography doppler and five-year survival analysis. Circulation 1999; 99:1325–1330.
25. McIntyre KM, Sasahara AA. Hemodynamic and ventricular responses to pulmonary embolism. Prog Cardiovasc Dis 1974; 17:175–190.
26. Bradley SP, Auger WR, Moser KM, Fedullo PF. Right ventricular pathology in chronic pulmonary hypertension. Am J Cardiol 1996; 78:584–587.
27. Auger WR, Permpikul P, Moser KM, et al. Lupus anticoagulant, heparin use, and thrombocytopenia in patients with chronic thromboembolic pulmonary hypertension. A preliminary report. Am J Med 1995; 99:392–396.
28. Wolf M, Boyer-Neumann C, Parent F, et al. Thrombotic risk factors in pulmonary hypertension. Eur Respir J 2000; 15:395–399.
29. Moser KM, Bloor CM. Pulmonary vascular lesions occurring in patients with chronic major-vessel thromboembolic pulmonary hypertension. Chest 1993; 103:684–692.
30. Moser KM, Daily PO, Peterson KL, et al. Thromboendarterectomy for chronic, major vessel thromboembolic pulmonary hypertension: Immediate and long-term results in 42 patients. Ann Intern Med 1987; 107:560–565.
31. Kim H, Yung GL, Marsh JJ, et al. Pulmonary vascular remodeling distal to

pulmonary artery ligation is accompanied by upregulation of endothelin receptors and nitric oxide synthase. Exp Lung Res 2000; 26:287–301.

32. Auger WR, Moser KM. Pulmonary flow murmurs: a distinctive physical sign found in chronic pulmonary thromboembolic disease [abstr]. Clin Res 1989; 37:145A.

33. D'Alonzo GE, Bower JS, Dantzker DR. Differentiation of patients with primary and thromboembolic pulmonary hypertension. Chest 1984; 85:457–461.

34. Gardeback M, Larsen FF, Radegran K. Nitric oxide improves hypoxaemia following reperfusion oedema after pulmonary thromboendarterectomy. Br J Anaesth 1995; 75:796–800.

35. Lisbona R, Kreisman H, Novales-Diaz J, et al. Perfusion lung scanning: differentiation of primary from thromboembolic pulmonary hypertension. Am J Roentgenol 1985; 144:27–30.

36. Moser KM, Page GT, Ashburn WL, Fedullo PF. Perfusion lung scans provide a guide to which patients with apparent primary pulmonary hypertension merit angiography. West J Med 1988; 148:167–170.

37. Rich S, Pietra GG, Kieras K, et al. Primary pulmonary hypertension: radiographic and scintigraphic patterns of histologic disease. Ann Intern Med 1986; 105:499–502.

38. Fishmann AJ, Moser KM, Fedullo PF. Perfusion lung scans vs pulmonary angiography in evaluation of suspected primary pulmonary hypertension. Chest 1983; 84:679–683.

39. Nagaya N, Uematsu M, Satoh T, et al. Serum uric acid levels correlate with the severity and the mortality of primary pulmonary hypertension. Am J Respir Crit Care Med 1999; 160:487–492.

40. Voelkel MA, Wynne KM, Badesch DB, et al. Hyperuricemia in severe pulmonary hypertension. Chest 2000; 117:19–24.

41. Woodruff WW III, Hoeck BE, Chitwood WR, et al. Radiographic findings in pulmonary hypertension from unresolved embolism. Am J Roentgenol 1985; 144:681–686.

42. Moser KM, Olson LK, Schlusselberg M, et al. Chronic thromboembolic occlusion in the adult can mimic pulmonary artery agenesis. Chest 1989; 95:503–508.

43. Morris TA, Auger WR, Ysrael MZ, et al. Parenchymal scarring is associated with restrictive spirometric defects in patients with chronic thromboembolic pulmonary hypertension. Chest 1996; 110:399–403.

44. Bernstein RJ, Ford RL, Clausen JL, Moser KM. Membrane diffusion and capillary blood volume in chronic thromboembolic pulmonary hypertension. Chest 1996; 110:1430–1436.

45. Steenhuis LH, Groen HJM, Koeter GH, van der Mark Th W. Diffusion capacity and haemodynamics in primary and chronic thromboembolic pulmonary hypertension. Eur Respir J 2000; 16:276–281.

46. Kapitan KS, Buchbinder M, Wagner D, et al. Mechanisms of hypoxemia in chronic thromboembolic pulmonary hypertension. Am Rev Respir Dis 1989; 139:1149–1154.

47. Kapitan KS, Clausen JL, Moser KM. Gas exchange in chronic thromboembolism after pulmonary thromboendarterectomy. Chest 1990; 98:14–19.
48. Bergin CJ, Rios G, King MA, et al. Accuracy of high-resolution CT in identifying chronic pulmonary thromboembolic disease. Am J Roentgenol 1996; 166:1371–1377.
49. Bergin CJ, Sirlin CB, Hauschildt JP, et al. Chronic thromboembolism: diagnosis with helical CT and MR imaging with angiographic and surgical correlation. Radiology 1997; 204:695–702.
50. King MA, Ysrael M, Bergin CJ. Chronic thromboembolic pulmonary hypertension: CT findings. Am J Roentgenol 1998; 170:955–960.
51. Rathbun SW, Raskob GE, Whitsett TL. Sensitivity and specificity of helical computed tomography in the diagnosis of pulmonary embolism: a systematic review. Ann Intern Med 2000; 132:227–232.
52. Moser KM, Fedullo PF, Finkbeiner WE, Golden J. Do patients with primary pulmonary hypertension develop extensive central thrombi? Circulation 1995; 91:741–745.
53. Russo A, De Luca M, Vigna C, et al. Central pulmonary artery lesions in chronic obstructive pulmonary disease. A transesophageal echocardiographic study. Circulation 1999; 100:1808–1815.
54. Bergin CJ, Hauschildt JP, Brown MA, et al. Identifying the cause of unilateral hypoperfusion in patients suspected to have chronic pulmonary thromboembolism: diagnostic accuracy of helical CT and conventional angiography. Radiology 1999; 213:743–749.
55. Bergin CJ, Sirlin C, Deutsch R, et al. Predictors of patient response to pulmonary thromboendarterectomy. Am J Roentgenol 2000; 174:509–515.
56. Auger WR, Fedullo PF, Moser KM, et al. Chronic major-vessel chronic thromboembolic pulmonary artery obstruction: Appearance of angiography. Radiology 1992; 183:393–398.
57. Nicod P, Peterson K, Levine M, et al. Pulmonary angiography in severe chronic pulmonary hypertension. Ann Intern Med 1987; 107:565–568.
58. Pitton MB, Duber C, Mayer E, Thelen M. Hemodynamic effects of nonionic contrast bolus injection and oxygen inhalation during pulmonary angiography in patients with chronic major-vessel thromboembolic pulmonary hypertension. Circulation 1996; 94:2485–2491.
59. Channick RN, Auger WR, Fedullo PF, et al. Angioscopy. In: Feinsilver SH, Fein AM, eds. Textbook of Bronchoscopy. Baltimore: Williams & Wilkins, 1995:477–485.
60. Shure D, Gregoratos G, Moser KM. Fiberoptic angioscopy: role in the diagnosis of chronic pulmonary artery obstruction. Ann Intern Med 1985; 103:844–850.
61. Sompradeekul S, Fedullo PF, Kerr KM, Channick RN, Auger WR. The role of pulmonary angioscopy in the preoperative assessment of patients with thromboembolic pulmonary hypertension (CTEPH) [abstr]. Am J Respir Crit Care Med 1999; 159(3):A456.
62. Decousus H, Leizorovicz A, Parent F, et al. A clinical trial of vena caval filters

in the prevention of pulmonary embolism in patients with proximal deep-vein thrombosis. N Engl J Med 1998; 338:409–415.

63. Addonizio VP Jr, Fisher CA, Kapp JR, Ellison N. Prevention of heparin-induced thrombocytopenia during open heart surgery with iloprost (ZK36374). Surgery 1987; 102:796–807.

64. Gitlin SD, Deeb GM, Yann C, Schmaier AH. Intraoperative monitoring of danaparoid sodium anticoagulation during cardiovascular operations. J Vasc Surg 1998; 27:568–575.

65. Rubens FD, Sabloff M, Wells PS, Bourke M. Use of recombinant-hirudin in pulmonary thromboendarterectomy. Ann Thorac Surg 2000; 69:1942–1943.

66. Koster A, Meyer O, Hausmann H, et al. In vitro cross-reactivity of danaparoid sodium in patients with heparin-induced thrombocytopenia type II undergoing cardiovascular surgery. J Clin Anesth 2000; 12:324–327.

67. Jamieson SW, Auger WR, Fedullo PF, et al. Experience and results with 150 pulmonary thromboendarterectomy operations over a 29-month period. J Thorac Cardiovasc Surg 1995; 106:116–127.

68. Kim HS, Fesler P, Channick RN, et al. Pre operative pulmonary artery occlusion measurements correlate with hemodynamic outcome following pulmonary thromboendarterectomy (PTE). Am J Repirir Crit Care Med 2002; 165:A24.

69. Yung GL, Channick RN, Fedullo PF, et al. Successful pulmonary thromboendarterectomy in two patients with sickle cell disease. Am J Respir Crit Care Med 1998; 157:1690–1693.

70. Zeebregts CJ, Dossche KM, Mosrhuis WJ, et al. Surgical thromboendarterectomy for chronic thromboembolic pulmonary hypertension using circulatory arrest with selective antegrade cerebral perfusion. Acta Chir Belg 1998; 98:95–97.

71. Zund G, Pretre R, Niederhauser U, et al. Improved exposure of the pulmonary arteries for thromboendarterectomy. Ann Thorac Surg 1998; 66:1821–1823.

72. Elliott CG, Colby TV, Hill T, Crapo. Pulmonary veno-occlusive disease associated with severe reduction of single breath carbon monoxide diffusing capacity. Respiration 1988; 53:262–266.

73. Olman MA, Auger WR, Fedullo PE, et al. Pulmonary vascular steal in chronic thromboembolic pulmonary hypertension. Chest 1990; 98:1430–1434.

74. Moser KM, Metersky ML, Auger WR, et al. Resolution of vascular steal after pulmonary thromboendarterectomy. Chest 1993; 104:1441–1444.

75. Kerr KM, Auger WR, Marsh J, et al. The use of Cylexin (CY-1503) in prevention of reperfusion lung injury in patients undergoing pulmonary thromboendarterectomy. Am J Respir Crit Care Med 2000; 162:14–20.

76. Levinson RM, Shure D, Moser KM. Reperfusion pulmonary edema after pulmonary thromboendarterectomy. Am Rev Respir Dis 1986; 134:1241–1245.

77. Ando M, Okita Y, Tagusari O, et al. Surgical treatment for chronic thromboembolic pulmonary hypertension under profound hypothermia and circulatory arrest in 24 patients. J Cardiol Surg 1999; 14:377–385.

78. Hartz RS, Byrne JG, Levitsky S, et al. Predictors of mortality in pulmonary thromboendarterectomy. Ann Thorac Surg 1996; 62:1255–1259.

79. Kramm T, Mayer E, Dahm M, et al. Long-term results after thromboendarter-

ectomy for chronic pulmonary embolism. Eur J Cardiothoracic Surg 1999; 15:579–583.

80. Mayer E, Dahm M, Hake U, et al. Mid-term results of pulmonary thromboendarterecomy for chronic thromboembolic pulmonary hypertension. Ann Thorac Surg 1996; 61:1788–1792.

81. Tanabe N, Odaka O, Nakagawa Y, et al. The efficacy of pulmonary thromboendarterectomy on long-term gas exchange. Eur Respir J 1997; 10:2066–2072.

82. Archibald CJ, Auger WR, Fedullo PF, et al. Long-term outcome after pulmonary thromboendarterectomy. Am J Respir Crit Care Med 1999; 160:523–528.

83. Mo M, Kapelanski DP, Mitruka SN, et al. Reoperative pulmonary thromboendarterectomy. Ann Thorac Surg 1999; 68:1770–1776.

16

Costs of Venous Thromboembolism in the United States

J. JAIME CARO

Caro Research Institute
and McGill University
Concord, Massachusetts, U.S.A.
and Montreal, Quebec, Canada

JUDITH A. O'BRIEN

Caro Research Institute
Concord, Massachusetts, U.S.A.

I. Introduction

This volume addresses in some detail the aspects of venous thromboembolism (VTE) of most interest to physicians—topics such as diagnosis, etiology, treatment, and prognosis. Not so long ago, this would have provided a comprehensive examination of a medical subject, touching on all the concerns of relevance to the management of patients. Now, however, additional demands are made by those who set health policy and control the available resources: physicians are required to consider the economic implications of their decisions. It is no longer enough to order a particular diagnostic test because it might provide useful information or to prescribe a treatment because it has been shown to be safe and effective. A key component of these decisions must now be their expected economic efficiency: Does the value of the expected benefit warrant the required consumption of resources compared to the expected efficiency of other interventions competing for the same scarce health care? Although much of the basic methodology involved in such judgments remains to be worked out (including whether efficiency is the sole economic criterion to consider), the demand for this type of information has soared.

Until recently, "cost" studies in a given illness took the form of compilations of all the financial consequences, typically in very broad categories. For example, the annual cost of treatment of thromboembolic disease in the United States has been estimated at $1.5 billion (1). Although impressive in their vastness, these types of estimates alone are not informative for health care decisions; they are too gross to be helpful by themselves. Full economic analysis of a particular intervention requires detailed mathematical representation (modeling) of the disease or condition in terms of what may occur, depending on what is done, and then valuation of the health consequences and of the resources consumed. As there are many factors that influence these assessments, they must be carried out in a specific context. Unlike estimates of efficacy and safety, there is no general "cost of" that will hold across time, place, and other aspects. Nevertheless, it is useful to quantify the economic implications provided this is done at the level of the relevant components of the illness (e.g., inpatient management of deep vein thrombosis), as these are the basic building blocks of the detailed economic analyses. If reported in sufficient detail, these estimates can be more meaningful to the clinician, as well as form the basis for inputs to an economic model, suitably modified to accord with the particular context at issue.

In this chapter, we provide current estimates of the costs of the various components of VTE and its management. Although these do not address the economic efficiency of any one intervention, they are the data required by anyone analyzing a strategy of managing VTE. We present the cost information in a manner that enables a clinician to understand the economic implications of a particular treatment plan on a per patient basis. We begin with a description of the key concepts. Next, we consider the costs of deep vein thrombosis, and then we do the same for pulmonary embolism. Deep vein thrombosis was selected for two reasons. First, it has a major impact on public health in the United States and the health care system. In 1996, it was estimated that it was the third most common cardiovascular disorder in the United States (2). Second, several therapeutic advances now provide physicians with more management options, all of which have implications for costs. Pulmonary embolism was selected because it is the most serious form of VTE and the most expensive thromboembolic complication. Each year, more than 200,000 people will develop pulmonary embolism and 10% will die as a result (3–6).

II. Elements of Cost Estimates

Four basic steps are required to estimate the costs of a condition: identification of the resources consumed, quantification of that consumption, valuation of each resource in terms of the cost per unit of consumption, and modeling all of it together to reflect properly the management of the condition in a specific context. Although, in principle, all of these steps could be carried out within a single data collection study, this is rarely possible in practice. Instead, it is usually necessary to gather cost-related pieces of information from a variety of sources. Determining which sources to use is always a balancing act between relevance, credibility, and availability.

A. Identification of the Resources Consumed

In general, the criterion for identifying the resources at issue is that the associated expenses be borne by the decision maker to whom the information is directed (i.e., the "perspective" of the analysis). Many guidelines advocate the so-called "societal" perspective as the one of choice for an economic analysis. This recommendation is based on the idea that a full analysis should encompass all possible implications. Thus, from this point of view, it is necessary to identify all changes in resource use—throughout the economy—possibly resulting from a disease or its management. Not only would obvious elements such as hospitalizations and physician's visits need to be counted, but also effects on employees (and employers) and even any consequences for other economic sectors beyond health care. Needless to say, this is an unattainable goal in any realistic time frame. Moreover, real decision makers are concerned, whether appropriately or not, with their own budgets and, thus, the perspective of a third-party payer responsible for the cost of health care is the more useful one. In the United States, this perspective is usually that of managed care organizations, Medicare, and other insurers.

Although many aspects of VTE might be considered under the rubric "costs" if a societal perspective were considered, and these may comprise a substantial portion of the overall costs of VTE, they are not relevant to a the third-party payer perspective in the United States. Lost wages and out-of-pocket expenditures are not factored into payers' decision making no matter how substantial they may be, as they are not responsible for those costs. Given the perspective, the focus is on the direct use of health care resources. This includes hospitalizations, professional services, laboratory and other tests, and drugs, and might extend to paramedical areas, such as stays in rehabilitation institutions or nursing homes. It does not encompass costs covered by patients and their families (e.g., transportation) nor the indirect costs of lost productivity and other such implications of VTE and its management.

There is no single payer in the United States that is responsible for health care coverage. It is a system of multiple third party payers, some funded by federal or state government, and others financed through employer contributions and privately paid premiums. The majority of patients older than 65 years have Medicare as the primary payer. Medicare can also be the primary insurer for those who qualify for Social Security Disability Insurance. Traditionally, policies relating to Medicare policies have also influenced other insurers.

This hodgepodge of health care coverage, and resulting multiplicity of regulations, makes it impossible to identify a resource-use profile that will be universally applicable in the United States. In principle, one could create a profile specific to each health care setting that properly accounts for all the particular coverage complexities, but this is clearly impractical and would, of course, have no merit for publication, as it would have no applicability elsewhere. Instead, most analysts loosely define the third-party payer perspective as that having to do with all medical resources regardless of who actually pays for them and ignoring such things as copays and deductibles. There is general agreement about the inclusion of some elements of these profiles—visits to the physician, acute hospitalizations, laboratory tests, for example—but not about others that may be viewed as more peripheral, such as nursing home stays and home services.

Another complication in developing these profiles is deciding the level at which they should be specified. At its most fundamental level, the profile could delve into the details of all the professionals involved, the amount of time they spend, the supplies they use, reagents that are consumed, and so on. This extreme microcosting is very rarely done, however, because it is very time consuming and many of the details are not readily available. The alternative most frequently employed is to accept the profile at whatever level of aggregation is accessible, and one of the most easily obtained is based on the Diagnosis Related Group (DRG). Unfortunately, although easier to find, this type of estimate has a serious deficiency for economic analysis: few (< 10%) DRGs are disease or procedure specific; they aggregate at a much higher level and any given DRG may reflect several conditions, some of which have little to do with the disease of interest. Pulmonary embolism, for example, can be grouped to a number of DRGs, none of which is specific to VTE. Even when the DRG is specific to a clinical condition, as is the case with deep vein thrombosis, taking the reported cost for that single DRG will not provide an accurate estimate of the overall hospital cost of managing the clinical condition, as cases where any significant surgical procedure was undertaken will be grouped to a different DRG. Thus, it is preferable to define the resource-use profile at a level somewhere between these two extremes: accept natural aggregation (e.g., an emergency room visit rather than all the people and materials involved individually) but avoid DRG-based estimates for specific conditions.

Definition of the resource-use profiles usually begins with the opinion of clinical experts—they are asked to identify the types of resources that are typically consumed in managing a given condition. As clinicians, like most people, are neither comprehensive nor unbiased in offering their opinions, these initial profiles must be supplemented by actual data obtained from whatever sources can be found: state hospital discharge data sets, other claims databases, government and other agency reports, practice guidelines, and peer-reviewed medical literature.

B. Quantification of Consumption

Once the resource-use profile has been identified, the consumption of each element must be quantified. As few resources get to be universally used, this quantification usually involves two steps: the proportion of people who will be users and, among those users, what will be the intensity of use. Both of these steps can be approached at several levels of detail.

The simplest, and most frequent, approach to quantification of the resources used is to provide a point estimate of each of the two elements, the probability of any use and the frequency if used. These point estimates are often obtained today by asking clinical experts to guess the value. This is a most unfortunate practice, as it leads to entire costing analyses based on the opinion of a few people whose expertise has nothing to do with resource use. The field seems oblivious, however, to this extraordinary weakness despite ample documentation of the inability of clinicians to properly estimate probabilities even when these are directly about the illness itself. Rather than take this expedient, but fundamentally flawed approach, some researchers expend the effort to obtain actual data for these estimates, typically using the same sources that were called upon to define the profile, such as claims databases and agency reports.

Depending on the sources used to estimate the resource uses and their intensity, it may be possible to provide additional detail beyond the point estimates. The next level is to describe the distributions of use. This may be done by expressing a mean and standard deviation or other measure of variability; or more comprehensively by reporting the entire distribution in terms of centiles or other such measures. As resource use usually has a very skewed (to the right) distribution, the measures that assume normality (e.g., mean and standard deviation) are often inappropriate.

The most thorough way to quantify the resource-use profile is to assess the determinants of occurrence—what factors influence the proportion of users and the intensity of use. As with any such epidemiological analysis, this can be done using a stratified approach (i.e., subgroups) or by using multivariate regression techniques. Although this chapter cannot address these in depth, it should be noted that this is an area very much in development and these regression models are complex because of the shape of the underlying distributions and the high degree of intercorrelation among the factors.

Regardless of the level to which the resource-use profile is quantified, several issues must be addressed. In most conditions, the resource use occurs over time, and this dependency may be difficult to work out, both because the underlying function is complicated and because the necessary data are scanty. Just as thorny is attribution of the resource use. Few elements are so unique that they can be attributed specifically to the condition of interest. For example, it may be obvious that a venogram is attributable to a deep vein thrombosis but is the next visit to the general practitioner similarly attributable? Researchers have tried to solve this emulating the approaches taken to other epidemiological problems by somehow creating a "control group." A seemingly natural method would be to use the relevant clinical trials that may be conducted. This is problematic, however, because the control group is usually defined by another intervention (e.g., placebo) rather than by the absence of the condition; and trials, through their protocols and selection criteria, substantially alter resource use. Prospective evaluations using cohort studies are usually marred by the changes in behavior that people manifest when they know they are being observed. Thus, most attempts at attribution are based on retrospective analyses; either using patients as their own controls (comparing resource use prior to and after a condition emerges) or using other patients. Needless to say both are very problematic—the former suffers from the dependency of resource use on time and the imprecisions inherent in pinning down the start of a condition; the latter from intractable confounding associated with the diagnosis of the condition at issue and those chosen as controls.

Sometimes, the resource-use profile cannot be quantified directly, because the frequency information is reported only in terms of its cost. In these cases, the gross cost (e.g., of a hospitalization) reflects both the resource-use frequencies and their unit costs but the parts cannot be extricated.

C. Valuation in Terms of Unit Costs

Assigning a unit cost is somewhat easier than quantifying the resource use, as lists of prices tend to exist in many places for most resources. These prices are rarely the actual cost of a resource, as they tend to reflect other add ons (e.g., a dispensing fee) and discounts (e.g., for bulk purchases), but they are used very frequently because of their availability. In some cases, it is possible to apply correction factors (e.g., a cost-to-charge ratio in the United States) to try to approximate the true cost-of-goods. Although the economist pursues these true costs, practical analyses designed to inform real decision makers may be better off addressing the prices actually faced by the payers.

Several aspects of estimating unit costs may also be problematic. When the source data are older than the reporting year of the analysis, most researchers choose to inflate the values. This practice, although perhaps unavoidable, can lead to severe distortions in the estimates, as the unit costs of individual items often fail to follow average inflation rates even if these are specific to health care. Indeed, the costs of some resources actually deflate over time. All estimates must be reported in terms of a particular currency and are thus subject to the fluctuations in that currency—the value of a dollar is not what it used to be! It is important, therefore, to cite both the year to which the source data correspond and the year used for the currency.

D. Putting It All Together

Once the elements of the resource-use profile have been identified, their frequency of use has been quantified and unit costs have been assigned, the analyst must combine this information to estimate the costs that are of interest. This is best done using a costing model—a calculational framework that structures the analysis and permits exploration of the variation in the results when assumptions or inputs are changed.

Apart from the costs per episode of VTE, there may be interest in the overall economic burden imposed in a particular region at a given time. To estimate this level of cost, it is necessary to bring together the individual cost estimates with information about the incidence of the condition. If the condition lasts for an appreciable time (and generates costs over that subsequent time), it is also necessary to consider the prevalence of patients with episodes in previous time periods.

III. Cost of Deep Vein Thrombosis

The cost of various approaches to managing deep vein thrombosis was estimated and reported in detail in 2001 (7). The estimates presented here reflect the published values.

As described above, the resource use profiles were defined using pertinent information from many sources. For deep vein thrombosis, they were derived from 1997 databases recording hospital discharges, emergency room visits, and ambulatory care (8–15), government and other agency reports (16–19), and peer-reviewed medical literature (20–27). The unit costs were often obtained from the same sources plus 1999 national physician (28) and laboratory fee schedules (29). The average daily drug costs were derived based on the amount recommended per kilogram of body weight using the mean weight (74.5 kg) of the U.S. adult population (30) and the average wholesale price (31) of the drugs available in the United States at the time of the analysis. The cost for injectables was based on the use of prefilled syringes. No allowances were made for wastage.

The management of deep vein thrombosis was considered according to the site where care is delivered and the type of treatment. Until recently, a deep vein thrombosis deemed to require treatment would be initially managed with intravenous unfractionated heparin and would result in hospitalization for several days in order to regulate the level of anticoagulation via frequent monitoring of activated partial thromboplastin times (32–34). This has changed with the advent of low molecular weight heparins, because these do not require monitoring nor frequent dose adjustments and, thus, can be employed in an outpatient setting in many cases (20,21,35–37). Despite the availability of these new drugs, some patients—those with complications or with a higher probability of hemorrhage—are still admitted. Even for those managed as outpatients, there are several approaches that can be taken (22,23,38,39).

All cost estimates in this chapter are reported in 1999 U.S. dollars (the original currency used in publications is given as well). Any older source data were inflated using the Medical Care Inflation Index reported by the Federal Bureau of Labor Statistics for the month of January for each of the relevant years. In the absence of a standard national cost-to-charge ratio, one calculated by the Commonwealth of Massachusetts Office of Health Care Finance and Policy was applied where relevant.

A. Inpatient Management

Data on the costs of admission (including all accommodation, laboratory, pharmacy, emergency room, operating room, diagnostic, and therapeutic procedures) for deep vein thrombosis were obtained from the inpatient databases that cover more than 1000 hospitals from California, Florida, Maine, Massachusetts, Maryland, and Washington. These databases contain demographic, clinical, and resource-use information pertaining to all discharges in a given year. Costs related to physician care during the hospital stay were calculated by developing an inpatient visit profile using various data elements (e.g., length of stay, special care unit stays, emergency room care, procedures) and applying unit costs from national fee schedules. They are included in the cost of hospital care.

There were nearly 30,000 discharges where the principal diagnosis (the condition after study that is deemed responsible for the hospital admission) contained an ICD-9-CM code (451.11, 451.19, 453.8) for deep vein thrombosis. Using the codes for other diagnoses and procedures, various types of admission were identified: uncomplicated, complicated by embolism or adverse drug effects (bleeding or thrombocytopenia), or complicated by other conditions.

The burden of deep vein thrombosis can be clearly seen when the types of admission are examined. Of the nearly 30,000 admissions for deep vein thrombosis that were recorded in the data sets of the six states, less than 5% were discharged home after a completely uncomplicated course with no further procedures or interventions. About 5% suffered either a pulmonary embolism or a bleeding event and the remainder was either not discharged home, required additional procedures, or suffered other complications (Fig. 1). Not surprisingly, the patients with no complications were younger, with a mean age of 52 years compared to 64 years overall, and in

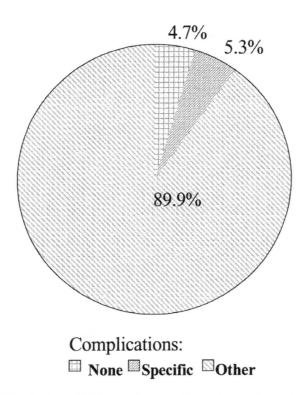

Complications:
⊞ **None** ▨**Specific** ◳**Other**

Figure 1 Distribution of 29,295 discharges with a primary diagnosis of deep vein thrombosis according to presence of complications.

the high 60s for some specific complications. The average length of stay was 5.8 days (range: 1–124 days), but again it varied considerably according to complications. Among patients with no complication whatsoever, the stay was on average 4.5 days, whereas a major bleed or pulmonary embolism brought this to 8.6 and 7.5 days, respectively.

The case-fatality rate during hospitalization was only 1% overall. This increased to 2% in those patients with drug-induced thrombocytopenia or a moderate bleed (epistaxis, hematuria, melena) to 4% when pulmonary embolism occurred and to 5% when there was a major bleed (intracranial or gastrointestinal). Of all patients discharged alive, four of five went home; 16% of whom were referred for home health care services. Among the remaining 20%, two-thirds of the patients required further subacute inpatient care (i.e., rehabilitation hospital, nursing facility). The other third of the patients includes those who signed out against medical advice and those discharged to prison, a mental health care facility, convalescent care, or unknown. These distributions do not vary by much depending on complications except for patients who survived a major bleed. Just under half of the patients went directly home, and one-third required further care (Fig. 2). Medicare was listed as the primary payer for 56% of the discharges. The second most frequent responsible payer was managed care organizations (22.5%).

The costs (actual charges adjusted downward by 0.61) for this inpatient care varied considerably according to complications. Admissions with no complication and a discharge home, cost on average $3500, with a 10-fold range from $900 to $9200. When examined per diem, a similar pattern emerges: a mean of $820 per day with a range of $360 to $3600. Admissions lasting only 1 day cost $1600, whereas the mean per diem cost dropped to $1000 for those who had a 2-day stay and to $840 per day for 3 days.

Early discharge (within 3 days) achieved some savings, as might be expected. The mean cost of the hospital care for these patients was more than $1000 less expensive ($2300, range: $600–$5,300). Even addition of the costs of additional therapy required upon discharge in order to continue anticoagulation for a full 6 days brought this cost to only $3000.

The occurrence of a major bleed during an admission for deep vein thrombosis almost quadruples the cost of the hospitalization to a mean of $11,200 and ranging up to $80,500 per stay. This results from both the longer length of stay (mean 8.6 days; range: 1–66) and the higher cost each day. The mean per diem cost for these patients was $1500; ranging from $330 to $10,200 per day. A complicating pulmonary embolism or drug-induced thrombocytopenia increases the costs almost threefold: a mean of $9500 (range: $795–$267,860) when a pulmonary embolism occurs and of $8700 (range: $1,350–$56,755) with the adverse effect. Even a moderate bleed doubles the cost to a mean of $8000 (range: $850–$78,150) (Table 1).

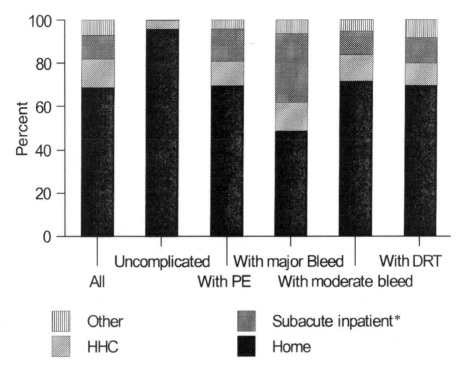

Figure 2 Disposition of survivors at hospital discharge by complication. *Subacute inpatient care includes rehabilitation, skilled nursing facilities, and nursing home care. PE, pulmonary embolus; DRT, drug-related thrombocytopenia.

Table 1 Characteristics and Costs of Hospitalizations for Deep Vein Thrombosis[a]

Complication	Cases	Mean age (yrs)	Mean LOS (days)	CFR (%)	Mean cost (/day)	Mean cost per stay
None[b]	1387	52	4.5	na	820	3486
Major bleed	287	66	8.6	4	1460	11,189
Moderate bleed	410	70	6.9	1	1174	7980
Pulmonary embolism	725	61	7.5	4	1320	9476
Thrombocytopenia	143	65	6.6	0	1378	8679
None of the four above	27,321	64	5.4	1	1020	5561
All deep vein thrombosis	29,295	64	5.8	1	1036	5779

LOS, length of stay; CFR, case fatality rate.
[a] All costs expressed in 1999 U.S. dollars.
[b] Patients with uncomplicated DVT had to survive the hospitalization, be discharged home, and have no comorbid conditions or complications.

B. Outpatient Management

Assuming that patients present, or are referred, to the emergency room for diagnosis of deep vein thrombosis, four resource-use profiles were developed. These account for variations in the way care is provided. Three of the profiles begin with a stay in a holding unit where patients are taught to self-inject and are educated about the treatment plan (14,19,22,38); the fourth assumes a 1-day stay in hospital for the same purpose. The profiles vary in whether a nurse visits the home to supervise or actually to inject low molecular weight heparin (26) or whether the patient visits a clinic for this (39). All outpatient profiles assume that 6 days of low molecular weight heparin treatment will be prescribed. The use of drugs, including the start of warfarin, and the associated monitoring are part of the profiles, as are physician visits.

The typical cost of managing a patient on low molecular weight heparin treated primarily in an outpatient setting ranges from $1400 to $2400 for the initial care period. Those who require a 1-night hospital stay to initiate anticoagulation therapy incur $2300 for acute management when they are discharged home on self-administered, daily low molecular weight heparin. For those never admitted, administration of low molecular weight heparin by a nurse at home is the most expensive approach to outpatient management, as might be expected. When the patient can self-inject, the cost of acute care is estimated at $1400 for once daily and $1700 for twice daily therapy. If a registered nurse is required to administer the low molecular weight heparin, the cost increases to $1700 for once daily and to $2400 for twice per day. In cases where a patient cannot self-administer the medication, no home health services are available, or there is a question of compliance, it may be necessary to have the patient receive the injections at the clinic. In this case, the cost of care would be $1500 for a daily injection of low molecular weight heparin and $2000 if twice-daily injections are required.

C. Subsequent Care

Care for the 6 months following acute treatment was also included in the cost estimates. In all patients, this included warfarin use and its associated monitoring (for two durations of use: 3 and 6 months (24)); follow-up physician visits; and the cost of care for those who had a recurrent deep vein thrombosis, pulmonary embolism, or major bleeding following initial acute therapy. For those patients admitted to the hospital for initial treatment of deep vein thrombosis, the disposition upon discharge relative to the source at admission was examined to determine continuing care (i.e., at home, at home with additional services, in skilled nursing care facility, in an intermediate care facility, in rehabilitation).

The cost of care subsequent to discharge for those with an uncomplicated course was estimated at $1600. The referral rate for additional services after discharge was highest for those who experienced a major bleed during their stay. Of those patients who survived this type of event, only 49% were discharged home. Thirty-two percent of the patients required subacute inpatient care and 13% were referred to home health care services. The remaining 6% of patients discharged alive were classified as "other." The 6-month cost of subsequent was estimated for those with a major bleeding event at about $6000. These costs are also higher when these complications arise during the initial hospitalization except in the case of moderate bleeding events.

For those treated as outpatients on low molecular weight heparin, the cost of subsequent care was estimated at $979. This estimate was developed based on typical resource use in this period for management of deep vein thrombosis in patients discharged early. In this analysis, all patients classified as "early discharge" had to be discharged to home, but 8% of them also had home health care services.

D. Episode Cost

Combining the acute and subsequent care for the various management approaches yields an estimate of the total costs for an episode of uncomplicated deep vein thrombosis treated primarily in an outpatient setting. This ranges from a low of $2400 for patients managed as outpatients on once daily self-administered low molecular weight heparin to $3370 for those treated with twice-daily injection at home by a nurse (Table 2). For patients who have an uncomplicated course treated in an inpatient setting initially, the cost of the episode of deep vein thrombosis rises to $5100. Complications increase this estimate considerably. A moderate bleed adds another $7000 to the average; drug-related thrombocytopenia increases the mean cost by $8400; the occurrence of pulmonary embolism does so by $9800, and a major hemorrhage adds more than $12,000, on average, compared with an uncomplicated case (Table 3).

Although these estimates are the most comprehensive published to date, they have some limitations. It may not always be the case that patients with deep vein thrombosis present via the emergency room. Thus, the average cost of outpatient management may be lower still if patients' diagnoses and management are entirely done from a physician's office. Although the inpatient cost estimates are based on extensive data with no selection bias in terms of payer, type of hospital, or other such characteristics, the administrative databases used are subject to their coding accuracy. ICD-9-CM codes may not be accurate and some conditions may not be reported. De-

Table 2 Cost of Deep Vein Thrombosis Managed Initially as Outpatient on Low Molecular Weight Heparin (LMWH)

Management approach	Acute care ($)	Subsequent care ($)	Total cost ($)
Hospital 1 day, home care, self	2267	979	3246
Home care			
LMWH twice daily			
Registered nurse administered	2390	979	3369
Self-administered	1734	979	2713
LMWH once daily			
Registered nurse administered	1707	979	2686
Self-administered	1415	979	2394
Clinic care			
LMWH twice daily	2015	979	2994
LMWH once daily	1520	979	2499

spite recent studies that have shown improving coding accuracy (40), the degree of miscoding or undercoding of complications of deep vein thrombosis in these databases is not known. Also, as severity is not noted in these databases, bleeding events were classified into moderate and major based on combinations of ICD-9-CM codes.

E. Total Cost

Some idea of the magnitude of the problem posed by deep vein thrombosis can be obtained by combining the estimates of the mean, per patient cost of

Table 3 Cost of Deep Vein Thrombosis When Initially Managed as Inpatient, According to Complications Occurring During Hospitalization

Complication	Acute care ($)	Subsequent care ($)	Total cost ($)
None	3486	1616	5102
Pulmonary embolism	9476	5173	14649
Major bleed	11189	5980	17168
Moderate bleed	7980	4162	12142
Drug-induced thrombocytopenia	8679	4790	13459
None of the four above	5561	4223	9785
All deep vein thrombosis	5779	4293	10072

managing an episode of deep vein thrombosis with the incidence of the condition. Based on detailed review of the health care records in Olmsted County, Minnesota, the incidence of deep vein thrombosis was estimated by age and sex (41). Applying these incidence rates (admittedly derived from a mostly white population) to the 1999 population of the United States (42) yields an estimated 210,555 cases of deep vein thrombosis per year. If all these cases are treated on a full inpatient basis, then the direct medical cost would amount to 2.1 billion dollars annually (95% confidence interval: 1.8–2.5 billion). This does not include the costs of diagnostic tests in suspected but ultimately unconfirmed cases, nor the costs of complications beyond the initial episode (e.g., postphlebitic syndrome in later years). Also left out are the indirect costs of lost productivity and the expenses to patients and their families. If it were possible to manage all of these cases as outpatients, the cost would drop significantly to about half a billion dollars annually (95% CI: 0.4–0.6 billion).

IV. Cost of Pulmonary Embolism

The costs of pulmonary embolism occurring as a complication of a diagnosed deep vein thrombosis are presented in Section III. This section addresses the costs of a primary episode of pulmonary embolism (a principal diagnosis of pulmonary embolus, ICD-9-CM codes: 415.11, 415.19). As almost all patients diagnosed with a pulmonary embolus are managed as inpatients initially, the resource-use estimates must include a hospital stay. The methodology and sources of data used to derive the cost estimates for pulmonary embolism were the same as described for deep vein thrombosis.

A. Inpatient Management

The estimates of the cost of the initial hospitalization were based on 14,434 cases with a principal diagnosis of pulmonary embolus. More than half (57%) were female and 64% presented through the emergency room. They tended to be slightly older than those cases where pulmonary embolus was listed as a secondary diagnosis (a mean age of 64 years compared to 61 years in the latter). On average, the length of stay was only 7 days, but it went as high as 85 days. The inpatient case fatality rate was 7%, which is almost double the 4% rate seen when patients were admitted for a deep vein thrombosis and developed a pulmonary embolus during their hospital stay. The mean age of those who died was 5 years older than that of those who survived to discharge. Less than one-quarter (21%) of those who survived spent time in a special care unit, whereas slightly more than half (55%) of those who died did. The mean hospital stay cost was $9970 (range: $210–

$319,500) with a mean per diem of $1500 (range: $218–$30,500). The cost of those who died during the stay was $3900 more, on average, than that of those discharged alive. Medicare was the largest primary payer (55%). Managed care organizations were the responsible payer for one-quarter of the admissions.

B. Subsequent Care

The costs of subsequent care of survivors depend on the site of care. About two-thirds of survivors were discharged home to outpatient care (69%); nearly equal proportions were transferred to subacute inpatient care followed by outpatient medical care (13%) or received home health care services along with outpatient medical care (14%). The remaining 4% had other discharge dispositions. As with the deep vein thrombosis cost, the cost of continuing warfarin therapy and its monitoring was included in the cost of subsequent care. Also incorporated in these estimates was the cost of additional hospital care for those readmitted within 6 months with another pulmonary embolus (6%), a deep vein thrombosis (3%), or a major bleeding event (<1%).

By weighting the costs accrued in each of the courses of subsequent care of those who survived hospitalization, an average cost for this portion of the episode can be derived. This amounts to an additional $5170 in subsequent care costs in the 6 months following diagnosis of a primary pulmonary embolus.

C. Episode Cost

Putting together the components of managing an episode of care for a pulmonary embolus when it is the admitting diagnosis leads to an estimated cost of $15,137. This is slightly higher than when pulmonary embolus is a complication of deep vein thrombosis ($14,649).

D. Total Cost

The total cost of managing pulmonary embolism can be estimated in the same way as for deep vein thrombosis. Based on the Olmsted County data (41) and the U.S. population of 1999 (42), it can be estimated that there would be 228,000 cases of pulmonary embolism reported annually. This includes both cases with a primary diagnosis of pulmonary embolism and those with deep vein thrombosis who also develop pulmonary embolism. If the appropriate weighted cost estimates for episodes of pulmonary embolism with and without deep vein thrombosis are applied, it can be estimated that this condition costs the health care system $3.4 billion dollars per year (95% CI: 2.8–4.1 billion) in direct medical expenditures alone.

V. Other U.S. Cost Estimates

There are several other reports in the literature that cover estimates of the cost related to various aspects of managing VTE. Several recent ones are reviewed in this section with a view to assessing the usefulness for clinicians of the cost estimates. As the costs are reported from several years, the inflated values expressed in 1999 U.S. dollars are given along with the original published values.

Many of the published estimates are part of analyses of the cost difference and potential cost savings of treating patients with low molecular weight heparin instead of unfractionated heparin (43–45). Others have addressed specific models of management (e.g., pharmacist-managed program) in the context of efforts to examine existing treatment plans in order to maintain or improve the quality of care while reducing the cost of that care (46,47). This concept is particularly relevant for VTE as an increasing number of facilities are instituting management programs coordinated through the pharmacy department with medical oversight. These programs are geared toward maximizing the steering of uncomplicated cases of deep vein thrombosis toward self-administered anticoagulation therapy in the home (22,23,38,48).

One economic analysis (45) was based on data from the American-Canadian Thrombosis Study, a multicenter randomized clinical trial of 432 patients that compared the use of subcutaneous low molecular weight heparin with intravenous heparin (49). The cost component of that study looked at the direct medical costs incurred in the acute care phase, excluding those related to the study process itself. These were examined from the perspective of a third-part payer and covered: anticoagulant therapy (warfarin, monitoring laboratory tests, and physician visits for 3 months), hospital stay (all patients were treated acutely as inpatients), treatment of recurrent venous thromboembolism for 12 months, and management of major bleeding complications. As minor bleeding events and nonhemorrhagic complications were reported infrequently in the trial; they were not included in the cost profile. Data on the resources used by each patient were collected as part of the trial. Unit costs for the United States were obtained from one urban midwestern hospital. The mean cost estimate for a patient treated with unfractionated heparin was $5005 ($3758 in 1992 U.S. dollars). Treatment with low molecular weight heparin in the trial lowered the cost slightly to $4470 per patient ($3357 in 1992 U.S. dollars).

Although these cost estimates are based on actual data, they reflect only inpatient management, which is no longer optimum. Despite attempts to exclude costs related to the study process, the data are still from a clinical trial and, thus, affected by the study itself (e.g., the degree of monitoring laboratory tests in the 3 month follow-up). Moreover, as the unit costs are from a single, urban, midwestern hospital, the estimates may not reflect the United States as a whole. For example, in 1998, the average Medicare payment of $6650 per hospital discharge in the Midwest was 20% and 16% lower than the average payments in the Northeast and West, respectively, and 3% higher than the average payment per discharge for those in the South (50).

Another study (44), reported results from a cost minimization analysis of a trial that randomized 339 hospitalized patients into three treatment arms: once daily subcutaneous low molecular weight heparin, twice daily low molecular weight heparin and dose-adjusted intravenous unfractionated heparin, all followed by oral anticoagulant therapy. The costs were estimated from a third-party payer perspective based on resource-use data collected during the trial that covered the hospital stay, laboratory tests, medications, and professional fees incurred during the 3 months following diagnosis. The frequency of anticoagulant monitoring was dictated by the trial. Unit costs were derived from billing data from 59 U.S. hospitals adjusted by cost-to-charge ratios, published professional fees, and drug prices. The per diem inpatient unit cost was calculated by removing charges for laboratory, pharmacy, and diagnostic services from the charge for DRG 128 (deep vein thrombophlebitis). This was then applied to the length of stay for each patient, and the ancillary charges were added back in based on the resources used by each patient in the trial. The average total cost of an episode was $12,928 ($12,166 in the original) for once-daily low molecular weight heparin. It decreased to $12,262 ($11,558 in the original) for twice daily. The cost for those treated initially with unfractionated heparin was similar at $12,886 ($12,146 in the original). Although these estimates are based on actual data and a more extensive source of unit costs, they are marred, as with the previous study, by the impact of the trial itself and protocol-driven costs. Thus, the applicability to current actual practice is questionable.

A more recently published study was based on a review of claims data from 37 U.S. health plans (43). The analysis was based on 3466 hospitalized cases with either a principal or secondary diagnosis of deep vein thrombosis. Payments were used as a proxy for costs that covered hospitalization for the acute care, outpatient treatment after discharge, and readmissions for deep vein thrombosis over a 1-year follow-up period. No year for cost values is supplied in the paper, so no conversion can be made to 1999 dollars. Although the paper presents comparative cost savings, it is possible to derive the underlying cost components. They are $5017 for the hospitalization, $711 for outpatient care, and $780 for readmissions, leading to total costs of $6508 for the episode of deep vein thrombosis.

Despite the large dataset used in that study, there are two important limitations. As cases with a secondary diagnosis of deep vein thrombosis were included in the study, the actual data could not be used, because it included care and procedures unrelated to VTE. Thus, the costs had to be deduced form the differences in length of stay and average per diem costs. The second limitation is that in nearly half the cases (46%), there was no documentation of any anticoagulation therapy in the medication claims. Although the investigators speculate on possible reasons, the outpatient care cost is very likely an underestimate.

Another published analysis focused on outpatient management of deep vein thrombosis in a group model HMO (48). The study compared the cost of managing 391 patients with deep vein thrombosis enrolled in the outpatient treatment program over 2 years to what it would have been had they been admitted for care. These outpatient enrollees comprised 91% of members of Kaiser Permanente Colorado Region diagnosed with deep vein thrombosis over that period. Services were provided in 15 medical offices throughout the Denver area, but the anticoagulation program was managed by a centralized team of pharmacy technicians and clinical pharmacists with special training. The estimates of direct medical costs from a payer perspective were based on resource-use data collected during the study and provider fees. Estimates reported in 1998 U.S. dollars covered medical office and emergency room visits, laboratory and medication costs, home health care visits, and telephone contacts. Hospitalization costs for the 16% of patients who had anticoagulation therapy initiated as inpatients were also included unless the patient required a longer stay because of a concurrent symptomatic disease, pulmonary embolism, bleeding, or pregnancy. Slightly more than half of the inpatient cases had a length of stay greater than 1 day. Anticoagulation therapy costs after the first 7 days were not included. This study reported that the average direct cost for treating a deep vein thrombosis in an outpatient setting was $1928 ($1868, 1998 U.S. dollars) compared to $4846 ($4696, 1998 U.S. dollars) if they had been hospitalized for acute management.

These estimates demonstrate the beneficial economic impact of managing deep vein thrombosis in the outpatient setting, but they have limited applicability given the single HMO setting and the highly specialized type of care involved. Applicability is further reduced by the exclusions of certain patients and various fees.

Another demonstration of the savings that can be obtained via outpatient management is provided by the analysis of a multidisciplinary outpatient program to treat deep vein thrombosis at a teaching institution in North Carolina (38). In that program, a clinical pharmacist reviews the case of patients with uncomplicated deep vein thrombosis either already admitted to the hospital or seen in the emergency room and, if eligible, orders discontinuation of existing anticoagulation therapies and alerts the case management services. Laboratory values are obtained and patients are started on low molecular weight heparin (a nurse administers the first dose and the patient is issued prefilled syringes for use at home) and concomitant oral warfarin. Patients are educated by the pharmacist and evaluated for successful compliance. The outpatient-monitoring program consists of blood work, drug counseling, outpatient warfarin therapy, and daily telephone follow-up for 90 days. The cost estimates in 1998 U.S. dollars were based on the resources consumed by 142 patients enrolled between April 1996 and May 1998, using payments as a proxy for costs. The average reimbursement for a hospitalized case was $3546 ($3436, 1998 U.S. dollars) at the time. It was estimated that switching management to the outpatient program would save $2550 ($2470, 1998 U.S. dollars). The report provides a good description of the program and a sample form for physician orders; the estimates, however, are limited to that one provider's experience during a period of research.

VI. Conclusions

In this chapter, the direct costs of the health care resources consumed in managing VTE in the United States have been addressed. The key methodological aspects of this type of assessment were also reviewed. There are four important steps: identification of the resources consumed, quantification of the consumption, valuation in terms of unit costs, and finally computation of the estimate by putting the pieces together. There are important methodological issues at all four steps but the most important ones concern the sources of data and the applicability of the estimates.

Patients admitted to hospital for initial management of deep vein thrombosis stayed an average of about 6 days and cost between $3500 and $11,200 depending on complications, with some patients accruing costs of more than $100,000. Initial outpatient management of patients without complications lowers the cost considerably to between $1400 and $2400 depending on how the care is delivered and the frequency of injections. Management following the acute phase generates costs of between $979 and $6000 depending on the course and site of treatment. The episode of care thus costs between $2400 for a patient treated entirely as an outpatient who self-administers low molecular weight heparin and $12,000 for those requiring inpatient care on average, but this cost can range to much higher levels in survivors with severe complications. Management of a primary episode of pulmonary embolism is estimated to cost about $15,000, with two-thirds being for the inpatient portion.

These estimates only address the direct cost of medical care. VTE, however, forces patients, their families, and employers to bear additional costs. The average lost wages associated with deep vein thrombosis were calculated at $850 and with pulmonary embolus at $2800 per episode, for example (51).

It is clear from the estimates presented here, that management of VTE can be a very costly activity. These estimates, and the shift in focus in the literature in the last decade, also convey the message that shifting inpatient care to outpatient management can achieve significant savings. Anticoagulation therapy for VTE has caught the attention of decision makers at both the clinical and financial levels and programs and guidelines are being developed and implemented, not only to accommodate, but also to facilitate changes in managing this condition.

References

1. Goldhaber SZ, Visani, De Rosa M. Acute pulmonary embolism: clinical outcomes in the International Cooperative Pulmonary Embolism Register (ICOPER). Lancet 1999; 353:1386–1389.
2. Hirsh J, Hoak J. Management of deep vein thrombosis and pulmonary embolism. Circulation 1996; 93:2212–2245.
3. Rubinstein I, Murray D, Hoffstein V. Fatal pulmonary emboli in hospitalized patients: an autopsy study. Arch Intern Med 1988; 148:1425–1426.
4. Dalen JE, Alpert JS. Natural history of pulmonary embolism. Prog Cardiovasc Dis 1975; 17:259–270.
5. Bell WR, Simon Tl. Current status of pulmonary thromboembolic disease, pathophysiology, diagnosis, prevention and treatment. Am Heart J 1982; 103: 239–262.
6. Kaunitz AM, Hughes JM, Grimes DA, Smith JC, Rochat RW, Kafrissen ME. Causes of maternal mortality in the United States. Obstet Gynecol 1985; 65: 605–612.
7. O'Brien JA, Caro JJ. Direct Medical costs of managing deep vein thrombosis according to the occurrence of complications. PharmacoEconomics 2002; 20:603–615.
8. California 1997 Discharge Data (Version A). Office of Statewide Health Planning and Development.
9. Florida 1997 Hospital Patient Data File. State of Florida, Agency for Health Care Administration, State Center for Health Statistics.
10. Maine 1997 Standard Hospital Inpatient Discharge Records, Unrestricted. Maine Health Data Organization.
11. Maryland 1997 Inpatient Public Use File. St. Paul Computer Center, Inc.
12. Massachusetts Fiscal Year 1997 Acute Hospital Case Mix Data Base, Massachusetts Division of Health Care Finance and Policy.

13. Washington 1997 CHARS (Comprehensive Hospital Abstract Reporting System) Public Data File. Washington State Department of Health, Office of Hospital and Patient Data.
14. Utah Emergency Department Encounter Database, 1997 Public-Use Data File. Bureau of Emergency Medical Services, Utah Department of Health.
15. Florida Medicaid Outpatient Database, 1997. Medicaid Program Analysis, State of Florida, Agency for Health Care Administration.
16. Health Care Financing Reviews: Medicare and Medicaid Statistical Supplement, 1999. Baltimore, MD, U.S. Dept. of Health and Human Services, HCFA, Office of Strategic Planning, November 1999 (HCFA publ. No. 03417).
17. Annual Report to Congress, 1996. Physician Payment Review Commission. Washington, DC, 1996.
18. Foundation for Healthy Communities. Specialty Hospital Standard Reports, January–December 1998. New Hampshire Hospital Association, Concord, NH September 1999.
19. The 1997 APG Handbook. HCIA, Inc. and 3M Health Care. Baltimore, MD, and Wallingford, CT, 1997.
20. Koopman MMW, Prandoni P, Piovella F, et al. Treatment of venous thrombosis with intravenous unfractionated heparin administered in the hospital as compared with subcutaneous low-molecular-weight heparin administered at home. N Engl J Med 1996; 334:682–687.
21. Levine M, Gent M, Hirsh J, et al. A comparison of low-molecular-weight heparin administered primarily at home with unfractionated heparin administered in the hospital for proximal deep-vein thrombosis. N Engl J Med 1996; 334:677–681.
22. Dedden P, Chang B, Nagel D. Pharmacy-managed program for home treatment of deep vein thrombosis with enoxaparin. Am J Health Syst Pharm 1997; 54:1968–1972.
23. Deitcher SR, Olin JW, Bartholomew J. How to use low-molecular-weight heparin for outpatient management of deep vein thrombosis. Cleve Clin J Med 1999; 56:329–331.
24. Blattler W. Ambulatory Care for Ambulant Patients with Deep Vein Thrombosis. J Mal Vasc 1991; 16:137–141.
25. Manton KG, Cornelius ES, Woodbury MA. Nursing home residents: a multivariate analysis of their medical, behavioral, psychosocial, and service use characteristics. J Gerontol Med Sci 1995; 30A:M242–M251.
26. Van den Belt AGM, Bossuy PMM, Prins MH, et al, for the TASMAN Study Group. Replacing inpatient care by outpatient care in the treatment of deep vein thrombosis—an economic evaluation. Thromb Haemost 1998; 78:259–263.
27. Gould MK, Dembitzer AD, Sanders GD, et al. Low-molecular-weight heparins compared with unfractionated heparin for treatment of acute deep venous thrombosis: a cost-effectiveness analysis. Ann Intern Med 1999; 130:789–799.
28. Annual Physician Fee Schedule Payment Amount File. Health Care Financing Agency, 1999. http://www.hcfa.gov/stats/pufiles.htm (accessed November 1999).
29. 1999 Clinical Diagnostic Laboratory Fee Schedule (CLAB) Public Use File (PUF) http://www.hcfa.gov/stats/pufiles.htm (accessed November 1999).

30. U.S. Bureau of the Census. Statistical Abstract of the United States, 1997. 117th ed. Washington, DC, 1997.
31. 1999 Drug Topics Red Book. Montvale, NJ: Medical Economics, 1999.
32. Hirsh J. Heparin. N Engl J Med 1991; 324:1565–1574.
33. Prandoni P. Unfractionated heparin and low-molecular-weight-heparin for the initial treatment of acute venous thromboembolism. Haemostasis 1998; 28:85–90.
34. Hull RD, Raskob GE, Hirsh J, et al. Continuous intravenous heparin compared with intermittent subcutaneous heparin in the initial treatment of proximal vein thrombosis. N Engl J Med 1986; 315:1109–1114.
35. Harrison L, McGinnis J, Crowther M, et al. Assessment of outpatient treatment of deep-vein thrombosis with low-molecular-weight heparin. Arch Intern Med 1998; 158:2001–2003.
36. Estrada CA, Mansfield CJ, Huedebert GR. Cost-effectiveness of low-molecular-weight heparin in the treatment of proximal deep vein thrombosis. J Gen Intern Med 2000; 15:108–115.
37. Lindmarker P, Holstrom M, and the Swedish Venous Thrombosis Dalteparin Trial Group. Use of low molecular weight heparin (dalteparin), once daily, for treatment of deep vein thrombosis. A feasibility and health economic study in an outpatient setting. J Intern Med 1996; 240:395–401.
38. Groce JB. Patient outcomes and cost analysis associated with an outpatient deep vein thrombosis treatment program. Pharmacotherapy 1998; 18:175S–180S.
39. Leong WA. Outpatient deep vein thrombosis treatment models. Pharmacotherapy 1998; 18:170S–174S.
40. Newton KM, Wagner EH, Ramsey SD, et al. The use of automated data to identify complications and comorbidities of diabetes: a validation study. J Clin Epidemiol 1999; 52:199–207.
41. Silverstein MD, Heit JA, Mohr DN, Petterson TM, O'Fallon WM, Melton LJ III. Trends in the incidence of deep vein thrombosis and pulmonary embolism. Arch Intern Med 1998; 158:585–593.
42. U.S. Census Bureau. Statistical Abstract of the United States: 2001. 121st ed. Washington, DC, 2001. Table 12.
43. Huse DM, Cummins G, Taylor DCA, Russell MW. Outpatient treatment of venous thromboembolism with low-molecular-weight heparin: an economic evaluation. Am J Manag Care 2002; 8:S10–S16.
44. de Lissovoy G, Yusen RD, Spiro TE, Krupski WC, Champion AH, Sorensen SV. Cost for inpatient care of venous thrombosis. Arch Intern Med 2000; 160:3160–3165.
45. Hull RD, Pineo GF, Raskob GE. The economic impact of treating deep vein thrombosis with low-molecular-weight heparin: outcomes of therapy and health economy aspects. Low-molecular-weight heparin versus unfractionated heparin. Haemostasis 1998; 28:8–16.
46. Vanscoy GJ. Outpatient management of venous thromboembolism. J Thromb Thrombol 1999; 7:109–112.
47. O'Brien JA, Jacobs LM, Pierce D. Clinical practice guidelines and the cost of care: a growing alliance. Intl J Technol Assess Health Care 2000; 16:1077–1091.

48. Tillman DJ, Charland SL, Witt DM. Effectiveness and economic impact associated with a program for outpatient management of acute deep vein thrombosis in a group model health maintenance organization. Arch Intern Med 2000; 160:2926–2932.

49. Hull RD, Raskob GE, Rosenbloom D, Pineo GF, Lerner RG, et al. Treatment of proximal vein thrombosis with subcutaneous low-molecular-weight heparin vs intravenous heparin. Arch Intern Med 1997; 157:289–294.

50. Medicare and Medicaid Statistical Supplement, 1999. Health Care Finance Review. US Dept. of Health and Human Services. HCFA Office of Strategic Planning, Baltimore, 2000.

51. Official Disability Guidelines. Work Loss Data Institute. Corpus Christi, TX; 1999–2001. www.stats.bls.gov/news.release, accessed May 2002.

INDEX